Design and Analysis of Cross-Over Trials

Third Edition

MONOGRAPHS ON STATISTICS AND APPLIED PROBABILITY

General Editors

F. Bunea, V. Isham, N. Keiding, T. Louis, R. L. Smith, and H. Tong

1. Stochastic Population Models in Ecology and Epidemiology *M.S. Barlett* (1960)
2. Queues *D.R. Cox and W.L. Smith* (1961)
3. Monte Carlo Methods *J.M. Hammersley and D.C. Handscomb* (1964)
4. The Statistical Analysis of Series of Events *D.R. Cox and P.A.W. Lewis* (1966)
5. Population Genetics *W.J. Ewens* (1969)
6. Probability, Statistics and Time *M.S. Barlett* (1975)
7. Statistical Inference *S.D. Silvey* (1975)
8. The Analysis of Contingency Tables *B.S. Everitt* (1977)
9. Multivariate Analysis in Behavioural Research *A.E. Maxwell* (1977)
10. Stochastic Abundance Models *S. Engen* (1978)
11. Some Basic Theory for Statistical Inference *E.J.G. Pitman* (1979)
12. Point Processes *D.R. Cox and V. Isham* (1980)
13. Identification of Outliers *D.M. Hawkins* (1980)
14. Optimal Design *S.D. Silvey* (1980)
15. Finite Mixture Distributions *B.S. Everitt and D.J. Hand* (1981)
16. Classification *A.D. Gordon* (1981)
17. Distribution-Free Statistical Methods, 2nd edition *J.S. Maritz* (1995)
18. Residuals and Influence in Regression *R.D. Cook and S. Weisberg* (1982)
19. Applications of Queueing Theory, 2nd edition *G.F. Newell* (1982)
20. Risk Theory, 3rd edition *R.E. Beard, T. Pentikäinen and E. Pesonen* (1984)
21. Analysis of Survival Data *D.R. Cox and D. Oakes* (1984)
22. An Introduction to Latent Variable Models *B.S. Everitt* (1984)
23. Bandit Problems *D.A. Berry and B. Fristedt* (1985)
24. Stochastic Modelling and Control *M.H.A. Davis and R. Vinter* (1985)
25. The Statistical Analysis of Composition Data *J. Aitchison* (1986)
26. Density Estimation for Statistics and Data Analysis *B.W. Silverman* (1986)
27. Regression Analysis with Applications *G.B. Wetherill* (1986)
28. Sequential Methods in Statistics, 3rd edition *G.B. Wetherill and K.D. Glazebrook* (1986)
29. Tensor Methods in Statistics *P. McCullagh* (1987)
30. Transformation and Weighting in Regression *R.J. Carroll and D. Ruppert* (1988)
31. Asymptotic Techniques for Use in Statistics *O.E. Bandorff-Nielsen and D.R. Cox* (1989)
32. Analysis of Binary Data, 2nd edition *D.R. Cox and E.J. Snell* (1989)
33. Analysis of Infectious Disease Data *N.G. Becker* (1989)
34. Design and Analysis of Cross-Over Trials *B. Jones and M.G. Kenward* (1989)
35. Empirical Bayes Methods, 2nd edition *J.S. Maritz and T. Lwin* (1989)
36. Symmetric Multivariate and Related Distributions *K.T. Fang, S. Kotz and K.W. Ng* (1990)
37. Generalized Linear Models, 2nd edition *P. McCullagh and J.A. Nelder* (1989)
38. Cyclic and Computer Generated Designs, 2nd edition *J.A. John and E.R. Williams* (1995)
39. Analog Estimation Methods in Econometrics *C.F. Manski* (1988)
40. Subset Selection in Regression *A.J. Miller* (1990)
41. Analysis of Repeated Measures *M.J. Crowder and D.J. Hand* (1990)
42. Statistical Reasoning with Imprecise Probabilities *P. Walley* (1991)
43. Generalized Additive Models *T.J. Hastie and R.J. Tibshirani* (1990)
44. Inspection Errors for Attributes in Quality Control *N.L. Johnson, S. Kotz and X. Wu* (1991)
45. The Analysis of Contingency Tables, 2nd edition *B.S. Everitt* (1992)
46. The Analysis of Quantal Response Data *B.J.T. Morgan* (1992)
47. Longitudinal Data with Serial Correlation—A State-Space Approach *R.H. Jones* (1993)
48. Differential Geometry and Statistics *M.K. Murray and J.W. Rice* (1993)
49. Markov Models and Optimization *M.H.A. Davis* (1993)

50. Networks and Chaos—Statistical and Probabilistic Aspects *O.E. Barndorff-Nielsen, J.L. Jensen and W.S. Kendall* (1993)
51. Number-Theoretic Methods in Statistics *K.-T. Fang and Y. Wang* (1994)
52. Inference and Asymptotics *O.E. Barndorff-Nielsen and D.R. Cox* (1994)
53. Practical Risk Theory for Actuaries *C.D. Daykin, T. Pentikäinen and M. Pesonen* (1994)
54. Biplots *J.C. Gower and D.J. Hand* (1996)
55. Predictive Inference—An Introduction *S. Geisser* (1993)
56. Model-Free Curve Estimation *M.E. Tarter and M.D. Lock* (1993)
57. An Introduction to the Bootstrap *B. Efron and R.J. Tibshirani* (1993)
58. Nonparametric Regression and Generalized Linear Models *P.J. Green and B.W. Silverman* (1994)
59. Multidimensional Scaling *T.F. Cox and M.A.A. Cox* (1994)
60. Kernel Smoothing *M.P. Wand and M.C. Jones* (1995)
61. Statistics for Long Memory Processes *J. Beran* (1995)
62. Nonlinear Models for Repeated Measurement Data *M. Davidian and D.M. Giltinan* (1995)
63. Measurement Error in Nonlinear Models *R.J. Carroll, D. Rupert and L.A. Stefanski* (1995)
64. Analyzing and Modeling Rank Data *J.J. Marden* (1995)
65. Time Series Models—In Econometrics, Finance and Other Fields *D.R. Cox, D.V. Hinkley and O.E. Barndorff-Nielsen* (1996)
66. Local Polynomial Modeling and its Applications *J. Fan and I. Gijbels* (1996)
67. Multivariate Dependencies—Models, Analysis and Interpretation *D.R. Cox and N. Wermuth* (1996)
68. Statistical Inference—Based on the Likelihood *A. Azzalini* (1996)
69. Bayes and Empirical Bayes Methods for Data Analysis *B.P. Carlin and T.A Louis* (1996)
70. Hidden Markov and Other Models for Discrete-Valued Time Series *I.L. MacDonald and W. Zucchini* (1997)
71. Statistical Evidence—A Likelihood Paradigm *R. Royall* (1997)
72. Analysis of Incomplete Multivariate Data *J.L. Schafer* (1997)
73. Multivariate Models and Dependence Concepts *H. Joe* (1997)
74. Theory of Sample Surveys *M.E. Thompson* (1997)
75. Retrial Queues *G. Falin and J.G.C. Templeton* (1997)
76. Theory of Dispersion Models *B. Jørgensen* (1997)
77. Mixed Poisson Processes *J. Grandell* (1997)
78. Variance Components Estimation—Mixed Models, Methodologies and Applications *P.S.R.S. Rao* (1997)
79. Bayesian Methods for Finite Population Sampling *G. Meeden and M. Ghosh* (1997)
80. Stochastic Geometry—Likelihood and computation *O.E. Barndorff-Nielsen, W.S. Kendall and M.N.M. van Lieshout* (1998)
81. Computer-Assisted Analysis of Mixtures and Applications—Meta-Analysis, Disease Mapping and Others *D. Böhning* (1999)
82. Classification, 2nd edition *A.D. Gordon* (1999)
83. Semimartingales and their Statistical Inference *B.L.S. Prakasa Rao* (1999)
84. Statistical Aspects of BSE and vCJD—Models for Epidemics *C.A. Donnelly and N.M. Ferguson* (1999)
85. Set-Indexed Martingales *G. Ivanoff and E. Merzbach* (2000)
86. The Theory of the Design of Experiments *D.R. Cox and N. Reid* (2000)
87. Complex Stochastic Systems *O.E. Barndorff-Nielsen, D.R. Cox and C. Klüppelberg* (2001)
88. Multidimensional Scaling, 2nd edition *T.F. Cox and M.A.A. Cox* (2001)
89. Algebraic Statistics—Computational Commutative Algebra in Statistics *G. Pistone, E. Riccomagno and H.P. Wynn* (2001)
90. Analysis of Time Series Structure—SSA and Related Techniques *N. Golyandina, V. Nekrutkin and A.A. Zhigljavsky* (2001)
91. Subjective Probability Models for Lifetimes *Fabio Spizzichino* (2001)
92. Empirical Likelihood *Art B. Owen* (2001)
93. Statistics in the 21st Century *Adrian E. Raftery, Martin A. Tanner, and Martin T. Wells* (2001)
94. Accelerated Life Models: Modeling and Statistical Analysis *Vilijandas Bagdonavicius and Mikhail Nikulin* (2001)
95. Subset Selection in Regression, Second Edition *Alan Miller* (2002)
96. Topics in Modelling of Clustered Data *Marc Aerts, Helena Geys, Geert Molenberghs, and Louise M. Ryan* (2002)
97. Components of Variance *D.R. Cox and P.J. Solomon* (2002)

98. Design and Analysis of Cross-Over Trials, 2nd Edition *Byron Jones and Michael G. Kenward* (2003)
99. Extreme Values in Finance, Telecommunications, and the Environment *Bärbel Finkenstädt and Holger Rootzén* (2003)
100. Statistical Inference and Simulation for Spatial Point Processes *Jesper Møller and Rasmus Plenge Waagepetersen* (2004)
101. Hierarchical Modeling and Analysis for Spatial Data *Sudipto Banerjee, Bradley P. Carlin, and Alan E. Gelfand* (2004)
102. Diagnostic Checks in Time Series *Wai Keung Li* (2004)
103. Stereology for Statisticians *Adrian Baddeley and Eva B. Vedel Jensen* (2004)
104. Gaussian Markov Random Fields: Theory and Applications *Håvard Rue and Leonhard Held* (2005)
105. Measurement Error in Nonlinear Models: A Modern Perspective, Second Edition *Raymond J. Carroll, David Ruppert, Leonard A. Stefanski, and Ciprian M. Crainiceanu* (2006)
106. Generalized Linear Models with Random Effects: Unified Analysis via H-likelihood *Youngjo Lee, John A. Nelder, and Yudi Pawitan* (2006)
107. Statistical Methods for Spatio-Temporal Systems *Bärbel Finkenstädt, Leonhard Held, and Valerie Isham* (2007)
108. Nonlinear Time Series: Semiparametric and Nonparametric Methods *Jiti Gao* (2007)
109. Missing Data in Longitudinal Studies: Strategies for Bayesian Modeling and Sensitivity Analysis *Michael J. Daniels and Joseph W. Hogan* (2008)
110. Hidden Markov Models for Time Series: An Introduction Using R *Walter Zucchini and Iain L. MacDonald* (2009)
111. ROC Curves for Continuous Data *Wojtek J. Krzanowski and David J. Hand* (2009)
112. Antedependence Models for Longitudinal Data *Dale L. Zimmerman and Vicente A. Núñez-Antón* (2009)
113. Mixed Effects Models for Complex Data *Lang Wu* (2010)
114. Intoduction to Time Series Modeling *Genshiro Kitagawa* (2010)
115. Expansions and Asymptotics for Statistics *Christopher G. Small* (2010)
116. Statistical Inference: An Integrated Bayesian/Likelihood Approach *Murray Aitkin* (2010)
117. Circular and Linear Regression: Fitting Circles and Lines by Least Squares *Nikolai Chernov* (2010)
118. Simultaneous Inference in Regression *Wei Liu* (2010)
119. Robust Nonparametric Statistical Methods, Second Edition *Thomas P. Hettmansperger and Joseph W. McKean* (2011)
120. Statistical Inference: The Minimum Distance Approach *Ayanendranath Basu, Hiroyuki Shioya, and Chanseok Park* (2011)
121. Smoothing Splines: Methods and Applications *Yuedong Wang* (2011)
122. Extreme Value Methods with Applications to Finance *Serguei Y. Novak* (2012)
123. Dynamic Prediction in Clinical Survival Analysis *Hans C. van Houwelingen and Hein Putter* (2012)
124. Statistical Methods for Stochastic Differential Equations *Mathieu Kessler, Alexander Lindner, and Michael Sørensen* (2012)
125. Maximum Likelihood Estimation for Sample Surveys *R. L. Chambers, D. G. Steel, Suojin Wang, and A. H. Welsh* (2012)
126. Mean Field Simulation for Monte Carlo Integration *Pierre Del Moral* (2013)
127. Analysis of Variance for Functional Data *Jin-Ting Zhang* (2013)
128. Statistical Analysis of Spatial and Spatio-Temporal Point Patterns, Third Edition *Peter J. Diggle* (2013)
129. Constrained Principal Component Analysis and Related Techniques *Yoshio Takane* (2014)
130. Randomised Response-Adaptive Designs in Clinical Trials *Anthony C. Atkinson and Atanu Biswas* (2014)
131. Theory of Factorial Design: Single- and Multi-Stratum Experiments *Ching-Shui Cheng* (2014)
132. Quasi-Least Squares Regression *Justine Shults and Joseph M. Hilbe* (2014)
133. Data Analysis and Approximate Models: Model Choice, Location-Scale, Analysis of Variance, Nonparametric Regression and Image Analysis *Laurie Davies* (2014)
134. Dependence Modeling with Copulas *Harry Joe* (2014)
135. Hierarchical Modeling and Analysis for Spatial Data, Second Edition *Sudipto Banerjee, Bradley P. Carlin, and Alan E. Gelfand* (2014)
136. Sequential Analysis: Hypothesis Testing and Changepoint Detection *Alexander Tartakovsky, Igor Nikiforov, and Michèle Basseville* (2015)
137. Robust Cluster Analysis and Variable Selection *Gunter Ritter* (2015)
138. Design and Analysis of Cross-Over Trials, Third Edition *Byron Jones and Michael G. Kenward* (2015)

Monographs on Statistics and Applied Probability 138

Design and Analysis of Cross-Over Trials

Third Edition

Byron Jones
Novartis Pharma AG
Basel, Switzerland

Michael G. Kenward
London School of Hygiene &
Tropical Medicine
London, UK

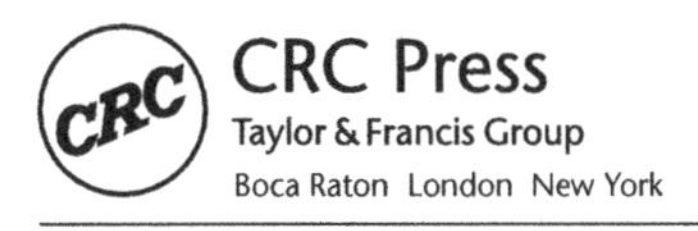
CRC Press
Taylor & Francis Group
Boca Raton London New York

CRC Press is an imprint of the
Taylor & Francis Group, an **informa** business
A CHAPMAN & HALL BOOK

CRC Press
Taylor & Francis Group
6000 Broken Sound Parkway NW, Suite 300
Boca Raton, FL 33487-2742

ISBN-13: 978-1-4398-6142-4 (hbk)

Library of Congress Cataloging-in-Publication Data

Jones, Byron.
Design and analysis of cross-over trials / Byron Jones, Michael G. Kenward. -- Third edition.
pages cm -- (Chapman & Hall / CRC monographs on statistics & applied probability ; 138)
Includes bibliographical references and index.
ISBN 978-1-4398-6142-4 (hardback)
1. Crossover trials. I. Kenward, Michael G., 1956- II. Title.

R853.C76J66 2014
610.72'7--dc23 2014028235

Visit the Taylor & Francis Web site at
http://www.taylorandfrancis.com

and the CRC Press Web site at
http://www.crcpress.com

This book is dedicated to Hilary
and to Pirkko.

Contents

List of Figures

List of Tables

Preface to the Third Edition

This book is concerned with a particular sort of comparative trial known as the cross-over trial, in which subjects receive different sequences of treatments. Such trials are widely used in clinical and medical research and in other diverse areas such as veterinary science, psychology, sports science and agriculture. The first edition of this book, which appeared in 1989, was the first to be wholly devoted to the subject. We remarked in the preface to the first edition that there existed a "large and growing literature." This growth has continued during the intervening years, and includes the appearance of several other books devoted to the topic. Naturally, the newer developments have not been spread uniformly across the subject, but have reflected both the areas where the design has remained in widespread use and new areas where it has grown in importance. Equally naturally, some of the literature also reflects the particular interests and idiosyncracies of key researchers. The second edition of the book, which appeared in 2003, reflected those areas of development. In the third edition we have kept to the structure of the second edition and have added some new chapters. Errors that we were aware of have been corrected and some of the software used has been revised to reflect the availability of new procedures in SAS, particularly `proc glimmix`.

In the first and second editions we started with a chapter wholly devoted to the two-period, two-treatment design. The aim was that this should be, to a large extent, self-contained and mostly at a level that was accessible to the less statistically experienced. It was intended that this chapter alone would be sufficient for those who had no need to venture beyond this simple design. We have not revised this chapter, other than to correct some known errors and to include the SAS procedure `proc mcmc` as an alternative to WinBUGS for the Bayesian analysis.

An important new development in this edition is the use of the R package *Crossover* written by Kornelius Rohmeyer, in collaboration with Byron Jones. This software has been written to accompany the book and provides a graphical user interface to locate designs in a large catalog and to search for new designs. This provides a convenient way of accessing all the designs tabulated in Chapter 4. It is intended that the catalog of designs contained in *Crossover* will be added to over time and become a unique and central depository for all useful cross-over designs.

Chapters 5 and 6, which were devoted to analysis, have been updated to include some recent methodological developments, in particular the use of period baselines and the analysis of data from very small trials. At the same time the opportunity has been taken to incorporate recent developments in the relevant SAS procedures, especially those in the procedures `proc glimmix` and `proc genmod`. All of the analyses for categorical data that were carried out in the second edition using `proc nlmixed` are now much more conveniently done in `proc glimmix`.

The two-treatment cross-over trial has been a standard design to use when testing for average bioequivalence. In the current edition we have removed the material on individual and population bioequivalence and refer the reader to Patterson and Jones (2006) for fuller coverage.

The final seven chapters of the book are completely new and are written in the form of short case studies. Three of these cover the topic of sample-size re-estimation when testing for average bioequivalence. The remaining new chapters cover important topics that we have also experienced in our daily consulting work: fitting a nonlinear dose response function, estimating a dose to take forward from Phase 2 to Phase 3, establishing proof of concept and recalculating the sample size using conditional power.

We are grateful to the following individuals who provided help in various ways during the writing of the new sections of the book: Bjoern Bornkamp, Frank Bretz, Yi Cheng, Tim Friede, Ekkehard Glimm, Ieuan Jones, Meinhard Kieser, Jeff Macca, Willi Maurer, Scott Patterson, James Roger, Ed Whalen, Kornelius Rohmeyer, Trevor Smart and Bernie Surujbally.

This book as been typeset using the LaTeX system, and we are grateful to the staff at Chapman & Hall/CRC for their help with this.

Of course, we take full responsibility for any errors or omissions in the text.

Chapter 1

Introduction

1.1 What is a cross-over trial?

In a completely randomized, or parallel groups, trial, each experimental unit is randomized to receive one experimental treatment. Such experimental designs are the foundation of much research, particularly in medicine and the health sciences. A good general introduction to experimental design is given by Cox and Reid (2000), while Pocock (1983), Friedman et al. (1998), Armitage (1996) and DeMets (2002) consider trial design and related issues in a clinical setting. A cross-over trial is distinguished from such a parallel groups study by each unit, or subject, receiving a *sequence* of experimental treatments. Typically, however, the aim is still to compare the effects of individual treatments, not the sequences themselves. There are many possible sets of sequences that might be used in a design, depending on the number of treatments, the length of the sequences and the aims of the trial. The simplest design is the *two-period two-treatment* or 2×2 design. In this design each subject receives two different treatments which we conventionally label as A and B. Half the subjects receive A first and then, after a suitably chosen period of time, **cross over** to B. The remaining subjects receive B first and then cross over to A. A typical example of such a trial is given in Example 1.1.

Example 1.1

The aim of this trial was to compare an oral mouthwash (treatment A) with a placebo mouthwash (treatment B). The 41 subjects who took part in the trial were healthy volunteers.

The trial, which lasted 15 weeks, was divided into two treatment periods of six weeks each, with a "wash-out" period of three weeks in between. One variable of interest was a subject's plaque score after using each of the two different mouthwashes. This was obtained for each subject by allocating a score of 0, 1, 2 or 3 to each tooth and averaging over all the teeth present in the mouth. The scores of 0, 1, 2 and 3 for each tooth corresponded, respectively, to no plaque, a film of plaque visible only by disclosing, a moderate accumulation of deposit visible to the naked eye and an abundance of soft matter. Prior to the first treatment period, an average plaque score was obtained for each subject.□□□

Some data obtained from the trial described in Example 1.1 will be analyzed in Chapter 2, which is devoted to the 2×2 trial. The definition of a

Table 1.1: Treatment sequences used in Example 1.2.

Subject	Period			
	1	2	3	4
1	B	D	C	A
2	A	C	B	D
3	C	A	D	B
4	D	B	A	C
5	B	A	D	C
6	A	D	C	B
7	C	B	A	D
8	D	C	B	A
9	B	C	D	A
10	C	D	A	B
11	C	A	B	D
12	A	C	D	B
13	B	D	A	C
14	A	B	D	C

wash-out period and the reasons for including it will be given in Section 1.3 below.

An example of a cross-over trial which compared four treatments is given in Example 1.2.

Example 1.2

The aims of this trial were to compare the effects of four treatments A, B, C and D on muscle blood flow and cardiac output in patients with intermittent claudication. Fourteen subjects took part in the trial and their treatment sequences are shown in Table 1.1. The seven weeks that the trial lasted were divided into four one-week treatment periods with a one-week wash-out period separating each pair of treatment periods.□□□

A notable feature of this trial is that every subject received the treatments in a different order. If 16 subjects could have been used, then an alternative design for four treatments might have used only four different treatment sequences, with four subjects on each sequence. With more than two treatments, there are clearly many more cross-over designs to choose from. How to choose an appropriate design is the topic of Chapter 4. In Chapter 5 we describe general methods for the analysis of continuous data, including an illustration using some data from the trial described in this example.

1.2 With which sort of cross-over trial are we concerned?

As might be guessed from the examples just given, the emphasis in this book is on cross-over trials as used in medical and pharmaceutical research, particularly research as undertaken within the pharmaceutical industry. With a few exceptions, most of the datasets we describe and analyse were obtained as part of trials undertaken by clinicians and statisticians working in the pharmaceutical industry. However, the theory, methods and practice we describe are applicable in almost any situation where cross-over trials are deemed appropriate. Such situations include, for example, sensory evaluation of food products, veterinary research, animal feeding trials and psychological experiments. Jones and Deppe (2001), for example, briefly reviewed the construction of cross-over designs for sensory testing. Cotton (1998), for example, describes designs and analyses as used in psychology. Parkes (1982), for example, has described the use of a cross-over trial to investigate occupational stress, and Raghavarao (1989) has described a potential application of cross-over trials in (the non-pharmaceutical) industry. Readers from these and other subject matter areas should have no difficulty in applying the contents of this book to their own individual situations.

1.3 Why do cross-over trials need special consideration?

The feature that distinguishes the cross-over trial from other trials which compare treatments is that measurements on different treatments are obtained from each subject. This feature brings with it advantages and disadvantages.

The main advantage is that the treatments are compared "within subjects." That is, every subject provides a direct comparison of the treatments he or she has received. In Example 1.1, for example, each subject provides two measurements: one on A and one on B. The difference between these measurements removes any "subject effect" from the comparison. Of course, this within-subject difference could also be thought of as a comparison between the two treatment periods. That is, even if the two treatments were identical, a large difference between the two measurements on a subject might be obtained if, for some reason, the measurements in one treatment period were significantly higher or lower than those in the other treatment period. The possibility of such a period difference has not been overlooked: it is the reason that one group of subjects received the treatments in the order AB and the other group received the treatments in the order BA.

The main aim of the cross-over trial is therefore to remove from the treatment (and period) comparisons any component that is related to the differences between the subjects. In clinical trials it is usually the case that the variability of measurements taken on different subjects is far greater than the variability of repeated measurements taken on the same subject. The cross-over trial aims to exploit this feature by making sure that, whenever possible, important comparisons of interest are estimated using differences obtained from the within-subject measurements. This is to be contrasted with another popular design: the "parallel groups trial." In this latter trial each subject receives only one of the possible treatments; the subjects are randomly divided into groups and each group is assigned one of the treatments being compared. Estimates of treatment differences are obtained from comparisons between the subject groups, i.e., are based on between-subject information.

Although the use of repeated measurements on the same subject brings with it great advantages, it also brings a *potential* disadvantage. We stress potential because, through appropriate choice of design and analysis, the impact of this disadvantage can be reduced, especially in trials with more than two periods. The disadvantage to which we refer is the possibility that the effect of a treatment given in one period might still be present at the start of the following period. Or more generally, that the treatment allocation in one period in some way, possibly indirectly, affects the outcomes differentially in later periods. Formally, previous treatment allocation is a *confounding* factor for later periods and means that we cannot justify our conclusions about the comparative effects of individual treatments (rather than sequences of treatments) from the randomization alone. In this way the cross-over trial has aspects in common with an observational study. The presence of carry-over is an empirical matter. It depends on the design, the setting, the treatment and response. This **carry-over** or **residual** effect can arise in a number of ways: for example, pharmacological carry-over occurs when the active ingredients of a drug given in one period are still present in the following period; psychological carry-over might occur if a drug produces an unpleasant response (e.g., total lack of pain relief) that might lead to a downgrading of the perceived response in the following period. The wash-out periods used in the trials described in Examples 1.1 and 1.2 were included to allow the active effects of a treatment given in one period to be washed out of the body before each subject began the next period of treatment. The type of measurements taken on the subjects during the treatment periods are usually also taken during the wash-out periods. These measurements, along with any **baseline** measurements taken prior to the start of the trial, can be of value at the data analysis stage. Quite often the trial is preceded by a **run-in** period which is used to familiarize subjects with the procedures they will follow during the trial and is also sometimes used as a screening period to ensure only eligible subjects proceed to the treatment periods.

The differences between the treatments as measured in one period might also be different from those measured in a later period because of a **treatment-by-period interaction**. Such an interaction might also be the result of treatments possessing different amounts of carry-over, or might be the result of a true interaction. That is, for some reason, the conditions present in the different periods affect the size of the differences between the treatments. Although in any well-planned trial the chance of treatments interacting with periods will be small, it may sometimes be desirable to use a design which permits the interaction to be detected and if possible to identify whether it is the result of carry-over or not. Generally, designs for more than two treatments can be constructed in such a way that they allow the interaction and carry-over to be estimated separately. Designs for two treatments however, require special attention and we consider these in Chapter 3.

1.4 A brief history

Although we concentrate on cross-over designs as used in clinical trials, the earliest uses of such designs were most likely in agriculture. Indeed, what may well be the first cross-over trial was started in 1853 and, in a much modified form, still exists today. It originated in one of the great nineteenth century controversies. John Bennett Lawes of Rothamsted, Hertfordshire, England, and Baron Justus von Liebig of Giessen, in Germany, disagreed about the nutrition of crop plants. Both were somewhat vague in classifying plant nutrients as either organic or mineral and Liebig sometimes contradicted himself. But in 1847 he wrote (Liebig, 1847) that cultivated plants received enough nitrogen from the atmosphere for the purpose of agriculture, though it might be necessary for the farmer to apply minerals. Lawes, a more practically minded man, but with no scientific qualifications, and much junior to Liebig, knew from the results of the first few seasons of his field experimental work that the yield of wheat was greatly improved by the application of ammoniacal salts. He noticed that yields varied greatly between seasons, but whenever one of his plots of wheat received ammoniacal salts it gave a good yield, but when minerals (i.e., phosphates, potash, etc.) were given the yield was much less. To separate the real effects of manures from the large differences between seasons, and to clinch his refutation of Liebig's argument, he allocated two plots to an alternation of treatments which continued long after his death. Each year one plot received ammonia without minerals, the other minerals without ammonia; the following season the applications were interchanged. The result was a total success: ammonia (after minerals in the preceding season) gave a full yield (practically equal to that given by the plot that received both every year) but minerals following ammonia gave about half as much (very little more than the plot that received minerals without ammonia every year). But Liebig never admitted his mistake.

Lawes and his co-worker J.H. Gilbert seem also to be the first to have been explicitly concerned with carry-over effects. Lawes (page 10 of a pamphlet published in 1846) gave advice on the use of artificial manures: Let the artificial manures be applied in greater abundance to the green crops, and the residue of these will manure the corn. Their interest in carry-over effects is further evident from Section II of Lawes and Gilbert (1864), which is entitled Effects of the unexhausted residue from previous manuring upon succeeding crops. The data collected in these classic experiments were among the first to occupy R. A. Fisher and his co-workers in the Statistics Department at Rothamsted. This department was created in 1919.

The particular design problems associated with long-term rotation experiments were considered by Cochran (1939). He seems to have been one of the first to formally separate out the two sorts of treatment effects (direct and carry-over) when considering which experimental plan to use.

Early interest in administering different treatments to the same experimental unit was not confined to agricultural experiments, however. Simpson (1938) described a number of cross-over trials which compared different diets given to children. In one trial he compared four different diets using 24 children. The plan of the trial was such that all possible permutations of the four diets were used, each child receiving one of the 24 different treatment sequences. He was aware of the possibility of carry-over effects and suggested that this might be allowed for by introducing a wash-out period between each pair of treatment periods. Yates (1938) considered in more detail one of the other designs suggested by Simpson (1938) and considered the efficiency of estimation of the direct, carry-over and cumulative (direct + carry-over) effects of three different sets of sequences for three treatments administered over three periods.

Cross-over trials have been used extensively in animal husbandry experiments since at least the 1930s. Indeed, some of the most important early contributions to the design theory came from workers like W. G. Cochran, H. D. Patterson and H. L. Lucas, who had an interest in this area.

Brandt (1938) described the analysis of designs which compared two treatments using two groups of cattle. Depending on the number of periods, the animals in one group received the treatments in the order ABAB..., and the animals in the other group received the treatments in the order BABA.... This type of design is usually referred to as the **switchback** or **reversal** design. In a now classic paper, Cochran et al. (1941) described a trial on Holstein cows which compared three treatments over three periods using two orthogonal Latin squares. They seem to have been the first to formally describe the least squares estimation of the direct and carry-over treatment effects. The design they used had the property of balance, which has been studied extensively ever since. Williams (1949, 1950) showed how balanced designs which used the minimum number of subjects could be constructed. He quoted an example taken from the milling of paper in which different pulp suspensions were compared using six different mills. We describe balanced and other sorts of design in Chapter 4.

Another early use of cross-over designs took place in the area of biological assay. Fieller (1940) described a 2×2 trial which used rabbits to compare the effects of different doses of insulin. Fieller also cites a very early paper (Marks, 1925) which described an application of the 2×2 design. Finney (1956) described the design and analysis of a number of different cross-over designs for use in biological assay. One sort of cross-over design with which we are not concerned here is when the whole trial is conducted on a single subject. These designs have also been used in biological assay. For further details see Finney and Outhwaite (1955, 1956) and Sampford (1957).

In this section we have given only a brief description of some of the early uses of cross-over trials that we are aware of. For more comprehensive reviews of the uses of cross-over trials see Bishop and Jones (1984), Hedayat and Afsarinejad (1975), Kenward and Jones (1988), Jones and Deppe (2001), Tudor et al. (2000) and Senn (1997a, 2000, 2002), for example.

1.5 Notation, models and analysis

For a cross-over trial we will denote by t, p and s, respectively, the number of treatments, periods and sequences. So, for example, in a trial in which each subject received three treatments A, B and C, in one of the six sequences ABC, ACB, BAC, BCA, CAB and CBA, we have $t = 3$, $p = 3$ and $s = 6$. In general, we denote by y_{ijk} the response observed on the kth subject in period j of sequence group i. It is assumed that n_i subjects are in sequence group i. To represent sums of observations we will use the dot notation, for example:

$$y_{ij\cdot} = \sum_{k=1}^{n_i} y_{ijk}, \quad y_{i\cdot\cdot} = \sum_{j=1}^{p} y_{ij\cdot}, \quad y_{\cdot\cdot\cdot} = \sum_{i=1}^{s} y_{i\cdot\cdot}.$$

In a similar way, the corresponding mean values will be denoted, respectively, as

$$\bar{y}_{ij\cdot} = \frac{1}{n_i}\sum_{k=1}^{n_i} y_{ijk}, \quad \bar{y}_{i\cdot\cdot} = \frac{1}{pn_i}\sum_{j=1}^{p} y_{ij\cdot}, \quad \bar{y}_{\cdot\cdot\cdot} = \frac{1}{p\sum n_i}\sum_{i=1}^{s} y_{i\cdot\cdot}.$$

To construct a statistical model we assume that y_{ijk} is the observed value of a random variable Y_{ijk}. For a continuous outcome we assume that Y_{ijk} can be represented by a linear model that, in its most basic form, can be written

$$Y_{ijk} = \mu + \pi_j + \tau_{d[i,j]} + s_{ik} + e_{ijk}, \tag{1.1}$$

where the terms in this model are

μ, an intercept;

π_j, an effect associated with period $j, j = 1,\ldots,p$;

$\tau_{d[i,j]}$, a direct treatment effect associated with the treatment applied in period j of sequence i, $d[i,j] = 1,\ldots,t$;

s_{ik}, an effect associated with the kth subject on sequence $i, i = 1,\ldots,s$, $k = 1,\ldots,n_i$;

e_{ijk}, a random error term, with zero mean and variance σ^2.

Sometimes we need to represent a potential carry-over effect in the model. A simple first-order carry-over effect (that is affecting the outcome in the following period only) will be represented by the term $\lambda_{d[i,j-1]}$ where it is assumed that $\lambda_{d[i,0]} = 0$. Additional terms such as second-order carry-over and direct treatment-by-period interaction effects can be added to this model, but such terms are rarely of much interest in practice.

An important distinction needs to be made between those models in which the subject effects (the s_{ik}) are assumed to be unknown fixed parameters and those in which they are assumed to be realizations of random variables, usually with zero mean and variance σ_s^2. The use of the former implies that the subsequent analysis will use information from within-subject comparisons only. This is appropriate for the majority of well-designed cross-over trials and has the advantage of keeping the analysis within the familiar setting of linear regression. There are circumstances, however, in which the subject totals contain relevant information and this can only be recovered if the subject effects are treated as random. Such a model is an example of a linear mixed model, and the use of these introduces some additional issues: properties of estimators and inference procedures are asymptotic (possibly requiring small-sample adjustments), and an additional assumption is needed for the distribution of the random subject effects.

Model fitting and inference for fixed subject-effect models will follow conventional ordinary least squares (OLS) procedures and for random subject-effect models we will use the now well-established REML analyses for linear mixed models (see, for example, Verbeke and Molenberghs (2000)). Throughout the book the necessary steps for accomplishing such analyses will be given for the `mixed` and `proc glimmix` procedures of SAS (Statistical Analysis System, SAS (2014)). Although most of these instructions will be common to earlier releases of the package, we do make, for linear mixed models, some small use of features that are only available in release 9.3 and later. Of course, many other statistical packages can be used for the ordinary linear model analyses, while some also include facilities for linear mixed models. Occasionally, we will also use the SAS `proc glm` procedure for fitting models with fixed subject effects.

The core modeling component of SAS `proc mixed` can be illustrated very simply for both fixed and random subject-effects models and these can be seen to be direct translations of model formulae of the form of (1.1). Suppose that the variates in the dataset representing sequence, subject, period, direct treatment and response are labeled accordingly. Then for a **fixed subject-effects** model we have the basic `proc mixed` commands

```
proc mixed;
  class sequence subject period treatment;
  model response = sequence(subject) period
                       treatment;
run;
```

If subjects each have individual identifiers, rather than being labeled within sequences as in model (1.1), then `sequence(subject)` is replaced by `subject`.

For a **random subject-effects** model, we can simply move the subject term from the `model` statement to a `random` statement:

```
proc mixed;
  class sequence subject period treatment;
  model response = period treatment;
  random sequence(subject);
run;
```

First-order carry-over effects can be added to the model in an obvious way, noting that the corresponding variate needs to be defined appropriately. The `class` statement identifies a variate as a factor, with a number of levels, for which indicator variables are generated. Factors should have a level defined for *all* observations, but we know that there cannot be a carry-over effect in the first period; hence there is no level. This problem can be avoided by ensuring that the carry-over variate takes the same level for each first period observation (any level can be used) and including period effect in the model.

The linear models described so far would not be appropriate for categorical or very non-normal data. A range of modeling approaches is available for the former, most of which maintain some aspect of model (1.1) through a **linear predictor**. Such models are the subject of Chapter 6.

1.6 Aims of this book

It is the purpose of this book to provide a thorough coverage of the statistical aspects of the design and analysis of cross-over trials. We have tried to maintain a practical perspective and to avoid those topics that are of largely academic interest. Throughout the book we have included examples of SAS code so that the analyses we describe can be immediately implemented using the SAS statistical analysis system. In particular, we have made extensive use of the `proc mixed` and `proc glimmix` procedures in SAS. Although our approach is practically oriented, we mean this in a statistical sense. The topic is a vast one and embraces planning, ethics, recruitment, administration, reporting, regulatory issues, and so on. Some, and occasionally, all of these aspects will have a statistical component but it must be borne in mind throughout this book that the statistical features of the design and analysis are but one aspect of the overall trial.

We have attempted to compromise in the level of statistical sophistication. Most of the discussion of the 2×2 trial in Chapter 2 is dealt with at a fairly elementary level and we hope this material will be accessible to those with limited statistical experience, including those whose primary role is not that of a statistician. The same is true of the introductory sections of Chapters 3, 4 and 7. To avoid over-lengthening the book, however, we have been somewhat briefer in other sections and expected more of the reader. This is particularly true of Chapters 5 and 6, where the most advanced material is to be found. Chapters 8 to 14 are brief case studies that give examples of interesting applications of cross-over trials. The practical aspects of these should be accessible to all. We do not believe, however, that any of the material should prove taxing to statisticians with some experience of the design and analysis of experiments.

1.7 Structure of the book

In the next chapter we cover in some detail the 2×2 cross-over trial with continuous observations and give some simple analyses for binary data. We also briefly describe some Bayesian analyses for continuous data and give a fairly lengthy discussion of nonparametric approaches. In Chapter 3 we continue to consider trials for two treatments, but now the trials have more than two periods or sequences. How to choose a design for a cross-over trial with three or more treatments is the topic of Chapter 4, where we give tables of useful designs and show how designs can be found using the R package *Crossover* that has been written to accompany this book. This software includes a facility to search a large catalog of designs as well as an option of finding an optimal design by using a search algorithm. Chapter 5 is devoted to a general coverage of the analysis of continuous data from a cross-over trial, including the situation where repeated measurements are taken within periods. Chapter 6 provides the equivalent of Chapter 5 for binary and categorical data. Average bioequivalence testing is the topic of Chapter 7. The remaining seven brief chapters are in the form of case studies and illustrate several novel applications of cross-over trials: fitting a dose–response function, searching for a dose to take forward for further development, use of conditional power at an interim analysis, evaluation of proof of concept and three variations on an interim analysis to recalculate the sample size of the trial after an interim analysis. Throughout the book, as already noted, we give the necessary computer software instructions for the reader to reproduce the analyses we describe.

Chapter 2

The 2 $\times$ 2 cross-over trial

2.1 Introduction

In this chapter we consider data obtained from the 2×2 trial. For most of this chapter we assume that the response measured in each period of the trial has been recorded on a continuous scale. However, simple analyses of binary data will be described in Section 2.13. The analysis of binary and categorical data is considered in more generality in Chapter 6.

After introducing an example we begin the chapter by describing two useful methods of plotting cross-over data. A linear model for the data is then introduced and used to derive two-sample t-tests for testing hypotheses about the direct treatment and carry-over effects. In addition, point and interval estimates of the difference between the direct treatments and between the carry-over effects are defined. A third useful plot is then described. The calculation of the sample size is considered next. Although all the hypothesis testing necessary for the 2×2 trial can be done using t-tests, we take the opportunity to describe the appropriate analysis of variance for the 2×2 trial. Following this we then define the residuals from our model and use them to check the assumptions made about the model. Some inherent difficulties associated with modeling data from 2×2 trials are then discussed. The consequences of using a preliminary test for a difference in carry-over effects are then discussed. Next, a Bayesian analysis of the 2×2 trial is described and then the use of run-in and wash-out baselines is considered. The use of covariates is described next. Then we give a fairly extensive discussion of nonparametric methods. Finally, simple testing methods for binary data, based on contingency tables, are described.

Example 2.1 To illustrate the various ways of analyzing 2×2 cross-over data we will use the data listed in Tables 2.1 and 2.2. These are data from a single-center, randomized, placebo-controlled, double-blind study to evaluate the efficacy and safety of an inhaled drug (A) given twice daily via an inhaler in patients with chronic obstructive pulmonary disease (COPD). Patients who satisfied the initial entry criteria entered a two-week run-in period. Clinic Visit 1 is used to denote the start of this period. After 13 days they returned to the clinic for a histamine challenge test (Clinic Visit 2). On the following day (Clinic Visit 3) they returned to the clinic and, following a methacholine challenge test, eligible patients were randomized to receive either Drug (A) or

Table 2.1: Group 1 (AB) mean morning PEFR (L/min).

Subject Number	Subject Label	Period 1	Period 2
1	7	121.905	116.667
2	8	218.500	200.500
3	9	235.000	217.143
4	13	250.000	196.429
5	14	186.190	185.500
6	15	231.563	221.842
7	17	443.250	420.500
8	21	198.421	207.692
9	22	270.500	213.158
10	28	360.476	384.000
11	35	229.750	188.250
12	36	159.091	221.905
13	37	255.882	253.571
14	38	279.048	267.619
15	41	160.556	163.000
16	44	172.105	182.381
17	58	267.000	313.000
18	66	230.750	211.111
19	71	271.190	257.619
20	76	276.250	222.105
21	79	398.750	404.000
22	80	67.778	70.278
23	81	195.000	223.158
24	82	325.000	306.667
25	86	368.077	362.500
26	89	228.947	227.895
27	90	236.667	220.000

matching Placebo (B) twice daily for four weeks. The patients then switched over at Clinic Visit 5 to the alternative treatment for a further four weeks. The patients also returned to the clinic a day before the end of each treatment period (Clinic Visits 4 and 6) when repeat histamine challenge tests were performed. There was a final clinic visit two weeks after cessation of all treatment (Clinic Visit 8). Patients were instructed to attend the clinic at approximately the same time of day for each visit.

The primary comparison of efficacy was based on the mean morning expiratory flow rate (PEFR) obtained from data recorded on daily record cards. Each day patients took three measurements of PEFR on waking in the morning, and at bed-time, prior to taking any study medication. On each occasion the highest of the three readings was recorded.

Of a total of 77 patients recruited into the study, 66 were randomized to treatment (33 per sequence group). Ultimately, data on the mean morning

Table 2.2: Group 2 (BA) mean morning PEFR (L/min).

Subject Number	Subject Label	Period 1	Period 2
1	3	138.333	138.571
2	10	225.000	256.250
3	11	392.857	381.429
4	16	190.000	233.333
5	18	191.429	228.000
6	23	226.190	267.143
7	24	201.905	193.500
8	26	134.286	128.947
9	27	238.000	248.500
10	29	159.500	140.000
11	30	232.750	276.563
12	32	172.308	170.000
13	33	266.000	305.000
14	39	171.333	186.333
15	43	194.737	191.429
16	47	200.000	222.619
17	51	146.667	183.810
18	52	208.000	241.667
19	55	208.750	218.810
20	59	271.429	225.000
21	68	143.810	188.500
22	70	104.444	135.238
23	74	145.238	152.857
24	77	215.385	240.476
25	78	306.000	288.333
26	83	160.526	150.476
27	84	353.810	369.048
28	85	293.889	308.095
29	99	371.190	404.762

PEFR (over the treatment days in each period) from 56 patients were obtained: 27 in the AB group and 29 in the BA group. The data from the patients in the AB sequence group are given in Table 2.1, and the data from the BA sequence group are given in Table 2.2.□□□

The general notation to be used in this chapter is as follows. The subjects are divided into two groups of sizes n_1 and n_2. The n_1 subjects in Group 1 receive the treatments in the order AB and the n_2 subjects in Group 2 receive the treatments in the order BA. As defined in Chapter 1, the response on subject k in period j of group i is denoted by y_{ijk}, where $i = 1,2$, $j = 1,2$ and $k = 1,2,\ldots,n_i$. The group-by-period means for the morning mean PEFR data are given in Table 2.3.

Table 2.3: Group-by-period means for the mean PEFR data.

Group	Period 1	Period 2	Mean
1 (AB) $n_1 = 27$	$\bar{y}_{11.} = 245.84$	$\bar{y}_{12.} = 239.20$	$\bar{y}_{1..} = 242.52$
2 (BA) $n_2 = 29$	$\bar{y}_{21.} = 215.99$	$\bar{y}_{22.} = 230.16$	$\bar{y}_{2..} = 223.08$
Mean	$\bar{y}_{.1.} = 230.38$	$\bar{y}_{.2.} = 234.52$	$\bar{y}_{...} = 232.45$

2.2 Plotting the data

As with the analysis of any set of data, it is always good practice to begin by drawing and inspecting graphs. A "feel" for the data can then be obtained and any outstanding features identified.

We begin by plotting for each patient, within each group, the mean PEFR in Period 2 vs the mean PEFR in Period 1. These plots are given in Figure 2.1. We have also added the line with slope 1 and intercept 0. It is clear that in each group there is a high positive correlation between the two responses

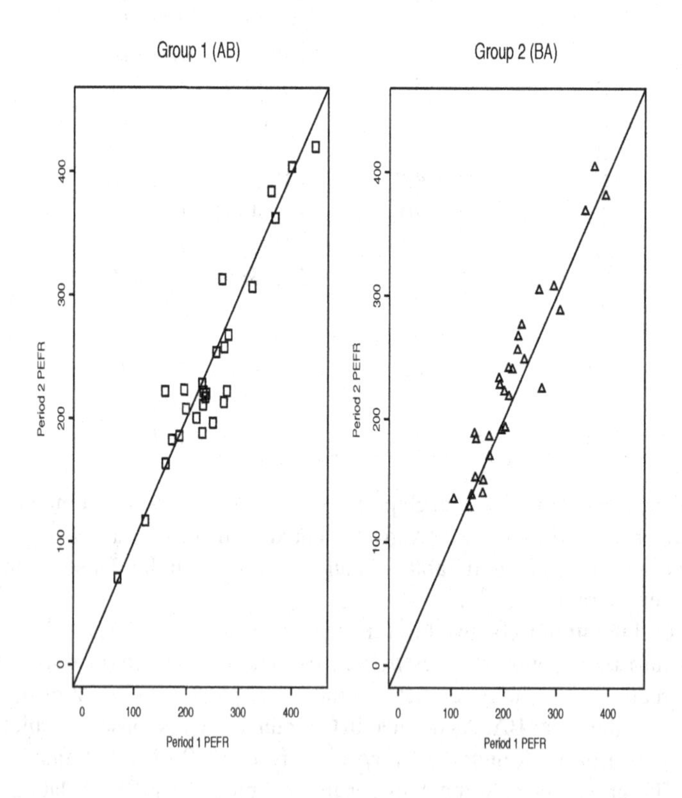

Figure 2.1: Period 2 vs Period 1 plots.

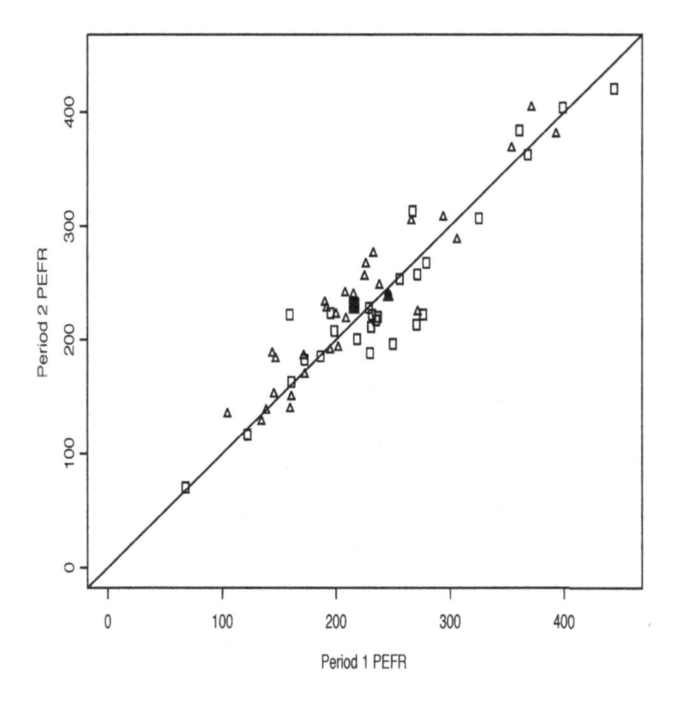

Figure 2.2: Period 2 vs Period 1 plot with centroids.

on the same patient. In Group 1 it is 0.943 and in Group 2 it is 0.949. There is a tendency for the plotted points to be below the line in Group 1 and above it in Group 2. Another way of describing the same feature is to note that in the direction parallel with the diagonal the points for each group are quite spread out, indicating high between-patient variability. We can also see that one patient in Group 1 has unusually low mean PEFR values.

The fact that the points from the two groups are almost symmetrically placed in relation to the diagonal line is evidence for the absence of a period effect. To determine evidence for a direct treatment effect we plot, in Figure 2.2, both sets of points on a single graph and indicate the centroid of each group with a solid enlarged character. The fact that the centroids are placed either side of the line with some vertical separation is evidence of a direct treatment effect. As a carry-over difference is hard to detect, even with a statistical test, we do not try to infer anything about it from the graphs.

The objective of a cross-over trial is to focus attention on within-patient treatment differences. A good plot for displaying these differences is the subject-profiles plot. Here we plot for each group the change in each patient's response over the two treatment periods. That is, for each value of k, the pairs

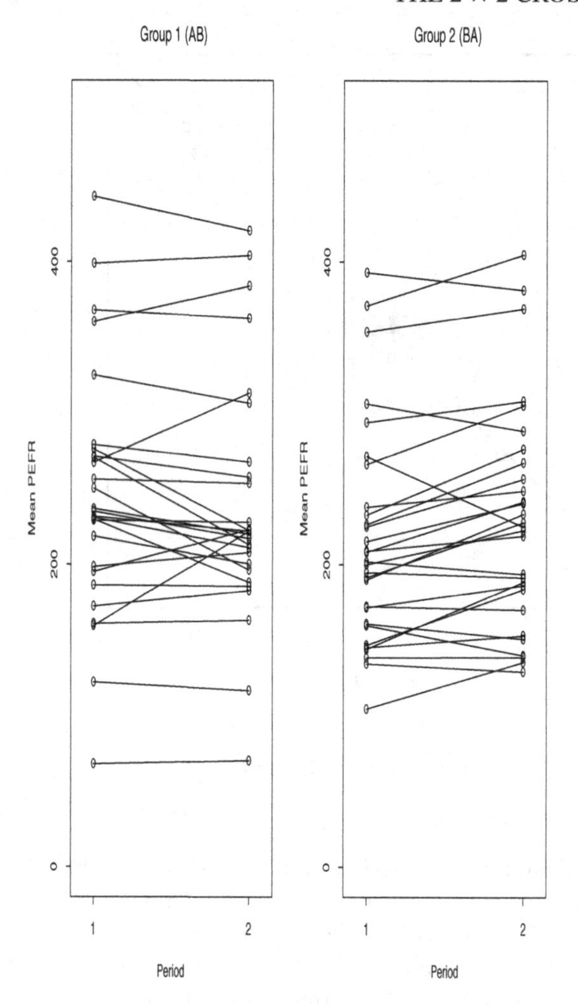

Figure 2.3: Profiles plot for PEFR data.

of points (y_{11k}, y_{12k}) and (y_{21k}, y_{22k}) are plotted and joined up. This plot is given in Figure 2.3.

Again, high between-patient variability is evident, as are the low mean PEFR values for one patient in Group 1. The within-patient (first period-second period) changes are generally positive (i.e., higher in Period 1) in Group 1 and negative in Group 2, although there are some notable exceptions. The absolute sizes of the changes are mostly quite small, though there are big changes for some patients. The general trend, however, implies a direct treatment effect in favor (i.e., higher mean PEFR) of treatment A.

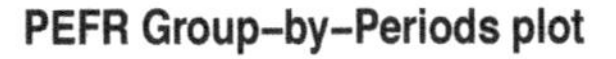

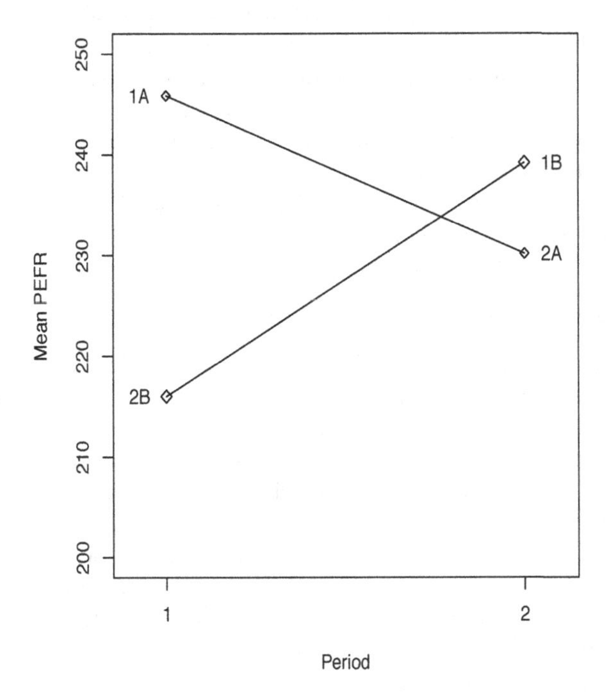

Figure 2.4: Group-by-periods plot for PEFR data.

Having looked at the PEFR values from individual patients, we now plot a graph that compares the average values over each group for each period. We refer to this as the groups-by-periods plot. We plot the four group-by-period means $\bar{y}_{11.}$, $\bar{y}_{12.}$, $\bar{y}_{21.}$ $\bar{y}_{22.}$ against their corresponding Period labels and join them up. On the graph it is convenient to label these means in terms of the group and treatment they represent, i.e., as 1A, 1B, 2B and 2A, respectively. It is also convenient to join 1A with 2A and 2B with 1B. For the data in Tables 2.1 and 2.2 the plot is given in Figure 2.4.

In Period 1, the treatment mean difference (A vs B) is 29.85, whereas in Period 2, the difference is negative and equal to 9.04. This is suggestive of a treatment-by-period interaction. The statistical significance of these features will be considered in the next section.

The graphs in this section provide an informal overview of the data. It is also very important to check that any assumptions made about the data are satisfied. This is best done after formally fitting a model to the data, and we therefore postpone our checks on the assumptions until Section 2.5. In that section we fit a model to the data and calculate residuals.

Before we fit the model, however, we will illustrate a general and useful technique for analyzing cross-over designs for two treatments with two sequence groups. This technique involves reducing the two responses on each subject to a single value and comparing the mean of this derived variate between the two groups. For normally distributed data, a two-sample t-test is used to compare the group means, and we illustrate this in the next section. For data that are not normally distributed, the Mann–Whitney–Wilcoxon rank-sum test can be used. We describe this latter test in Section 2.12.

2.3 Analysis using t-tests

Although the general approach we will adopt in the remainder of the book is to fit linear models to cross-over data, the 2×2 cross-over trial provides a simple illustration of a general technique for two-group designs with two treatments. For normally distributed data the estimation and testing can be done entirely using two-sample t-tests. This approach was first suggested by Hills and Armitage (1979). (See also Chassan (1964).) To compare the direct effects of the two treatments, the estimation and testing make use of the difference of the measurements taken in Periods 1 and 2 for each subject. To compare carry-over effects, the total of the two measurements on each subject is used. These derived variates are given in Tables 2.4 and 2.5. We will make use of this general technique again in Chapter 3, when we consider designs for two treatments that have more than two periods.

The linear model on which the t-tests are based is as defined in Section 1.5 of Chapter 1 with $s = 2$, $p = 2$ and s_{ik} a *random* subject effect. In general, this model contains terms for the direct treatment and carry-over effects. As noted earlier, we do not recommend testing for a carry-over difference in the AB/BA design. However, in order to explain why, we first have to consider a model that does contain carry-over effects.

The fixed effects associated with each subject in each period in each of the two groups are displayed in Table 2.6, where τ_1 and τ_2 are the direct effects of treatments A and B, respectively, and λ_1 and λ_2 are the corresponding carry-over effects.

The subject effects, s_{ik}, are assumed to be independent and identically distributed (i.i.d.) with mean 0 and variance σ_s^2. Similarly, the random errors are assumed to be i.i.d. with mean 0 and variance σ^2. In order to derive hypothesis tests, it will be further assumed, unless stated otherwise, that the observed data are random samples from normal (Gaussian) distributions.

The linear model contains parameters to account for possible differences between the carry-over effects, if these exist, but no parameters to account for any direct-by-period interaction. This interaction would occur if the difference between the direct treatment effects was not the same in each period. The

Table 2.4: Group 1 (AB) subject totals and differences.

Subject Number	Subject Label	Total	Differences
1	7	238.572	5.238
2	8	419.000	18.000
3	9	452.143	17.857
4	13	446.429	53.571
5	14	371.690	0.690
6	15	453.405	9.721
7	17	863.750	22.750
8	21	406.113	−9.271
9	22	483.658	57.342
10	28	744.476	−23.524
11	35	418.000	41.500
12	36	380.996	−62.814
13	37	509.453	2.311
14	38	546.667	11.429
15	41	323.556	−2.444
16	44	354.486	−10.276
17	58	580.000	−46.000
18	66	441.861	19.639
19	71	528.809	13.571
20	76	498.355	54.145
21	79	802.750	−5.250
22	80	138.056	−2.500
23	81	418.158	−28.158
24	82	631.667	18.333
25	86	730.577	5.577
26	89	456.842	1.052
27	90	456.667	16.667

reason we have omitted the interaction parameters is that, as there are only four sample means $\bar{y}_{11.}$, $\bar{y}_{12.}$, $\bar{y}_{21.}$ and $\bar{y}_{22.}$, we can include only three parameters at most to account for the differences between these means. Of the three degrees of freedom between the means, two are associated with differences between the periods and direct treatments, leaving only one to be associated with the carry-over and interaction. In other words, the carry-over and the direct-by-period interaction parameters are intrinsically aliased with each other. Indeed, there is a third possibility, that of including a parameter to account for the difference between the two groups of subjects. If this parameter is included, however, it too will be found to be aliased with the carry-over and direct-by-period interaction. This is one disadvantage of the 2×2 cross-over trial: several important effects are aliased with each other. This point will be taken up again

Table 2.5: Group 2 (BA) subject totals and differences.

Subject Number	Subject Label	Total	Difference
1	7	276.904	−0.238
2	8	481.250	−31.250
3	9	774.286	11.428
4	13	423.333	−43.333
5	14	419.429	−36.571
6	15	493.333	−40.953
7	17	395.405	8.405
8	21	263.233	5.339
9	22	486.500	−10.500
10	28	299.500	19.500
11	35	509.313	−43.813
12	36	342.308	2.308
13	37	571.000	−39.000
14	38	357.666	−15.000
15	41	386.166	3.308
16	44	422.619	−22.619
17	66	330.477	−37.143
18	71	449.667	−33.667
19	76	427.560	−10.060
20	79	496.429	46.429
21	68	332.310	−44.690
22	80	239.682	−30.794
23	81	298.095	−7.619
24	82	455.861	−25.091
25	86	594.333	17.667
26	89	311.002	10.050
27	90	722.858	−15.238
28	85	601.984	−14.206
29	99	775.952	−33.572

Table 2.6: The fixed effects in the full model.

Group	Period 1	Period 2
1 (AB)	$\mu+\pi_1+\tau_1$	$\mu+\pi_2+\tau_2+\lambda_1$
2 (BA)	$\mu+\pi_1+\tau_2$	$\mu+\pi_2+\tau_1+\lambda_2$

in Section 2.6. For the moment, however, we will present our analyses in terms of the model given previously, which includes the carry-over effect parameters λ_1 and λ_2.

We should point out that the test for a carry-over difference is likely to have low power to detect a significant difference. In addition, the testing of direct treatment effects in the presence of carry-over effects is problematic. We will ignore this for now, leaving a more considered discussion until Section 2.7.

Testing $\lambda_1 = \lambda_2$

The first test we consider is the test of equality of the carry-over effects. We note that even though we may wish to test the more specific hypothesis that $\lambda_1 = \lambda_2 = 0$, this cannot be done if the period effects are retained in the model.

In order to derive a test of the null hypothesis that $\lambda_1 = \lambda_2$, we note that the subject totals

$$t_{1k} = y_{11k} + y_{12k} \quad \text{for the } k\text{th subject in Group 1}$$

and

$$t_{2k} = y_{21k} + y_{22k} \quad \text{for the } k\text{th subject in Group 2}$$

have expectations

$$E[t_{1k}] = 2\mu + \pi_1 + \pi_2 + \tau_1 + \tau_2 + \lambda_1$$

and

$$E[t_{2k}] = 2\mu + \pi_1 + \pi_2 + \tau_1 + \tau_2 + \lambda_2.$$

If $\lambda_1 = \lambda_2$, these two expectations are equal. Consequently, to test if $\lambda_1 = \lambda_2$, we can apply the familiar two-sample t-test to the subject totals. With this in mind, we define $\lambda_d = \lambda_1 - \lambda_2$ and $\hat{\lambda}_d = \bar{t}_{1.} - \bar{t}_{2.}$ and note that

$$\begin{aligned} E[\hat{\lambda}_d] &= \lambda_d \\ \text{Var}[\hat{\lambda}_d] &= 2(2\sigma_s^2 + \sigma^2)\left(\frac{1}{n_1} + \frac{1}{n_2}\right) \\ &= \sigma_T^2 m, \text{ say, where} \end{aligned}$$

$$\sigma_T^2 = 2(2\sigma_s^2 + \sigma^2) \ \text{ and } m = \frac{n_1 + n_2}{n_1 n_2}.$$

To estimate σ_T^2, we will use

$$\hat{\sigma}_T^2 = \sum_{i=1}^{2} \sum_{k=1}^{n_i} (t_{ik} - \bar{t}_{i.})^2 / (n_1 + n_2 - 2),$$

the pooled sample variance which has $(n_1 + n_2 - 2)$ degrees of freedom (d.f.). On the null hypothesis that $\lambda_1 = \lambda_2$, the statistic

$$T_\lambda = \frac{\hat{\lambda}_d}{(\hat{\sigma}_T^2 m)^{\frac{1}{2}}}$$

has a Student's t-distribution on $(n_1 + n_2 - 2)$ d.f.

In order to illustrate this test, let us refer back to Example 2.1 and the data displayed in Tables 2.4 and 2.5. Using these data, we obtain $\bar{t}_{1.} = 485.042$, $\bar{t}_{2.} = 446.154$ and $\hat{\lambda}_d = 38.89$. Also $\sum_{k=1}^{27}(t_{1k} - \bar{t}_{1.})^2 = 683497.9$ and $\sum_{k=1}^{29}(t_{2k} - \bar{t}_{2.})^2 = 586233.2$. The pooled estimate of σ_T^2 is $\hat{\sigma}_T^2 = (683497.9 + 586233.2)/54 = 23513.54$ and the t statistic is

$$T_\lambda = \frac{38.89}{\left(\frac{56}{783} \times 23513.54\right)^{\frac{1}{2}}} = 0.948 \quad \text{on 54 d.f.}$$

The observed P-value is 0.347.

As we mentioned earlier, this test has low power and so we cannot assert that the lack of significance implies lack of effect. We have to rely on other explanations why a carry-over difference is unlikely, e.g., adequate wash-out periods or, in the absence of wash-out periods, that the primary endpoint measurements are taken from times within the treatment periods when carry-over is unlikely to be present.

Prior to Freeman (1989), it was common practice to follow the advice of Grizzle (1965) when testing for a carry-over difference. Grizzle suggested that the test should be done as a preliminary to testing for a direct treatment difference, and to base the carry-over test on a 10% two-sided significance level. If the test was significant, Grizzle suggested that only the data from Period 1 should be used to compare the direct treatments, as in a parallel groups design. If the test was not significant, he suggested using the data from both periods to test for a direct treatment difference. Freeman (1989) showed that this two-stage procedure of testing for a carry-over difference in the first stage and then for a direct treatment difference in the second stage not only inflated the probability of making a Type I error, but also produced a biased estimate of the direct treatment difference. We will give more details of Freeman's results in Section 2.7.

For the mean PEFR data, a carry-over difference was not expected and we consider a nonsignificant test result as being supportive of this. When we have good reason to suppose that $\lambda_1 = \lambda_2$, then we can proceed to test for a direct treatment difference in the following way.

Testing $\tau_1 = \tau_2$ *(assuming* $\lambda_1 = \lambda_2$ *)*

If we can assume that $\lambda_1 = \lambda_2$, then the period differences

$$d_{1k} = y_{11k} - y_{12k} \quad \text{for the } k\text{th subject in Group 1}$$

and

$$d_{2k} = y_{21k} - y_{22k} \quad \text{for the } k\text{th subject in Group 2}$$

have expectations

$$E[d_{1k}] = \pi_1 - \pi_2 + \tau_1 - \tau_2$$

and

$$E[d_{2k}] = \pi_1 - \pi_2 + \tau_2 - \tau_1.$$

On the null hypothesis that $\tau_1 = \tau_2$ these two expectations are equal and so we can test the null hypothesis by applying the two-sample t-test to the period differences.

In particular, if we define $\tau_d = \tau_1 - \tau_2$, then $\hat{\tau}_d = \frac{1}{2}[\bar{d}_{1.} - \bar{d}_{2.}]$ is such that

$$E[\hat{\tau}_d] = \tau_d$$

and

$$\begin{aligned}\text{Var}[\hat{\tau}_d] &= \frac{2\sigma^2}{4}\left(\frac{1}{n_1} + \frac{1}{n_2}\right) \\ &= \frac{\sigma_D^2}{4} m \text{ say,}\end{aligned}$$

where

$$\sigma_D^2 = 2\sigma^2.$$

The pooled estimate of σ_D^2 is

$$\hat{\sigma}_D^2 = \sum_{i=1}^{2} \sum_{k=1}^{n_i} (d_{ik} - \bar{d}_{i.})^2 / (n_1 + n_2 - 2).$$

On the null hypothesis that $\tau_1 = \tau_2$, the statistic

$$T_\tau = \frac{\hat{\tau}_d}{(\hat{\sigma}_D^2 m/4)^{\frac{1}{2}}}$$

has a Student's t-distribution on $(n_1 + n_2 - 2)$ d.f.

Continuing our analysis of the data in Tables 2.4 and 2.5, we obtain $\bar{d}_{1.} = 6.6354$, $\bar{d}_{2.} = -14.1698$ and $\hat{\tau}_d = 10.40$. Also $\sum_{k=1}^{27} (d_{1k} - \bar{d}_{1.})^2 = 19897.1$ and $\sum_{k=1}^{29} (d_{2k} - \bar{d}_{2.})^2 = 15337.2$. Therefore $\hat{\sigma}_D^2 = (19897.1 + 15337.2)/54 = 652.486$ on 54 d.f.

The t-statistic is

$$T_\tau = \frac{10.40}{\left(\frac{56}{783} \times \frac{652.486}{4}\right)^{\frac{1}{2}}} = 3.046 \text{ on } 54 \text{ d.f.}$$

The observed P-value is 0.0036. There is strong evidence to reject the null hypothesis at the (two-sided) 5% level.

A $100(1-\alpha)\%$ confidence interval for the direct treatment difference $\tau_d = \tau_1 - \tau_2$ is

$$\hat{\tau}_d \pm t_{\alpha/2,(n_1+n_2-2)} \left(\frac{m\sigma_D^2}{4}\right)^{\frac{1}{2}}$$

where $t_{\alpha/2,(n_1+n_2-2)}$ is the upper $(100\alpha/2)\%$ point of the t-distribution on $(n_1 + n_2 - 2)$ d.f.

Putting in our observed values and a t-value of 2.005, we have that $(3.56 \leq \tau_d \leq 17.25)$ is a 95% confidence interval for τ_d.

If it is of interest to test for a difference between the period effects, we proceed as follows.

Testing $\pi_1 = \pi_2$ (assuming $\lambda_1 = \lambda_2$)

In order to test the null hypothesis that $\pi_1 = \pi_2$, we use the "cross-over" differences

$$c_{1k} = d_{1k} = y_{11k} - y_{12k} \text{ for the } k\text{th subject in Group 1}$$

and

$$c_{2k} = -d_{2k} = y_{22k} - y_{21k} \text{ for the } k\text{th subject in Group 2.}$$

Note that because any carry-over effect that is common to both treatments is part of the period effect, we can set

$$\lambda_1 = -\lambda_2.$$

Then, if $\lambda_1 = \lambda_2$, both must be zero,

$$E[c_{1k}] = \pi_1 - \pi_2 + \tau_1 - \tau_2$$

and

$$E[c_{2k}] = \pi_2 - \pi_1 + \tau_1 - \tau_2.$$

If $\pi_1 = \pi_2$, these expectations are equal and consequently to test the null hypothesis we apply the two-sample t-test to the cross-over differences. That is, if $\pi_d = \pi_1 - \pi_2$ and $\hat{\pi}_d = \frac{1}{2}(\bar{c}_{1.} - \bar{c}_{2.})$, then, on the null hypothesis,

$$T_\pi = \frac{\hat{\pi}_d}{(\hat{\sigma}_D^2 m/4)^{\frac{1}{2}}}$$

has a Student's $t-$distribution on $(n_1 - n_2 - 2)$ d.f.

For our example data, $\hat{\pi}_d = \frac{1}{2}(6.635 - 14.170) = -3.77$ and $T_\pi = -1.103$ on 54 d.f. The observed P-value is 0.275. At the 5% level there is insufficient evidence to reject the null hypothesis of equal period effects.

What if $\lambda_1 \neq \lambda_2$?

If $\lambda_1 \neq \lambda_2$, then we cannot proceed to test $\tau_1 = \tau_2$ and $\pi_1 = \pi_2$ in the same way as done above. To see this we note that if $\lambda_d = \lambda_1 - \lambda_2 \neq 0$, then

$$E[\hat{\tau}_d] = E[(\bar{d}_{1.} - \bar{d}_{2.})/2] = \tau_d - \frac{\lambda_d}{2}.$$

That is, $\hat{\tau}_d$ is no longer an unbiased estimator of τ_d if $\lambda_d \neq 0$.

By noting that

$$\hat{\lambda}_d = \bar{y}_{11.} + \bar{y}_{12.} - \bar{y}_{21.} - \bar{y}_{22.}$$

and

$$\hat{\tau}_d = \frac{1}{2}[\bar{y}_{11.} - \bar{y}_{12.} - \bar{y}_{21.} + \bar{y}_{22.}]$$

we see that an unbiased estimator of τ_d, given that $\lambda_d \neq 0$, is

$$\hat{\tau}_d|\lambda_d = \frac{1}{2}[\bar{y}_{11.} - \bar{y}_{12.} - \bar{y}_{21.} + \bar{y}_{22.}] + \frac{1}{2}[\bar{y}_{11.} + \bar{y}_{12.} - \bar{y}_{21.} - \bar{y}_{22.}] = \bar{y}_{11.} - \bar{y}_{21.}.$$

That is, $\hat{\tau}_d|\lambda_d$ is the difference between the groups in terms of their first-period means. Also, $\text{Var}[\hat{\tau}_d|\lambda_d] = m\,(\sigma_s^2 + \sigma^2)$, in our previous notation.

In other words, if $\lambda_d \neq 0$, then the estimator of τ_d is based on *between-subject* information and is the estimator we would have obtained if the trial had been designed as a parallel-groups study. Whether or not this between-subjects estimator of τ_d will be sufficiently precise to detect a direct treatment difference of the size envisaged when the trial was planned will now be in doubt. At the planning stage, the size of the trial was probably determined on the assumption that the within-subjects estimator $\hat{\tau}_d$ was going to be used.

To test the null hypothesis that $\tau_d = 0$ given that $\lambda_d \neq 0$, we would still use a two-sample t-test, but would estimate $\sigma_s^2 + \sigma^2$ using only the first-period data.

One useful benefit of using derived variates to estimate and test effects is that they can be plotted in an informative way. The totals contain information on the carry-over effects and the differences contain information on the direct treatment effects. The larger the difference between $\bar{t}_{1.}$ and $\bar{t}_{2.}$ the more evidence there is to reject the hypothesis that $\lambda_d = 0$. Similarly, given $\lambda_d = 0$, the larger the difference between $\bar{d}_{1.}$ and $\bar{d}_{2.}$ the more evidence there is to reject the hypothesis that $\tau_d = 0$.

We can visually portray what the data have to tell us about $\hat{\lambda}_d$ and $\hat{\tau}_d$ if we plot for each subject the mean difference $d_{ik}/2$ against the total t_{ik} and use a different plotting symbol for each group. This plot is given in Figure 2.5. To aid the comparison of the groups, we have also added the outermost and innermost convex hulls of each group. The outermost convex hull of a set of points is that subset that contains all the other points. If we were to remove these points from consideration and repeat the process, we would obtain the next inner convex hull. If this removal process is repeated, we will eventually get to the innermost convex hull. The innermost convex hull of each group is shaded in Figure 2.5, with a different shading for each group. A separation of the groups along the horizontal (t_{ik}) axis would suggest that $\lambda_d \neq 0$ and (assuming $\lambda_d = 0$) a separation of the groups along the vertical ($d_{ik}/2$) axis would suggest that $\tau_d \neq 0$. For our data there is a clear separation of the two groups in the vertical direction, indicating a direct treatment difference. The centroids of each group have been plotted in Figure 2.5 using open and filled diamond shapes. The vertical difference between them is the size of the estimated direct treatment difference, which in this case is about 10 L/min. There is no apparent separation in the horizontal direction, indicating there is no difference in the carry-over effects. The size of the horizontal separation of the centroids is an estimate of the carry-over difference.

In addition to giving visual information about the direct treatment and carry-over effects, Figure 2.5 also gives information about the distribution of

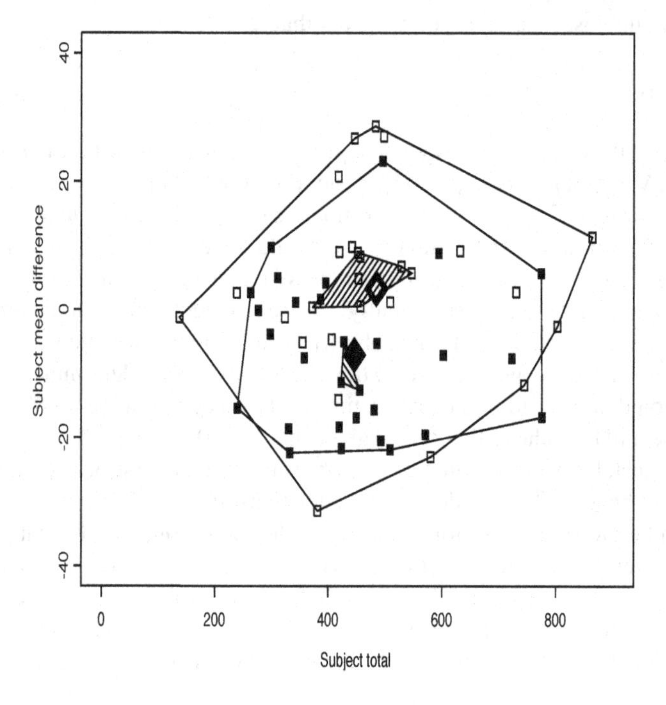

Figure 2.5: Mean differences vs totals.

the subject mean differences and totals. Looking at the plot we can see that there are more extreme values in Group 1, both for the mean differences and the totals. Perhaps the distribution of the mean differences and totals is not the same in the two groups.

A simple way to compare the distributions of the derived variates is to draw a histogram for each variate in each group and to compare them. The results of doing this are given in Figure 2.6.

The shapes of the histograms do seem to differ markedly between the groups, with those for Group 2 having shapes that might suggest the derived variates for that group are not normally distributed. A useful plot for assessing the normality of a set of data is the quantile-quantile plot (or qq-plot). The qq-plots for the subject mean totals and mean differences for each group are given in Figure 2.7. If the data in a plot are sampled from a normal distribution, the plotted points should lie close to a straight line. It would appear from Figure 2.7 that while none of the sets of points follow the line closely, the subject totals and mean differences for Group 2 have large deviations near the end of the lines. A formal test of normality can be done using the Shapiro–Wilk test. For the subject totals and mean differences in Group 1, the P-values for this test are 0.1438 and 0.2505, respectively. For Group 2, the corresponding P-values

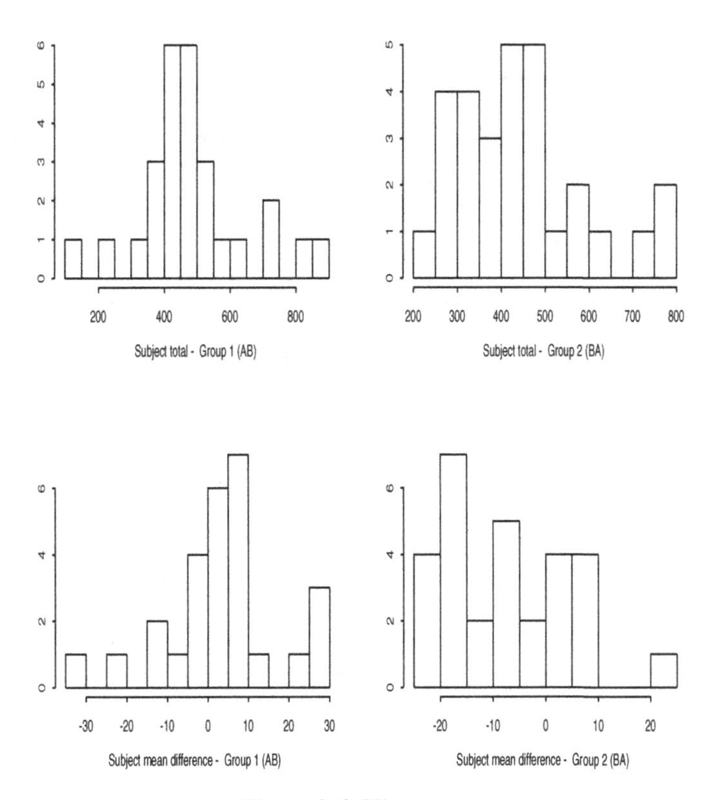

Figure 2.6: Histograms.

are 0.0428 and 0.1009, respectively. There is therefore some evidence that the subject totals in Group 2 are not sampled from a normal distribution. For the moment we merely note these features of the data and proceed to fit a linear model to the mean PEFR values obtained on each subject in each period.

2.4 Sample size calculations

In any clinical trial it is important for ethical and economic reasons that only the minimum number of subjects that are absolutely necessary are enrolled into the trial. When deciding from the results of a clinical trial if a significantly large direct treatment difference has been detected, it is possible to make two errors: the Type I error and the Type II error. If H_0 denotes the null hypothesis of no direct treatment difference and H_a denotes the alternative hypothesis that the difference between the direct treatments is Δ, then the Type I error is the mistake of rejecting H_0 when H_0 is true and the Type II error is the mistake of failing to reject H_0 when H_a is true. The probabilities of making these errors

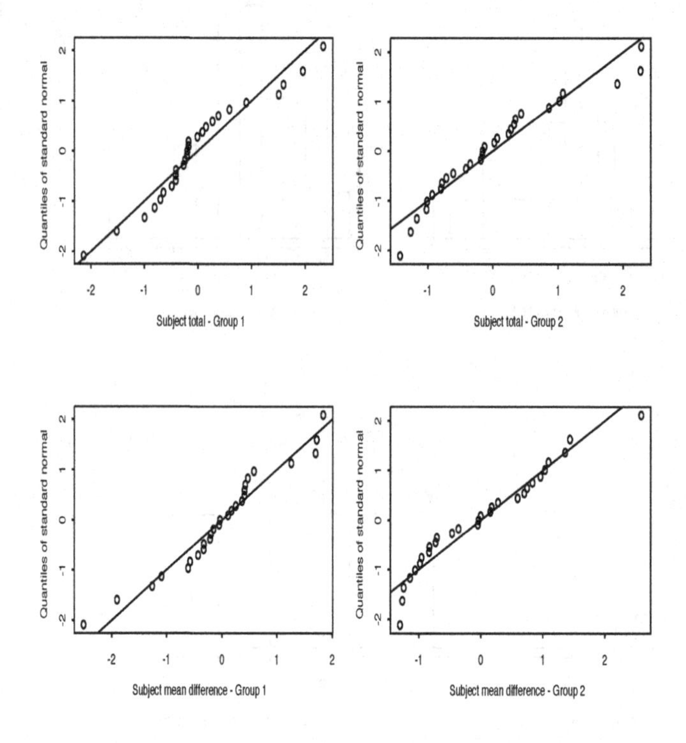

Figure 2.7: Quantile-quantile plots.

will be denoted by α and β, respectively. That is,

$$P(\text{reject } H_0|H_0) = \alpha$$

$$P(\text{accept } H_0|H_a) = \beta.$$

In this situation the significance level of the test is α. The power of the test is

$$\text{Power } = P(\text{reject } H_0|H_a) = 1 - \beta.$$

While it would be desirable to simultaneously minimize α and β, this is not possible, as we will illustrate shortly. In practice α is fixed at some small value, usually 0.05, and then the sample size is chosen so that the power $1-\beta$ is large enough to be acceptable, e.g., 0.8 or 0.9.

Here we assume that the observations on each subject are normally distributed. If there are $n/2$ subjects on each sequence and the (known)

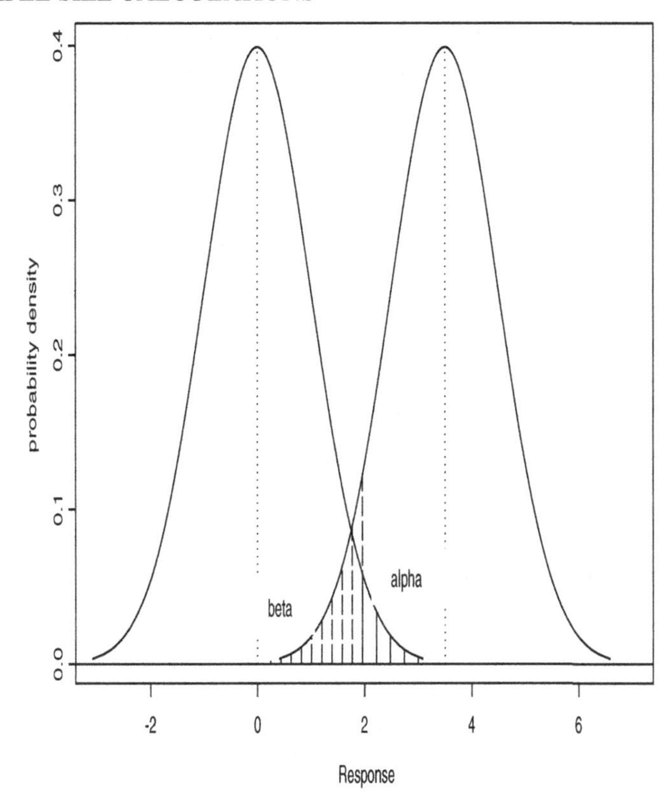

Figure 2.8: Probabilities of Type I and Type II errors.

within-subject variance is σ^2, the variance of the estimated treatment difference is

$$\text{Var}[\hat{\tau}_d] = \frac{2\sigma^2}{4}\left(\frac{2}{n}+\frac{2}{n}\right) = \frac{2\sigma^2}{n} = \sigma_d^2 \text{ say.}$$

We reject H_0 at the two-sided α level if $|\hat{\tau}_d|/\sqrt{\sigma_d^2} \geq z_{\alpha/2}$, where $z_{\alpha/2}$ is such that $P(z > z_{\alpha/2}) = \alpha/2$ and $z \sim N(0,1)$. If $\alpha = 0.05$, then $z_{0.025} = 1.96$.

In Figure 2.8 we illustrate the situation for the case where $\Delta = 3.5$ and $\sigma_d^2 = 1$. Here the distribution on the left is the distribution of the estimated direct treatment difference under the null hypothesis and the distribution on the right is the corresponding distribution under the alternative hypothesis, i.e., $\Delta = 3.5$. The shaded area to the right of 1.96 is $\alpha/2 = 0.025$ and the shaded area to the left of 1.96 is β. We can see that if we change $z_{\alpha/2}$ to a value greater than 1.96, then α will decrease and β will increase. The only way we can reduce β for a given α is to reduce the variance of the estimated treatment difference. For a fixed value of σ^2 this can only be done by increasing n, the number of subjects. We will now explain how to choose n for given values of Δ, σ^2, α and

β. Suppose for the moment that the alternative hypothesis is one-sided, $\Delta > 0$, and the significance level is α. Then, for example, $z_\alpha = z_{0.05} = 1.64$.

$$\begin{aligned}
1-\beta &= \mathrm{P}(\hat{\tau}_d/\sigma_d > z_\alpha | H_a) \\
&= \mathrm{P}(\hat{\tau}_d > z_\alpha \sigma_d | H_a) \\
&= \mathrm{P}\left(\frac{\hat{\tau}_d - \Delta}{\sigma_d} > \frac{z_\alpha \sigma_d - \Delta}{\sigma_d} \mid \frac{\hat{\tau}_d - \Delta}{\sigma_d}\right) \sim N(0,1) \\
&= \mathrm{P}\left(Z > \frac{-\Delta}{\sigma_d} + z_\alpha\right)
\end{aligned}$$

where $Z \sim N(0,1)$. In other words,

$$z_\beta = -(z_\alpha - \frac{\Delta}{\sigma_d})$$

and hence

$$\Delta = (z_\alpha + z_\beta)\sigma_d.$$

For a two-sided test the corresponding equation is

$$|\Delta| = (z_{\alpha/2} + z_\beta)\sigma_d.$$

Putting in the full expression for σ_d gives

$$|\Delta| = (z_{\alpha/2} + z_\beta)\frac{\sqrt{2}\sigma}{\sqrt{n}}.$$

That is,

$$n = \frac{(z_{\alpha/2} + z_\beta)^2 2\sigma^2}{\Delta^2}, \qquad (2.1)$$

i.e., $n/2$ subjects per group.

To improve the approximation, $\frac{1}{2}z^2_{\alpha/2}$ may be added to n, i.e.,

$$n = \frac{(z_{\alpha/2} + z_\beta)^2 2\sigma^2}{\Delta^2} + \frac{1}{2}z^2_{\alpha/2}. \qquad (2.2)$$

As an example, let us consider the trial described in Example 2.1. Suppose at the planning stage it was decided that a difference of at least $\Delta = 10$ units in the mean PEFR score was important to detect and that the within-patient variance in mean PEFR scores was $\sigma^2 = 326$. To detect a difference of this size with power 0.8 and two-sided significance level $\alpha = 0.05$ would require $n = (1.96+0.84)^2(2 \times 326)/100 + (1.96^2)/2 = 53$ subjects. As we require an even integer number of subjects, this would be rounded up to 54, i.e., 27 in each sequence group. In Table 2.7 we give the total sample size (n) required to detect a standardized difference Δ/σ with power at least 0.8 or 0.9 and each for two significance levels $\alpha = 0.05$ and 0.1. The usefulness of this table is that

Table 2.7: Total number of subjects required for 2 × 2 cross-over.

	Power = 0.8		Power = 0.9	
Δ/σ	$\alpha = 0.05$	$\alpha = 0.10$	$\alpha = 0.05$	$\alpha = 0.10$
0.1	1572	1238	2104	1716
0.2	396	312	528	430
0.3	178	140	236	192
0.4	102	80	134	110
0.5	66	52	88	70
0.6	46	36	62	50
0.7	34	28	46	38
0.8	28	22	36	30
0.9	22	18	28	24
1.0	18	14	24	20
1.1	16	12	20	16
1.2	14	12	18	14
1.3	12	10	16	12
1.4	12	10	14	12
1.5	10	8	12	10
1.6	10	8	12	10
1.7	8	8	10	8
1.8	8	6	10	8
1.9	8	6	10	8
2.0	8	6	8	8
2.1	8	6	8	6
2.2	6	6	8	6
2.3	6	6	8	6
2.4	6	6	8	6
2.5	6	6	8	6
2.6	6	6	6	6
2.7	6	6	6	6
2.8	6	6	6	6
2.9	6	4	6	6
3.0	6	4	6	6

it does not depend on the actual sizes of Δ and σ, but on their ratio, which is a dimensionless quantity. Therefore Table 2.7 is applicable in general.

A check on the sample size can be made by calculating the power using the noncentral t-distribution, which is the distribution of our test statistic under the alternative hypothesis. This distribution has noncentrality parameter $\gamma = \sqrt{n}(\Delta/\sqrt{2\sigma^2})$ and $n-2$ degrees of freedom. For the trial in Example 2.1 and assuming $n = 54$, $\gamma = \sqrt{54}(10/\sqrt{2 \times 326}) = 2.88$.

As an example, let us return to the sample size calculation for Example 2.1. Here $\Delta/\sigma = 10/\sqrt{(326)} = 0.554$. If $\alpha = 0.05$ and a power of 0.8 is required for a two-sided test, then from Table 2.7 we see that the total sample size should be about 56: we linearly interpolate between 46 and 66 and round up to an even integer, i.e., $n \approx 66 - (20/0.1) \times 0.054 = 56$, which is slightly higher than that obtained using formula (2.1).

The following SAS code (based on Senn (1993), Table 9.3) can be used to calculate the power using the noncentral t-distribution. For 54 patients the power is 0.8063, i.e., at least 0.8 as required.

SAS code for 2×2 *cross-over power calculation*

```
data sampsize;
* alpha (two-sided);
alpha=0.05;
* sample size (total number of patients);
n=54;
* within-patient variance;
sigma2=326;
* standard error of a difference;
stderrdiff=sqrt(2*sigma2/n);
* size of difference to detect;
delta=10;
* degrees of freedom for t-test;
df=n-2;
* critical value of t-distribution;
* (two-sided alpha level);
t1=tinv(1-alpha/2,df);
* noncentrality parameter;
gamma=delta/(stderrdiff);
* power;
power=1-probt(t1,df,gamma);
run;
proc print data=sampsize;
var alpha n delta  sigma2 stderrdiff
    gamma power;
run;
```

An alternative is to use the sample-size calculations provided in commercial software, for example, nQuery Advisor 7.0 (Elashoff, J.D.). For the above example, this software gives 27 subjects per group.

2.5 Analysis of variance

Although we can test all the hypotheses of interest by using two-sample t-tests, it is important to note that we can also test these hypotheses using *F-tests* obtained from an analysis of variance table. The analysis of variance approach is also the one that is most convenient to follow for the higher-order designs that we will describe in later chapters. As a reminder, the linear model assumed for the 2×2 trial is

$$\begin{aligned} Y_{11k} &= \mu + \pi_1 + \tau_1 + s_{1k} + \varepsilon_{11k} \\ Y_{12k} &= \mu + \pi_2 + \tau_2 + \lambda_1 + s_{1k} + \varepsilon_{12k} \\ Y_{21k} &= \mu + \pi_1 + \tau_2 + s_{2k} + \varepsilon_{21k} \\ Y_{22k} &= \mu + \pi_2 + \tau_1 + \lambda_2 + s_{2k} + \varepsilon_{22k} \end{aligned} \quad (2.3)$$

where the terms in the model were defined in Section 2.3. The analysis of variance table for the 2×2 cross-over design has been a source of confusion in the past. Although Grizzle (1965) was the first to present the table, his results were only correct for the special case of $n_1 = n_2$. Grieve (1982) pointed out that Grizzle's later correction (Grizzle, 1974) did not clarify the situation and went on to present the correct table. A correct table had earlier been given by Hills and Armitage (1979) in an appendix to their paper. The correct table is presented in Table 2.8, where SSW-S $= \sum_{i=1}^{2}\sum_{j=1}^{2}\sum_{k=1}^{n_i} y_{ijk}^2 - \sum_{i=1}^{2}\sum_{k=1}^{n_i}\frac{y_{i.k}^2}{2} - \sum_{i=1}^{2}\sum_{j=1}^{2}\frac{y_{ij.}^2}{n_i} + \sum_{i=1}^{2}\frac{y_{i..}^2}{2n_i}$.

The columns in Table 2.8 are for the source of variation (Source), degrees of freedom (d.f.) and sums of squares (SS). In Table 2.9 we give the expected mean squares (EMS). It is clear for the EMS column that, as noted before, it is only sensible to test the hypothesis that $\tau_1 = \tau_2$ if it can first be assumed that $\lambda_1 = \lambda_2$.

It will be noted that the total corrected SS has been partitioned into an SS between subjects and an SS within subjects. The between-subjects SS is further partitioned into an SS for carry-over and an SS for residual. This residual we refer to as the Between-Subjects Residual or B-S Residual for short. The SS

Table 2.8: Analysis of variance for full model: sums of squares.

Source	d.f.	SS
Between-subjects:		
Carry-over	1	$\frac{2n_1n_2}{(n_1+n_2)}(\bar{y}_{1..} - \bar{y}_{2..})^2$
B-S Residual	(n_1+n_2-2)	$\sum_{i=1}^{2}\sum_{k=1}^{n_i}\frac{y_{i.k}^2}{2} - \sum_{i=1}^{2}\frac{y_{i..}^2}{2n_i}$
Within-subjects:		
Treatments	1	$\frac{n_1n_2}{2(n_1+n_2)}(\bar{y}_{11.} - \bar{y}_{12.} - \bar{y}_{21.} + \bar{y}_{22.})^2$
Periods	1	$\frac{n_1n_2}{2(n_1+n_2)}(\bar{y}_{11.} - \bar{y}_{12.} + \bar{y}_{21.} - \bar{y}_{22.})^2$
W-S Residual	(n_1+n_2-2)	SSW-S
Total	$2(n_1+n_2)-1$	$\sum_{i=1}^{2}\sum_{j=1}^{2}\sum_{k=1}^{n_i} y_{ijk}^2 - \frac{y_{...}^2}{2(n_1+n_2)}$

Table 2.9: Analysis of variance for full model: expected mean squares.

Source	EMS
Between-subjects:	
Carry-over	$\frac{2n_1n_2}{(n_1+n_2)}(\lambda_1 - \lambda_2)^2 + 2\sigma_s^2 + \sigma^2$
B-S Residual	$2\sigma_s^2 + \sigma^2$
Within-subjects:	
Treatments	$\frac{2n_1n_2}{(n_1+n_2)}\left[(\tau_1 - \tau_2) - \frac{(\lambda_1-\lambda_2)}{2}\right]^2 + \sigma^2$
Periods	$\frac{2n_1n_2}{(n_1+n_2)}\left[(\pi_1 - \pi_2) - \frac{(\lambda_1+\lambda_2)}{2}\right]^2 + \sigma^2$
W-S Residual	σ^2

within-subjects is partitioned into (i) an SS for direct treatments (adjusted for periods), (ii) an SS for periods (adjusted for direct treatments) and (iii) an SS for residual. This residual we refer to as the Within-Subjects Residual or the W-S Residual for short. The 2 × 2 cross-over is a simple example of a split-plot design: subjects form the main plots and the time points at which repeated measurements are taken are the subplots. It will be convenient to use the split-plot analysis of variance in the analyses of the more complicated designs to be described in later chapters.

In the following, $F_{1,v}$ denotes the F-distribution on 1 and v degrees of freedom.

The analysis of variance table for the mean PEFR data is given in Table 2.10. Also given in the table is an F column and a P-value column. The F column contains the calculated values of the F-ratios which we define below and the P-value column contains the corresponding P-values obtained by testing the null hypotheses of no carry-over difference, no period difference and

Table 2.10: Analysis of variance for the PEFR data.

Source	d.f.	SS	MS	F	P-value
Between-subjects:					
Carry-over	1	10572.680	10572.680	0.899	0.347
B-S Residual	54	634865.580	11756.770		
Within-subjects:					
Treatments	1	3026.120	3026.120	9.28	0.004
Periods	1	396.858	396.858	1.22	0.275
W-S Residual	54	17617.134	326.243		
Total	111	666561.119			

no direct treatment difference, respectively. Again we include the test of no carry-over difference for illustration only.

To test the null hypothesis that $\lambda_1 = \lambda_2$, we calculate the F-ratio

$$\begin{aligned} \text{FC} &= \frac{\text{Carry-over MS}}{\text{B-S Residual MS}} \\ &= \frac{10572.680}{11756.770} \\ &= 0.899 \text{ on } (1, 54) \text{ d.f.} \end{aligned}$$

On the null hypothesis, FC is an observed value from the $F_{1,(n_1+n_2-2)}$ distribution. The P-value corresponding to this observed value is 0.347. As before (of course), there is insufficient evidence to reject the null hypothesis.

To test the null hypothesis that $\tau_1 = \tau_2$, we calculate the F-ratio

$$\begin{aligned} \text{FT} &= \frac{\text{Direct Treatment MS}}{\text{W-S Residual MS}} \\ &= \frac{3026.120}{326.243} \\ &= 9.28 \text{ on } (1, 54) \text{ d.f.} \end{aligned}$$

On the null hypothesis, FT is an observed value from the $F_{1,(n_1+n_2-2)}$ distribution. The corresponding P-value is 0.004. As before, there is strong evidence to reject the null hypothesis.

To test the null hypothesis that $\pi_1 = \pi_2$, we calculate the F-ratio

$$\begin{aligned} \text{FP} &= \frac{\text{Period MS}}{\text{W-S Residual MS}} \\ &= \frac{396.858}{326.243} \\ &= 1.22 \text{ on } (1, 54) \text{ d.f.} \end{aligned}$$

On the null hypothesis, FP is an observed value from the $F_{1,(n_1+n_2-2)}$ distribution. The corresponding P-value is 0.275, indicating that there is insufficient evidence to reject the null hypothesis. The numerical values displayed in Table 2.10 can be obtained using SAS `proc glm` with the following statements:

COPD Example — SAS `proc glm` *code:*

```
data d1;
input patient group treat period response;
datalines;
03  2  2  1  138.333
03  2  1  2  138.571
07  1  1  1  121.905
07  1  2  2  116.667
 .  .  .  .     .
 .  .  .  .     .
 .  .  .  .     .
90  1  1  1  236.667
90  1  2  2  220.000
99  2  2  1  371.190
99  2  1  2  404.762;
proc glm data=d1;
class patient group period treat;
model response= group patient(group)
      period treat;
random patient(group)/test;
lsmeans treat/pdiff;
estimate 'Trt1 -Trt2'
treat 1 -1;
run;
```

It will be noted that in order to obtain the correct F-test for the carry-over difference, the `random patient(group)/test` statement has been used. In later chapters we will fit models using SAS `proc mixed` rather than `proc glm`, as there will be advantages in fitting models where the subject effects are formally assumed to be random effects in the fitting process. The `random` statement in `proc glm` does not fit models that contain random effects. We will give a more considered and detailed introduction to fitting mixed models to cross-over data in Chapter 5. A general description of how to fit mixed models using SAS is given by Littell et al. (1996). To use `proc mixed` for our example, we should use the following statements:

COPD Example — `proc mixed` *code:*

```
proc mixed data=d1;
class patient group period treat;
model response = group period treat/s;
random patient(group);
lsmeans treat/pdiff;
estimate 'Trt1 - Trt2' treat 1 -1;
estimate 'Car1- Car2' group  2 -2;
run;
```

Edited output from using these commands is given below. We note that the output from `proc mixed` is quite different to that of `proc glm`. `proc mixed` uses residual (or restricted) maximum likelihood (REML) to fit the model and estimate the variance parameters σ_s^2 and σ^2. For our data

COPD Example — `proc mixed` *output:*

```
Covariance Parameter Estimates
Cov Parm     Estimate
patient(group) 5715.26
Residual       326.24

Type 3 Tests of Fixed Effects
Effect Num DF Den DF F Value  Pr > F
group   1       54      0.90     0.3472
period  1       54      1.22     0.2749
treat   1       54      9.28     0.0036

Estimates
Label          Estimate Std Err DF  t   Pr > |t|
Trt1 - Trt2 10.4026  3.4156  54 3.05 0.0036
Car1- Car2  38.8885  41.0083 54 0.95 0.3472
```

these estimates are $\hat{\sigma}_s^2 = 5715.263$ and $\hat{\sigma}^2 = 326.243$. The `proc mixed` output does not contain an analysis of variance table, but the results of applying the F-tests to test the null hypotheses for carry-over, period and direct treatment effects are given. Of course, for the 2×2 trial without missing data on one or other of the treatments, all the information on the direct treatment and period differences is wholly within subjects, and so the values of the test statistics and estimates are exactly as would be obtained by fitting a model with fixed subject effects using `proc glm`. This will not be the case for some of the designs to be met in later chapters.

2.6 Aliasing of effects

Perhaps the most important advantage of formally fitting a linear model is that diagnostic information on the validity of the assumed model can be obtained. This information resides primarily in the residuals, which we consider in Section 2.8. Here we show that the part of the linear model that concerns the carry-over effects can be expressed in three alternative ways: as carry-over effects, as group effects and as direct treatment-by-period interaction effects. In fact, we made use of this when fitting the model to the mean PEFR data: we included a factor for Group with levels 1 and 2, rather than a factor for Carry-over. We have already emphasized the power of the test for equal carry-over effects is likely to have low power and we do not recommend using it as a preliminary to testing for a direct treatment difference. This aliasing of effects (i.e., when a single numerical estimate can be interpreted in a number of alternative ways) is another reminder of the limitations of the basic 2×2 design.

To illustrate this aliasing, consider writing the fixed effects in the full model as given below:

Group	Period 1	Period 2
1 (AB)	$\mu+\pi_1+\tau_1+(\tau\pi)_{11}$	$\mu+\pi_2+\tau_2+(\tau\pi)_{22}$
2 (BA)	$\mu+\pi_1+\tau_2+(\tau\pi)_{21}$	$\mu+\pi_2+\tau_1+(\tau\pi)_{12}$

Here $(\tau\pi)_{ij}$ is the interaction parameter associated with treatment i and period j and allows the model to account for a treatment effect that is not the same in each of the two periods. If the usual constraints $\pi_1+\pi_2=0$ and $\tau_1+\tau_2=0$ are applied to the parameters, and we set $\pi_1=-\pi$ and $\tau_1=-\tau$, the model can be written as

Group	Period 1	Period 2
1 (AB)	$\mu-\pi-\tau+(\tau\pi)_{11}$	$\mu+\pi+\tau+(\tau\pi)_{22}$
2 (BA)	$\mu-\pi+\tau+(\tau\pi)_{21}$	$\mu+\pi-\tau+(\tau\pi)_{12}$

If the usual constraints $(\tau\pi)_{11}+(\tau\pi)_{12}=0$, $(\tau\pi)_{21}+(\tau\pi)_{22}=0$, $(\tau\pi)_{11}+(\tau\pi)_{21}=0$ and $(\tau\pi)_{12}+(\tau\pi)_{22}=0$ are applied to the interaction parameters, and we set $(\tau\pi)_{11}=(\tau\pi)$, the model becomes

Group	Period 1	Period 2
1 (AB)	$\mu-\pi-\tau+(\tau\pi)$	$\mu+\pi+\tau+(\tau\pi)$
2 (BA)	$\mu-\pi+\tau-(\tau\pi)$	$\mu+\pi-\tau-(\tau\pi)$

Using these constraints therefore reveals the aliasing of the interaction and the group effects. If, however, we use the less familiar constraints $(\tau\pi)_{11}=0$, $(\tau\pi)_{21}=0$, $(\tau\pi)_{12}+(\tau\pi)_{22}=0$ and set $(\tau\pi)_{22}=-(\tau\pi)$, the model becomes

Group	Period 1	Period 2
1 (AB)	$\mu-\pi-\tau$	$\mu+\pi+\tau-(\tau\pi)$
2 (BA)	$\mu-\pi+\tau$	$\mu+\pi-\tau+(\tau\pi)$

That is, the interaction effects are now associated with the carry-over effects. (See Cox (1984) for further, related discussion.)

The constraints applied do not affect the numerical values obtained for the sums of squares in an analysis of variance or the estimates of any treatment contrasts. Therefore, whichever constraints are applied, the same numerical values will be obtained: it is their interpretation that will differ.

If the null hypothesis of equal carry-over effects is rejected, there are, as suggested above, a number of possible causes and additional information must be used to decide between them. The main point to note, however, is that if the null hypothesis of equal carry-over effects is rejected, *we have evidence of a treatment difference*. Because of the intrinsic aliasing, the problem left to sort out is that of deciding on a meaningful estimate and a meaningful interpretation of the difference between the treatments. The solution to this problem cannot be obtained from the results of the trial alone: additional background information on the nature of the treatments and periods must be used.

2.7 Consequences of preliminary testing

Prior to the Freeman (1989) paper, it was common practice for the test for a direct treatment difference to be preceded by a test for equal carry-over effects. Depending on the result of the carry-over test, one of two different tests for a direct treatment difference was then done, as suggested by Grizzle (1965). If the test for a carry-over difference was not significant, then the t-test based on the within-subject differences, as described in Section 2.3, was used. If the carry-over test was significant, then the two treatments were compared using only the Period 1 data, as in a parallel groups design. That is, a two-sample t-test comparing the mean of A in Period 1 with the mean of B in Period 1 was done. This test uses between-subject information, and so negates the advantages of using a cross-over design. Freeman (1989) showed that using such a preliminary test not only leads to a biased estimate of the direct treatment difference but also increases the probability of making a Type I error. In other words, the actual significance level of the direct treatment test is higher than the nominal one chosen for the test. In this section we review and illustrate Freeman's results and evaluate their consequences for typical trials. In this section we consider the special case where there are n subjects on each treatment in each sequence group.

Let $s_{ik} = y_{i1k} + y_{i2k}$, $f_{ik} = y_{i1k}$ and $d_{ik} = y_{i1k} - y_{i2k}$ be the total of the two responses, the first period response and the difference of the two responses, respectively, on subject k in Group i. If $\rho = \frac{\sigma_s^2}{\sigma_s^2+\sigma^2}$, then the following results hold:

$$S = \bar{s}_1 - \bar{s}_2 \sim N(\lambda_d, \frac{4\sigma^2}{n}\frac{1+\rho}{1-\rho})$$

$$F = \bar{f}_1 - \bar{f}_2 \sim N(\tau_d, \frac{2\sigma^2}{n}\frac{1}{1-\rho})$$

$$D = \frac{\bar{d}_1 - \bar{d}_2}{2} \sim N(\tau_d - \frac{\lambda_d}{2}, \frac{\sigma^2}{n}),$$

where s_i is the mean of the s_{ik}, f_i is the mean of the f_{ik} and d_i is the mean of the d_{ik}, respectively, for Group i. It is worth noting that the correlation between S and F is $\sqrt{(1+\rho)/2}$.

Freeman referred to using the test based on F as procedure PAR and using the test based on D as CROSS. The Grizzle (1965) two-stage procedure corresponds to first using the test for carry-over based on S and then using PAR if the test is significant and using CROSS otherwise. Freeman referred to this two-stage procedure as TS.

Depending on the procedure used, there are three alternative estimators of τ_d:

$$\hat{\tau}_{dPAR} = F$$

$$\hat{\tau}_{dCROS} = D$$

$$\hat{\tau}_{dTS} = D \text{ with probability } p \text{ or } F \text{ with probability } 1-p,$$

where p equals the probability that the carry-over test based on S is not significant at level α_1. Grizzle (1965) suggested setting $\alpha_1 = 0.1$, rather than 0.05 to compensate for the lack of power of the test based on S. Estimator PAR is unbiased, and has variance $\frac{2\sigma^2}{n}(\frac{1}{1-\rho})$. Estimator CROSS has bias $-\frac{\lambda_d}{2}$ and variance $\frac{\sigma^2}{n}$. If it is assumed that σ_s^2 and σ^2 are known, Freeman showed that estimator TS has bias

$$-\frac{\lambda_d p}{2} + \frac{\sigma_1}{\sqrt{2\pi}} \exp\left[-\frac{1}{2}\left(z_{\alpha_1}^2 + \frac{\lambda_d^2}{\sigma_1^2}\right)\right] \sinh\frac{z_{\alpha_1}\lambda_d}{\sigma_1},$$

where $\sigma_1^2 = \frac{4\sigma^2}{n}\left(\frac{1+\rho}{1-\rho}\right)$.

The variance $\hat{\tau}_{dTS}$ is

$$\begin{aligned}
\text{Var}(\hat{\tau}_{dTS}) &= \frac{\lambda_d^2}{4}p(1-p) + \frac{\sigma^2}{n}(4-3p) \\
&+ \frac{z_{\alpha_1}\sigma_1^2}{2\sqrt{2\pi}} \exp\left[-\frac{1}{2}\left(z_{\alpha_1}^2 + \frac{\lambda_d^2}{\sigma_1^2}\right)\right] \cosh\frac{z_{\alpha_1}\lambda_d}{\sigma_1} \\
&- \frac{\lambda_d\sigma_1}{2\sqrt{2\pi}}(1-2p) \exp\left[-\frac{1}{2}\left(z_{\alpha_1}^2 + \frac{\lambda_d^2}{\sigma_1^2}\right)\right] \sinh\frac{z_{\alpha_1}\lambda_d}{\sigma_1} \\
&- \frac{\sigma_1^2}{2\pi} \exp\left[-\frac{1}{2}\left(z_{\alpha_1}^2 + \frac{\lambda_d^2}{\sigma_1^2}\right)\right] \sinh^2\frac{z_{\alpha_1}\lambda_d}{\sigma_1}.
\end{aligned}$$

To compare the three estimators, we use the mean squared error (MSE), which equals variance + bias^2. The MSEs of the three estimators are

$$\begin{aligned}
MSE_{PAR} &= \frac{2\sigma^2}{n}\left(\frac{1}{1-\rho}\right) \\
MSE_{CROSS} &= \frac{\lambda_d^2}{4} + \frac{\sigma^2}{n} \\
MSE_{TS} &= \frac{\lambda_d^2 p}{4} + \frac{\sigma^2}{n}(4-3p) \\
&+ \frac{\sigma_1^2}{2\sqrt{2\pi}} \exp\left[-\frac{1}{2}\left(z_{\alpha_1}^2 + \frac{\lambda_d^2}{\sigma_1^2}\right)\right] \\
&\times \left[z\cosh\frac{z_{\alpha_1}\lambda_d}{\sigma_1} - \frac{\lambda_d}{\sigma_1}\sinh\frac{z_{\alpha_1}\lambda_d}{\sigma_1}\right],
\end{aligned}$$

where $\sigma_1^2 = \frac{4\sigma^2}{n}(\frac{1+\rho}{1-\rho})$.

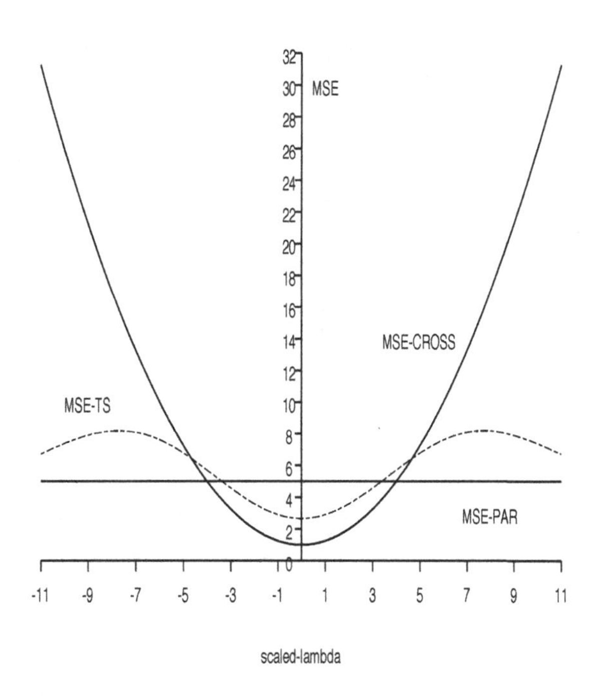

Figure 2.9: Mean squared errors of PAR, CROSS and TS.

To provide an illustration, we consider the situation with $\sigma = \sqrt{(n)}$ (to simplify the forthcoming plots), $\alpha = 0.05$, $\alpha_1 = 0.1$ (as suggested by Grizzle (1965)), $\rho = 0.6$ and $\frac{\lambda_d \sqrt{(n)}}{\sigma}$ taking values from -11 to $+11$. For these values, the MSE values corresponding to each of the three types of estimator (PAR, CROSS, TS) are plotted in Figure 2.9. It can be seen that the MSE for TS is always between that of the other two estimators. For relatively small values of the carry-over difference, TS performs much better than PAR and not much worse than CROSS. But even though TS is not as good as PAR for larger values of the carry-over difference, TS has a smaller MSE than CROSS, whose MSE keeps on increasing.

A second way of comparing the properties of the three estimators, as also done by Freeman, is to calculate the coverage probability of the confidence interval for the true treatment difference τ_d. If $\alpha = 0.05$, the nominal coverage probability of the confidence interval should be 0.95. For PAR it is 0.95 for all values of λ_d, but not for CROSS or TS. The actual values of the coverage probability (again assuming the values for α, α_1, n and σ as used for the MSE calculations) are plotted in Figure 2.10. The coverage probability at $\lambda_d = 0$ is, of course, 0.95 for PAR and CROSS, but for TS it is only 0.9152, i.e., the actual

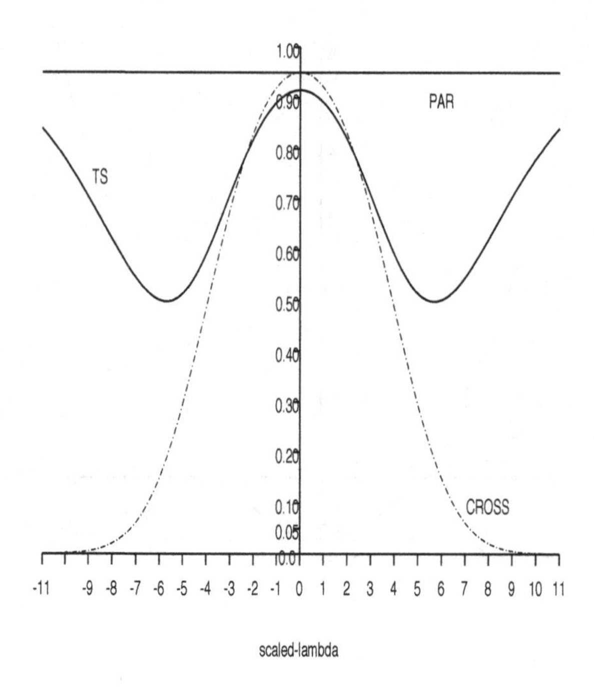

Figure 2.10: Coverage probability.

significance level is 0.0848. The minimum coverage probability is 0.4974 and occurs at $|\lambda_d \sqrt(n)/\sigma| = 5.7$. (The actual significance level at these points is therefore 0.5026.)

Figure 2.11 shows the power of each procedure for three values of λ_d (left panel $\lambda_d = 0$, middle panel $\lambda_d = 5\sigma/\sqrt(n)$, right panel $\lambda_d = \sigma/\sqrt(n)$). We can see for $\lambda_d = 0$ that, as expected, both TS and CROSS do better than PAR, although TS does this at the expense of an increased significance level (0.0848) at $\tau_d = 0$. For $\lambda_d = 0$, TS does not do very much worse than CROSS. When $\lambda_d = 5\sigma/\sqrt(n)$, there are some values of $\tau_d \sqrt(n)/\sigma$ for which TS has higher power than CROSS and some where it is lower. The power (i.e., significance level) at $\tau_d = 0$ is high for both TS and CROSS (0.4865 and 0.7054, respectively). The contours of the rejection probabilities for TS are given in Figure 2.12.

Another disturbing feature of the TS procedure has been pointed out by Senn (1996). That is, in the absence of a carry-over difference, significant values of the SEQ test imply that the PAR test will be biased. This is because in the absence of a carry-over difference (and a direct treatment-by-period interaction) a significant SEQ test implies a significant difference between the two

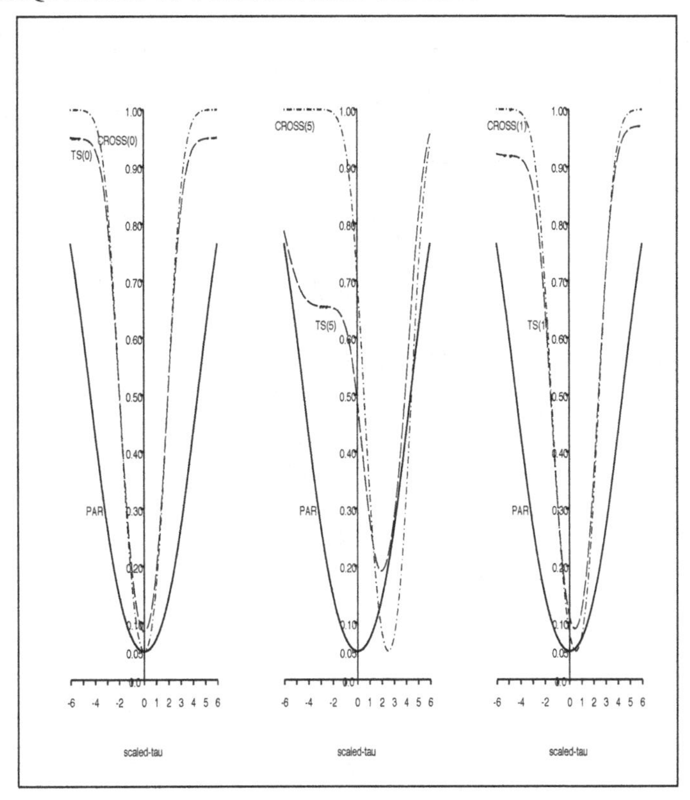

Figure 2.11: Power curves for PAR, CROSS and TS (left panel $\lambda_d = 0$, middle panel $\lambda_d = 5\sigma/\sqrt(n))$, right panel $\lambda_d = \sigma/\sqrt(n))$.

sequence groups. This difference will introduce a bias in the PAR test, because it compares the treatments using a between-group test. See Senn (1996, 1997b) for further discussion.

Our advice therefore is to avoid having to test for a carry-over difference by doing all that is possible to remove the possibility that such a difference will exist. This requires using wash-out periods of adequate length between the treatment periods. This in turn requires a good working knowledge of the treatment effects, which will most likely be based on prior knowledge of the drugs under study, or ones known to have a similar action. In Section 2.12 we give an alternative approach that avoids the problems of preliminary testing.

Freeman recommended using a Bayesian analysis to overcome the disadvantages of preliminary testing. We consider Bayesian approaches in Section 2.9.

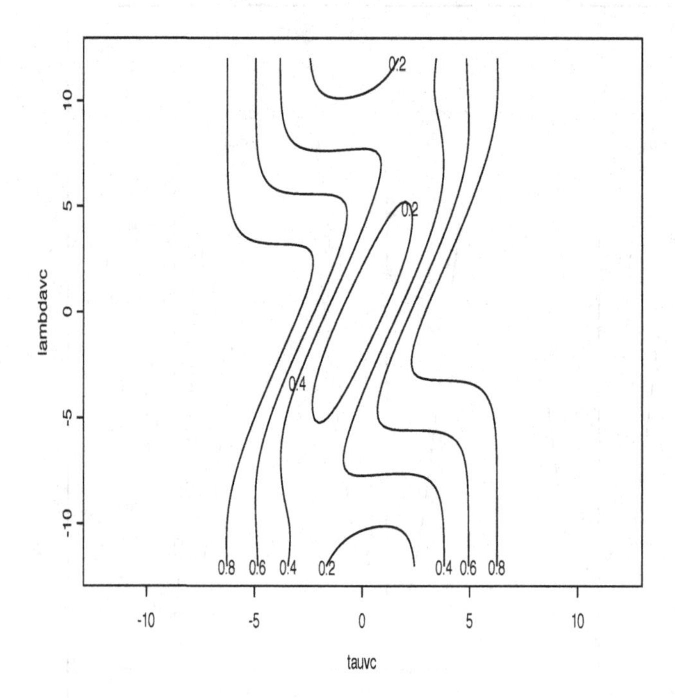

Figure 2.12: Contours of power for TS ($\rho = 0.6$).

2.8 Analyzing the residuals

Any analysis is incomplete if the assumptions which underlie it are not checked. Among the assumptions made above are that the repeated measurements on the each subject are independent, normally distributed random variables with equal variances. These assumptions can be most easily checked by analyzing the residuals. If $\hat{y}_{ijk}$ denotes the estimated value of the response based on the full model, then the residual r_{ijk} is defined as

$$r_{ijk} = y_{ijk} - \hat{y}_{ijk} = y_{ijk} - \bar{y}_{i.k} - \bar{y}_{ij.} + \bar{y}_{i..}.$$

The r_{ijk} are estimators of the ε_{ijk} terms in the full model and, if the model is correct, should share similar properties. However, although the r_{ijk} are normally distributed with mean 0, they are not independent and do not have equal variances. Their variances and covariances are given below, where k is not equal to q:

$$\text{Var}(r_{i1k}) = \text{Var}(r_{i2k}) = \frac{(n_i - 1)}{2n_i}\sigma^2,$$

$$\text{Cov}(r_{i1k}, r_{i1q}) = \text{Cov}(r_{i2k}, r_{i2q}) = -\text{Cov}(r_{i1k}, r_{i2q}) = -\frac{\sigma^2}{2n_i}$$

and

$$\text{Cov}(r_{i1k}, r_{i2k}) = -\frac{(n_i - 1)}{2n_i}\sigma^2.$$

All other covariances are zero.

It can be seen that if n_1 and n_2 are large and approximately equal, the r_{ijk} are approximately independent with equal variances. Rather than use these raw residuals, however, it is more convenient to work with the following "studentized" residuals:

$$t_{ijk} = \frac{r_{ijk}}{\left(\widehat{\text{Var}}(r_{ijk})\right)^{\frac{1}{2}}}$$

where $\widehat{\text{Var}}(r_{ijk})$ is the estimated value of $\text{Var}(r_{ijk})$ obtained by replacing σ^2 by the W-S Residual MS. Each t_{ijk} has mean 0 and variance 1. Although their joint distribution is complicated, little is lost in practice if the studentized residuals are treated as standard normal variables. The distribution of such residuals obtained from regression models is discussed by Cook and Weisberg (1982), pp.18–20.

The values of t_{ijk} for our mean PEFR data are given in Tables 2.11 and 2.12, for each group, respectively, where it will be noted that only the residual from Period 1 is given for each subject, because $r_{i.k} = 0$.

It can be seen that two largest residuals, ignoring the sign, occur for Subject 36 in Group 1 and Subject 59 in Group 2. If the model and assumptions are correct, we should not expect to see "large" studentized residuals. Lund (1975) has tabulated critical values for determining if the largest studentized residual is significantly large (at the 10%, 5% and 1% levels). The response values corresponding to unusually large studentized residuals are called outliers or discordant values. The larger the residual the more discordant is the corresponding response. If outliers are found in a set of data, then their response values should be carefully examined. After such an examination, it might be decided to remove these values and to reanalyze the depleted data set. For our data the largest studentized residual (-2.77) should not be considered an outlier.

More often than not, plotting residuals in various ways can be most informative. Figure 2.13 shows two useful diagnostic plots of the studentized residuals for the first period mean PEFR values. (We could equally well have plotted those for the second period. However, as these are the negative of those in the first period, only the residuals from one of the periods should be plotted.) In the left panel the residuals t_{ijk} are plotted against the fitted values $\hat{y}_{ijk}$ and in the right panel is a q-q plot. If the model assumptions are satisfied, there should be no relationship between the t_{ijk} and the $\hat{y}_{ijk}$. The plot in the left panel of Figure 2.13 does not suggest any nonrandom pattern, except perhaps for a suggestion that the variance of the residuals is larger for subjects with average-sized fitted values. The plot in the right panel of Figure 2.13 shows that the plotted points lie close to a straight line, giving no reason to doubt the assumption that the residuals are normally distributed.

Table 2.11: PEFR data: studentized residuals for Group 1, Period 1.

Subject	y_{ijk}	$\hat{y}_{ijk}$	t_{ijk}
7	121.90	122.60	−0.06
8	218.50	212.82	0.45
9	235.00	229.39	0.45
13	250.00	226.53	1.87
14	186.19	189.16	−0.24
15	231.56	230.02	0.12
17	443.25	435.19	0.64
21	198.42	206.37	−0.63
22	270.50	245.15	2.02
28	360.48	375.56	−1.20
35	229.75	212.32	1.39
36	159.09	193.82	−2.77
37	255.88	258.04	−0.17
38	279.05	276.65	0.19
41	160.56	165.10	−0.36
44	172.10	180.56	−0.67
58	267.00	293.32	−2.10
66	230.75	224.25	0.52
71	271.19	267.72	0.28
76	276.25	252.50	1.90
79	398.75	404.69	−0.47
80	67.78	72.35	−0.36
81	195.00	212.40	−1.39
82	325.00	319.15	0.47
86	368.08	368.61	−0.04
89	228.95	231.74	−0.22
90	236.67	231.65	0.40

2.9 A Bayesian analysis of the 2 × 2 trial

2.9.1 *Bayes using approximations*

Here we describe the Bayesian analysis of the 2 × 2 trial as presented by Grieve (1985, 1986). A Bayesian analysis of the 2 × 2 trial as used in bioequivalence testing, and for equal group sizes, was earlier given by Selwyn et al. (1981). Other related references are Dunsmore (1981) and Fluehler et al. (1983). Some examples of the use of Bayesian methods in the pharmaceutical industry (with discussion) have been given by Racine et al. (1986).

The model we shall assume is for the two-period design without baselines and is as given in Section 2.5, with the addition of the constraints $T = \tau_1 = -\tau_2$ and $R = \lambda_1 = -\lambda_2$. In other words, the difference between the carry-over effects is $\lambda_1 - \lambda_2 = 2R$ and the difference between the treatment effects

Table 2.12: PEFR data: studentized residuals for Group 2, Period 1.

Subject	y_{ijk}	$\hat{y}_{ijk}$	t_{ijk}
3	138.33	131.37	0.56
10	225.00	233.54	−0.68
11	392.86	380.06	1.02
16	190.00	204.58	−1.16
18	191.43	202.63	−0.89
23	226.19	239.58	−1.07
24	201.90	190.62	0.90
26	134.29	124.53	0.78
27	238.00	236.17	0.15
29	159.50	142.67	1.34
30	232.75	247.57	−1.18
32	172.31	164.07	0.66
33	266.00	278.42	−0.99
39	171.33	171.75	−0.03
43	194.74	186.00	0.70
47	200.00	204.22	−0.34
51	146.67	158.15	−0.92
52	208.00	217.75	−0.78
55	208.75	206.70	0.16
59	271.43	241.13	2.41
68	143.81	159.07	−1.22
70	104.44	112.76	−0.66
74	145.24	141.96	0.26
77	215.38	220.85	−0.44
78	306.00	290.08	1.27
83	160.53	148.42	0.96
84	353.81	354.34	−0.04
85	293.89	293.91	0.00
99	371.19	380.89	−0.77

is $\tau_1 - \tau_2 = 2T$. It will be recalled that $\hat{T} = [\bar{y}_{11.} - \bar{y}_{12.} - \bar{y}_{21.} + \bar{y}_{22.}]/4$ and $\hat{R} = [\bar{y}_{11.} + \bar{y}_{12.} - \bar{y}_{21.} - \bar{y}_{22.}]/2$. Also we will define $\sigma_A^2 = 2\sigma_s^2 + \sigma^2$ and note that $m = (n_1 + n_2)/(n_1 n_2)$.

The joint (uninformative) prior distribution for our model parameters is assumed to be proportional to $(\sigma_A^2 \times \sigma^2)^{-1}$. The following posterior distributions are then obtained, where $\mathbf{y}$ denotes the observed data:

$$P(T,R|\mathbf{y}) \propto \left(\frac{Q_1\,Q_2}{SSE\;SSP}\right)^{-(n_1+n_2-1)/2} \tag{2.4}$$

$$P(R|\mathbf{y}) \propto \left(\frac{Q_2}{SSP}\right)^{-(n_1+n_2-1)/2} \tag{2.5}$$

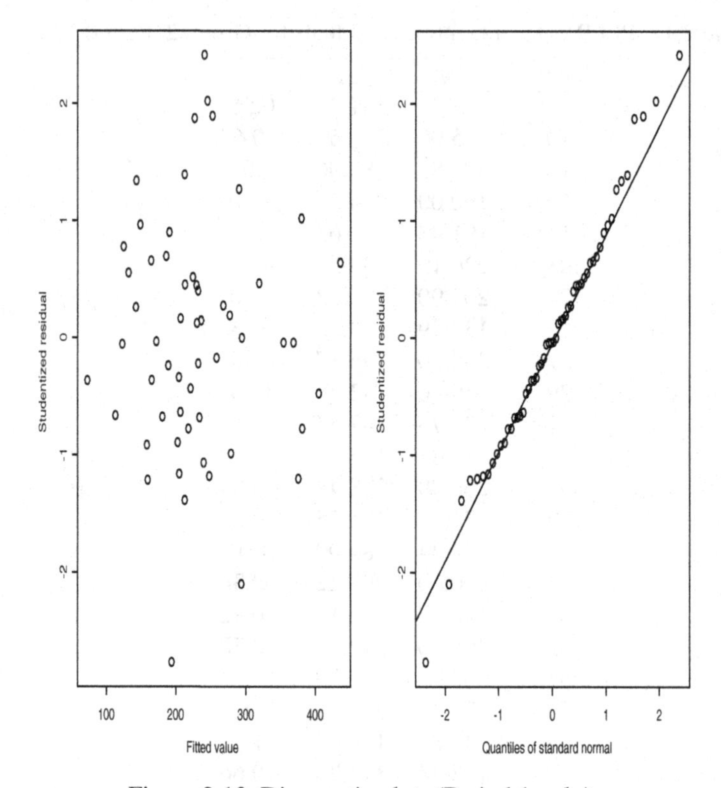

Figure 2.13: Diagnostic plots (Period 1 only).

$$P(T|R,\mathbf{y}) \propto \left(\frac{Q_1}{SSE}\right)^{-(n_1+n_2-1)/2}. \tag{2.6}$$

Here

$$SSE = \text{Within-subjects residual SS},$$

$$SSP = \text{Between-subjects residual SS},$$

$$Q_1 = \frac{8(T-R/2-\hat{T})^2}{m} + SSE$$

and

$$Q_2 = \frac{2(R-\hat{R})^2}{m} + SSP.$$

In fact, from the above it can be seen that

$$P(R|\mathbf{y}) = t\left[\hat{R}, \frac{m\,SSP}{2(n_1+n_2-2)}, n_1+n_2-2\right], \tag{2.7}$$

where $t[a,b,c]$ denotes a shifted and scaled t-distribution with c d.f., location parameter a and scale parameter $b^{\frac{1}{2}}$.

The marginal distribution of T, $P(T|\mathbf{y})$, does not have a convenient form and must be obtained by numerically intergrating out R from the joint posterior distribution for T and R given in equation (2.4). However, Grieve (1985) has shown that, to a very good approximation,

$$P(T|\mathbf{y}) = t\left[\hat{T} + \frac{\hat{R}}{2}, \frac{m\, b_0}{8\, b_1}, b_1\right] \tag{2.8}$$

where

$$b_1 = \frac{(SSE + SSP)^2(n_1 + n_2 - 6)}{(SSE)^2 + (SSP)^2} + 4$$

and

$$b_0 = \frac{(b_1 - 2)(SSE + SSP)}{(n_1 + n_2 - 4)}.$$

Also,

$$P(T|R, \mathbf{y}) = t\left[\hat{T} + \frac{R}{2}, \frac{m\, SSE}{8(n_1 + n_2 - 2)}, n_1 + n_2 - 2\right]. \tag{2.9}$$

Grieve also considered the effect of including the extra constraint $\sigma_A^2 > \sigma^2$ in the prior information and concluded that it makes very little difference.

To provide an illustration of the Bayesian approach, we give in Figure 2.14 the posterior distributions obtained for the mean PEFR data.

The posterior distribution, $P(R|\mathbf{y})$, has mean 19.44 and variance 436.6 on 54 d.f. The 90% credible (confidence) interval for R is $(-21.66, 60.55)$ and does therefore support the null hypothesis that $R = 0$.

If we assume that $R = 0$, then the appropriate posterior distribution for T is $P(T|R = 0, \mathbf{y})$. The difference between $P(T|R = 0, \mathbf{y})$ and $P(T|\mathbf{y})$ is quite dramatic, however, and it is important to make a sensible choice between them. The distribution $P(T|R = 0, \mathbf{y})$ has mean 5.20 and variance 3.03 on 54 d.f. The 95% credible interval for T is (1.78, 8.63), i.e., the 95% credible interval for $\tau_1 - \tau_2$ is (3.55, 17.25). If we assume that $R \neq 0$, the posterior is $P(T|\mathbf{y})$, which has mean 14.92 and variance 112.18 on 56.77 d.f. The 95% credible interval for $\tau_1 - \tau_2$ is then $(-9.09, 68.79)$.

Further examples of a Bayesian analysis are given by Grieve (1985, 1987, 1990, 1994a) and Racine et al. (1986).

In the analysis so far, we have assumed an uninformative prior for the parameters. Naturally, in the Bayesian approach it is appealing to make use of informative prior information which may be subjective or may have been obtained in earlier trials. Selwyn et al. (1981) show how an informative prior distribution on R can be included in the analysis. While this is a step forward, it does seem to us that if prior information on R is available, there must be prior information on T also. As regards the period parameters, it is unlikely that any prior information on these will be available, except perhaps the fact that they are not needed. The period effects are going to be difficult to predict

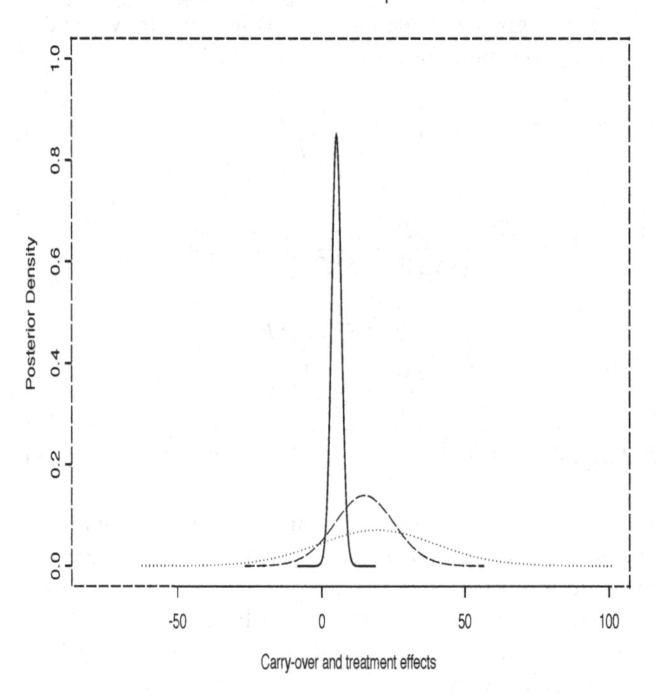

Figure 2.14: Posterior distributions for treatment and carry-over effects for the PEFR data: $P(R|y)$, dotted curve; $P(T|R,y)$, solid curve; $P(T|y)$, dashed curve.

a priori because they depend on two future time points and the effects of these are likely to be quite capricious.

Grieve (1985) and Racine et al. (1986) have also considered the approach of Selwyn et al. (1981) and conclude that it is likely to be difficult to put into practice: they prefer an approach which uses a Bayes factor to assess the significance of the carry-over effect.

In order to explain the Bayes factor approach, we let M_1 denote the model (as defined in Section 2.3) which includes the carry-over parameters and let M_0 denote the model with the carry-over parameters omitted.

The prior odds on no carry-over difference is then defined as $P = P(M_0)/P(M_1)$, where $P(M_i)$ denotes the prior probability of model M_i, $i = 0, 1$. The posterior probabilities for the two models are then

$$P(M_0|\mathbf{y}) = \frac{P\,B_{01}}{1 + P\,B_{01}}$$

and

$$P(M_1|\mathbf{y}) = \frac{1}{1+P\,B_{01}}$$

where B_{01} is the Bayes factor obtained from

$$B_{01} = \left(\frac{P(M_0|\mathbf{y})}{P(M_1|\mathbf{y})}\right) / \left(\frac{P(M_0)}{P(M_1)}\right) = \frac{P(\mathbf{y}|M_0)}{P(\mathbf{y}|M_1)}.$$

Inference on T is then based on the mixture posterior form:

$$P_M(T|\mathbf{y}) = \frac{PB_{01}}{1+P\,B_{01}} P(T|\mathbf{y}, M_0) + \frac{1}{1+P\,B_{01}} P(T|\mathbf{y},\, M_1)$$

where $P(T|\mathbf{y},\, M_0)$ is given by (2.9) with $R = 0$, and $P(T|\,\mathbf{y},\, M_1)$ is obtained by either integrating out R from (2.4) or by using the approximation (2.8). For the 2×2 trial

$$B_{01} = \left(\frac{3}{2m}\right)^{\frac{1}{2}} \left(1 + \frac{FC}{n_1+n_2-2}\right)^{-(n_1+n_2)/2}$$

where FC is as defined in Section 2.5

The sensitivity of the conclusions to the prior belief of a carry-over difference can then be obtained by displaying summaries of $P_M(T|\mathbf{y})$ as a function of $P(M_1) = 1/(1+P)$. Examples of doing this are given in (Grieve, 1985, 1990) and Racine et al. (1986).

2.9.2 *Bayes using Gibbs sampling*

Instead of using Grieve's approximations, we can obtain the necessary posterior distributions using Markov Chain Monte Carlo (MCMC) sampling. This is conveniently done using Gibbs sampling via the WinBUGS software (Spiegelhalter et al., 2000). Details of how MCMC works can be found, for example, in Gilks et al. (1996). In effect, the required posterior distributions are obtained by repeatedly sampling in turn from a series of appropriate and simple conditional distributions. Under suitable conditions the series of samples converges to a state where the samples are being taken from the required posterior distributions. For additional reading see, for example, Carlin and Louis (1996), Gelman et al. (1995), Gamerman and Lopes (2006) and Lunn et al. (2013).

A WinBUGS doodle which defines the model for the 2×2 cross-over trial with carry-over effects is given Figure 2.15.

The corresponding WinBUGS code to analyze the PEFR data is given in the following box. Here seq[j] is a variable that is 1 for an observation in the AB group and -1 otherwise. The precision parameters precs and prece are the inverses of between-subjects and within-subjects variances, respectively. Vague priors for the parameters are specified. The output from WinBUGS includes plots of the posterior distributions and values of particular percentiles of the sampled posterior distributions. We do not reproduce the plots of the posterior distributions here, but they were not unlike those shown already in Figure 2.14. There was no evidence to suggest that the carry-over difference was anything other than zero. For the model without carry-over effects, the posterior mean for the treatment parameter was 5.20 and the 2.5% and 97.5% percentiles of the posterior distribution were 1.76 and 8.60, respectively. Looking back, we see that these are almost identical to the estimate and confidence interval obtained using Grieve's approximation.

WinBUGS code for 2×2 *cross-over trial:*

```
model;
{ for( k in 1 : P )
{ for( j in 1 : N )
{ Y[j , k] ~ dnorm(m[j , k],prece)}}
for( k in 1 : P )
{ for( j in 1 : N ) {
m[j , k] <- mu + equals(k,1) * pi +
seq[j] * tau) + equals(k,2) *
( -pi - seq[j] * ( tau - lambda)) + s[j]}}
for( j in 1 : N ) {
s[j] ~ dnorm( 0.0,precs)}
prece ~ dgamma(0.001,0.001)
precs ~
dgamma(0.001,0.001)
pi ~ dnorm( 0.0,0.001)
tau ~ dnorm( 0.0,0.001)
mu ~ dnorm( 0.0,0.001)
sigma2e <- 1 / prece
sigma2A <- 2 / precs + 1 / prece
lambda ~ dnorm( 0.0,0.001)}
list(N=56,P=2, seq =
c(1,1,1,1,1,1,1, 1,1,1,1,1,1,1,1,
1,1,1,1,1,1,1,1,1,1,1,1,-1,-1,-1,
-1,-1,-1,-1,-1,-1,-1,-1, -1,-1,-1,
-1,-1,-1,-1,-1,-1,-1,-1,-1,-1,-1,-1,-1,-1,-1),
Y = structure(.Data = c(121.905,116.667, ...,
371.190,404.762), .Dim = c(56, 2)))
list(mu=232, tau=5, lambda=20, pi=-2,
prece=0.00252, precs=0.0001761)
```

A similar analysis can be done using `proc mcmc` in SAS, using the following example code:

`proc mcmc` *code for* 2×2 *cross-over trial:*

```
data crossover;
  input index patient seq trt period carry y;
datalines;
  1        3      2          2       1    1 138.333
  2        3      2          1       2    1 138.571
  3        7      1          1       1    1 121.905
  4        7      1          2       2    2 116.667
  .        .      .          .       .
109       90      1          1       1    1 236.667
110       90      1          2       2    2 220.000
111       99      2          2       1    1 371.190
112       99      2          1       2    1 404.762
;
run;

proc mcmc data=crossover seed=27513
     nmc=100000 monitor=( _parms_ );
   random trt_ ~ normal(0,sd=1000)
   subject=trt zero=last monitor=(trt_);
   random period_ ~ normal(0,sd=1000)
   subject=period  monitor=(period_);
   parms residual 1;
   parms sg  1;
   prior residual ~ igamma(0.01, scale=0.01);
   prior sg ~ igamma(0.001,scale=0.001);
   random u ~ normal(0,var=sg) subject=patient ;
   model y ~ normal( trt_ + period_ + u, var=residual);
run;
```

From the resulting output (not shown) we can see that the posterior estimate and standard deviation of the treatment difference are 10.2914 and 3.6283, respectively. The corresponding, equal-tailed, credible interval is (3.015 17.509).

One advantage of using Bayesian analysis is that data with missing values can be analyzed easily. As an illustrative example, the second period responses from the first two subjects in each group were removed and the analysis (with no carry-over effects) was repeated. Posterior distributions of the variates corresponding to the missing values were obtained. The means of these can be used as estimates of the missing values if required. In our case the estimates of the missing values, obtained from WinBUGS, with actual values in parentheses, were 120.8 (116.7), 212.3(200.5), 156.0 (138.6) and 238.0 (256.25). The estimate of the treatment parameter was 5.02 with percentiles of 1.39 (2.5%)

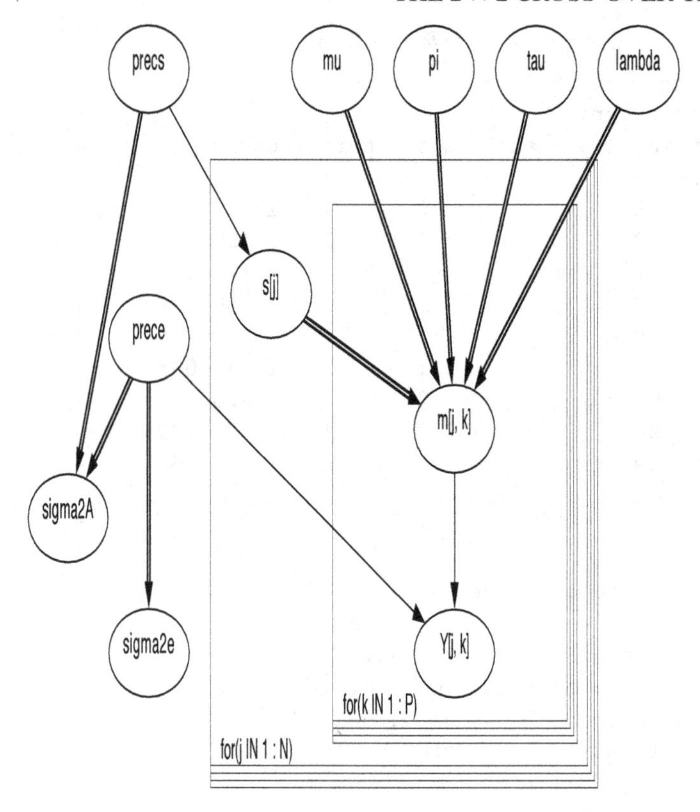

Figure 2.15: WinBUGS doodle for 2×2 cross-over trial.

and 8.67 (97.5%), which gives a slightly wider 95% confidence interval compared to the results from the complete data set.

2.10 Use of baseline measurements

It will be recalled that the test for the presence of a direct-by-period interaction (or different carry-over effects) uses the subject totals from which the subject differences have not been eliminated. Hence this test will generally be less powerful than that for a direct treatment difference. Although, in the presence of a direct-by-period interaction, we can still get an estimate of the direct treatment difference from the first period data, this again uses between-subject comparisons. One way to increase the power of these tests is to use baseline measurements taken during the run-in and wash-out periods. Sometimes, for ethical reasons, for example, a wash-out period is not possible and only the first of the baseline measurements is taken. The analysis in this case is straightforward since the first baseline can be treated as a genuine covariate (see Section 2.11). We shall concentrate here on the case where both baseline measurements

Table 2.13: Patel's (1983) data FEV_1 measurements.

Subject	Run-in	Period 1	Wash-out	Period 2
Group 1 (AB)				
	x_1	y_1	x_2	y_2
1	1.09	1.28	1.24	1.33
2	1.38	1.60	1.90	2.21
3	2.27	2.46	2.19	2.43
4	1.34	1.41	1.47	1.81
5	1.31	1.40	0.85	0.85
6	0.96	1.12	1.12	1.20
7	0.66	0.90	0.78	0.90
8	1.69	2.41	1.90	2.79
Group 2 (BA)				
1	1.74	3.06	1.54	1.38
2	2.41	2.68	2.13	2.10
3	3.05	2.60	2.18	2.32
4	1.20	1.48	1.41	1.30
5	1.70	2.08	2.21	2.34
6	1.89	2.72	2.05	2.48
7	0.89	1.94	0.72	1.11
8	2.41	3.35	2.83	3.23
9	0.96	1.16	1.01	1.25

are available and the appropriate analysis is not so obvious. (See Chapter 5 for further information on analyses that include baselines.)

To illustrate the analysis, we will use the data given in Table 2.13. These data, which were originally given by Patel (1983), were reported as being taken from the results of a trial involving subjects with mild to acute bronchial asthma. The treatments were single doses of two active drugs and we will label them as A and B, respectively. The response of interest was the forced expired volume in one second (FEV_1). Table 2.13 contains four FEV_1 values (in liters) for each subject and these are labeled as x_1,y_1,x_2 and y_2, respectively. It will be noted that we have deviated slightly from the notation defined in Chapter 1 in order to distinguish between the responses observed in the run-in and wash-out periods and the active treatment periods. The baseline FEV_1 measurement x_1 was taken during the run-in period immediately prior to giving the first treatment. Then two and three hours later FEV_1 measurements were taken again and the average of these is the y_1 value given in Table 2.13. A suitable period of time was then left before a second (wash-out) baseline measurement x_2 was taken. The second treatment was then administered and measurements taken at two and three hours to give the average value y_2.

We have four periods and two sequence groups, hence a total of six within-subject degrees of freedom from which to estimate effects. Three of these

Table 2.14: Expectations of the responses in each group.

Group 1 (AB)	Group 2 (BA)
$E(x_{11k}) = \mu - \gamma + \pi_1$	$E(x_{21k}) = \mu + \gamma + \pi_1$
$E(y_{11k}) = \mu - \gamma + \pi_2 - \tau$	$E(y_{21k}) = \mu + \gamma + \pi_2 + \tau$
$E(x_{12k}) = \mu - \gamma + \pi_3 - \theta$	$E(x_{22k}) = \mu + \gamma + \pi_3 + \theta$
$E(y_{12k}) = \mu - \gamma + \pi_4 + \tau - \lambda$	$E(y_{22k}) = \mu + \gamma + \pi_4 - \tau + \lambda$

correspond to the period effects. The remaining three correspond to the group-by-period interaction and contain information on the direct treatment effects, carry-over effects and direct-by-period interaction. There are two possible carry-over effects, a difference in treatment carry-over at the time of the second baseline measurement (first-order carry-over) and a difference in treatment carry-over at the time of the second period (second-order carry-over). This second carry-over is aliased with the direct-by-period interaction. The way in which we partition the three degrees of freedom of the group-by-period interaction depends on the order in which we examine these various effects. In order to illustrate this we first define a linear model for the expectations of the observations. Let $[x_{i1k}, y_{i1k}, x_{i2k}, y_{i2k}]$ represent the four observations, in order of collection, from the kth subject in the ith group. That is, the baseline and treatment measurements are represented by x_{ijk} and y_{ijk}, respectively. We can write the expectations of these as in Table 2.14. The parameter μ represents an overall mean, π_j the jth period effect ($\pi_1 + \pi_2 + \pi_3 + \pi_4 = 0$) and γ the group effect. Given correct randomization, there is no real reason to expect a group effect, and the inclusion of γ from this point of view is rather artificial. However, its role in the model is rather to ensure that the least squares estimators of the other effects will all be within-subject contrasts. The remaining three parameters, τ, θ and λ, represent, respectively, direct treatment and first- and second-order carry-over effects. (It should be noted that $-2\tau = \tau_d$ as defined in Section 2.3.) In more general terms, θ represents any difference between groups of the second baseline means and λ any direct-by-period interaction, whether due to carry-over differences or not. There are many ways in which effects can arise which are aliased with these two parameters. Our aim is to produce appropriate ways of isolating the two degrees of freedom which will include any such effects, should they exist. Some authors, for example, Willan and Pater (1986), set $\pi_1 = \pi_2$ and $\pi_3 = \pi_4$. Unless the treatment periods are very short compared with the wash-out period, there seems little justification for this.

We now need to consider the assumptions to be made about the covariance structure of the four observations from each subject. This has really been unnecessary previously when we had only two observations from each subject. Conventional split-plot analyses of variance are based on the so-called compound symmetry covariance structure in which the variances of the observations on a subject are constant and the covariances between pairs of observations on the same subject are constant. Observations from different subjects are independent. In other words, the pattern of the dispersion matrix of the four repeated measurements on each subject is

$$\sigma^2 \begin{bmatrix} 1 & \rho & \rho & \rho \\ \rho & 1 & \rho & \rho \\ \rho & \rho & 1 & \rho \\ \rho & \rho & \rho & 1 \end{bmatrix}.$$

This is the structure generated by a model which includes a random subject effect with variance $\sigma^2\rho$ and an error term with variance $\sigma^2(1-\rho)$. In spite of the conventional adoption of this structure, we have found it to be too restrictive for general applications in the 2×2 trial with baselines (Kenward and Jones (1987), Section 3). For this reason the analyses in this section have been constructed in such a way that they are valid under any covariance structure. However, although we make no requirements about the covariance structure, we shall still use ordinary least squares (OLS) estimates of the parameters defined in Table 2.14. Strictly, these are only optimal under the uniform structure (and some other less practically important structures) but they have the great advantage of simplicity, and it is unlikely in practice that they will be much less efficient than alternatives.

We want to make inferences about the effects represented by τ, θ and λ, and we shall always allow for possible period effects, i.e., the parameters π_j will always be retained in any model. We shall get a different least squares estimator of each of τ, θ and λ, depending on the assumptions made about the other two, but in all cases the estimators will take the form $\hat{c}_1 - \hat{c}_2$ where $\hat{c}_i$ is a contrast among the four means from group i, that is,

$$\hat{c}_i = w_1\bar{x}_{i1.} + w_2\bar{y}_{i1.} + w_3\bar{x}_{i2.} + w_4\bar{y}_{i2.}$$

where

$$\sum_{i=1}^{4} w_i = 0, \qquad \bar{x}_{ij.} = \frac{1}{n_i}\sum_{k=1}^{n_i} x_{ijk}$$

and similarly for $\bar{y}_{ij.}$. This means that any of the estimators can be defined using the set (w_1, w_2, w_3, w_4).

In the following we test hypotheses using t-tests. If a nonparametric analysis of the data is thought to be appropriate, then these t-tests should be replaced by Wilcoxon rank-sum tests (see Section 2.12).

If the linear model is fitted with all parameters present, then the estimators of the three effects of interest are defined by the following contrasts:

$$\tau|\theta,\lambda \ : \ \frac{1}{2}(1,-1,0,0)$$

$$\theta|\tau,\lambda \ : \ \frac{1}{2}(1,0,-1,0)$$

and

$$\lambda|\tau,\theta \ : \ \frac{1}{2}(2,-1,0,-1)$$

where the notation $\psi_1|\psi_2,\psi_3$ indicates the contrast for parameter ψ_1, given that ψ_2 and ψ_3 are in the model. It is assumed that the other parameters (μ, γ, and π_j, $i = 1,2,3$) are always included.

We can interpret these estimators as follows. By including both θ and λ in the model we are in effect saying that the second pair of measurements cannot be used to compare the direct treatments. Hence the estimator of τ is based on the first treatment and baseline difference. This is standard practice (see, for example, Hills and Armitage (1979)), although using first baseline as a covariate is preferable.

The simple baseline differences, $x_{i1k} - x_{i2k}$, are used to estimate θ. This has also been suggested by Wallenstein (1979), Patel (1983) and Hills and Armitage (1979).

Finally, the difference between the average of the two treatment measurements and the first baseline measurement, $\bar{y}_{i..} - \bar{x}_{i1.}$, is used in the estimator of the direct-by-period interaction, λ. The average alone, $\bar{y}_{i..}$, is used in a 2×2 trial without baseline measurements, and here we use the first baseline measurement to remove the between-subject variation from the comparison based on this average.

The estimator of λ under the assumption that $\theta = 0$ is defined by $\lambda|\tau : \frac{1}{2}(1,-1,1,-1)$. In this case we use the standard estimator of the direct-by-period interaction from a 2×2 trial without baselines, but replace the treatment measurements, y_{ijk}, by the (treatment minus baseline) differences, $y_{ijk} - x_{ijk}$.

The only remaining model of interest is the one in which both θ and λ are zero. We then get the estimator of τ defined by $\tau : \frac{1}{4}(0,-1,0,1)$. This does not involve the baseline measurements at all, and is the same estimator as we would use in a 2×2 trial without baseline measurements. In the absence of a carry-over effect or direct-by-period interaction, this defines, under the split-plot covariance structure, the optimal (i.e., least squares) estimator of τ. Hence an appropriate estimator of τ does not necessarily use baseline measurements, as some authors have implied, for example, Willan and Pater (1986).

In order to produce a simple and robust analysis, we confine ourselves to the comparison between groups of the contrasts for the effects defined above. For each effect, a particular contrast is calculated from each subject and the mean of this contrast is compared between groups using standard two-sample procedures, typically t-tests or corresponding confidence intervals. In this way it is not necessary to make any assumptions about the covariance structure, apart from the fact that the contrast has the same variance in each group. The values of the contrasts for $\theta|\tau$, λ, $\lambda|\tau$ and τ are given in Table 2.15.

It will be noted that Subject 1 in Group 2 has been removed prior to analysis. This is because the usual analysis of the active periods data (not shown), as in Sections 2.5 and 2.8, indicates this subject is an outlier.

We will illustrate the calculation of the contrasts using the data from the asthma trial. Some SAS code to calculate the appropriate contrasts and perform the t-tests is given in the following two boxes. We estimate θ using the

Table 2.15: Contrasts for effects of interest.

	Group 1 (AB)		
Subject	$\theta\|\tau,\lambda$	$\lambda\|\tau$	τ
1	−0.0750	−0.1400	0.0125
2	−0.2600	−0.2650	0.1525
3	0.0400	−0.2150	−0.0075
4	−0.0650	−0.2050	0.1000
5	0.2300	−0.0450	−0.1375
6	−0.0800	−0.1200	0.0200
7	−0.0600	−0.1800	0.0000
8	−0.1050	−0.8050	0.0950
Mean	−0.0469	−0.2469	0.0294
Variance	0.0193	0.0055	0.0078
	Group 2 (BA)		
2	0.1400	−0.1200	−0.1450
3	0.4350	0.1550	−0.0700
4	−0.1050	−0.0850	−0.0450
5	−0.0255	−0.2550	0.0650
6	−0.0800	−0.6300	−0.0600
7	0.0850	−0.7200	−0.2075
8	−0.2100	−0.6700	−0.0300
9	−0.0250	−0.2200	0.0225
Mean	−0.0019	−0.3181	−0.0588
Variance	0.0490	0.1019	0.0075

contrast defined by $\frac{1}{2}(1,0,-1,0)$, i.e., we use the differences $\frac{1}{2}(x_{i1k}-x_{i2k})$ from each subject. From the SAS output (not shown), we have $\hat{\theta}=-0.045$ with a standard error on 14 degrees of freedom of 0.092. The 90% interval for θ is $(-0.208, 0.118)$, indicating that the effect is far from statistical significance, even at the 10% level.

We next examine the direct treatment-by-period interaction using the contrast defined by $\frac{1}{2}(1,-1,1,-1)$. Here $\hat{\lambda}=0.071$ with a standard error of 0.140. A 90% confidence interval is given by $(-0.176, 0.318)$. As with θ, the effect is far from statistical significance. Note that the confidence interval for λ is somewhat longer than that for θ. However, in comparison to the estimate of λ we would have used if we had not first assumed that $\theta=0$, we have gained in precision: the standard error for the estimate corresponding to $\frac{1}{2}(2,-1,0,-1)$ is 0.201. If we had no baseline measurements at all, we would have had to estimate λ using the subject totals $y_{i.k}=y_{i1k}+y_{i2k}$. The corresponding standard error is 0.672, more than four times that of $\hat{\lambda}$, indicating the importance of using within-subject comparisons.

In the absence of the two effects corresponding to θ and λ, we use the estimator for the direct treatment effect τ defined by $\frac{1}{4}(0,-1,0,1)$. For the example we get $\hat{\tau}=0.088$, with a standard error of 0.044. The confidence intervals for θ and λ tests were at the 90% level. We change the level to 95% for τ, giving a confidence interval of $(-0.006, 0.182)$. Multiplying by 2 to get the estimate and confidence interval for the treatment difference B-A gives 0.176 and (−0.012, 0.364), respectively. The three contrasts defined by $\frac{1}{2}(1,0,-1,0)$, $\frac{1}{2}(1,-1,1,-1)$ and $\frac{1}{4}(0,-1,0,1)$ are orthogonal and hence the contrasts comprise a complete decomposition of the three degrees of freedom of the group-by-period interaction, although the usual analysis of variance decomposition into independent sums of squares is not appropriate under a general covariance structure. If the observations have a distribution which is very non-normal, the two-sample t-tests can be replaced, as noted earlier, by appropriate nonparametric tests: the analysis is still based on the same three contrasts. If it is believed that either θ or λ is not zero, the treatment effect should be estimated using only the first two observations, i.e., using the contrast $\frac{1}{2}(1,-1,0,0)$. In the example the resulting estimate of τ is 0.101, with a standard error of 0.094, about twice the standard error of $\hat{\tau}$ obtained using both treatment observations from each subject.

One criticism of the analyses just described is that we have not taken account of their sequential nature. We have discussed in Section 2.7 the potentially serious consequences of sequential testing in the 2×2 trial without baselines, and similar issues apply here. An alternative view of the set of tests is that they show how the information in the sets of observations can be partitioned and how information in one partition can be dependent on assumptions made about one or more of the others.

SAS code for 2×2 cross-over trial with baselines — set up contrasts

```
data d1;
input group pat base1 resp1 base2 resp2;
datalines;
1 1 1.09 1.28 1.24 1.33
1 2 1.38 1.60 1.9  2.21
. .  .    .    .    .
. .  .    .    .    .
2 8 2.41 3.35 2.83 3.23
2 9 0.96 1.16 1.01 1.25
run;
data d1;
set d1;
if group = 2 and pat = 1 then delete;
* Calculate values of contrasts;
* for each subject;
c1 = 0.5*(base1-base2);
c2 = 0.5*(base1-resp1+base2-resp2);
c3 = 0.25*(resp2-resp1); run;
```

SAS code for 2×2 cross-over trial with baselines — estimate contrast

```
* t-test for carry-over to 2nd baseline;
* given treatment and carry-over to 2nd;
* period treatment;
proc ttest alpha=0.10;
 title1 'Test with contrast
 0.5*(base1-base2):
 1st carry / treat, 2nd carry';
 class group;
 var c1;
run;
* t-test for direct x period interaction;
* given treatment and assuming 1st carry-over;
*  is 0;
proc ttest alpha=0.10;
 title1 'Test with contrast
 0.5*(base1-resp1+base2-resp2):
 2nd carry / treat';
 class group;
 var c2;
run;
* t-test for treatment effect assuming;
* no direct x period interaction given;
* treatment and or carry-overs;
proc ttest;
 title1 'Test with contrast 0.25*(resp2-resp1):
 treat';
 class group;
 var c3;
run;
```

The Bayesian analysis of the 2×2 design with baselines has been described by Grieve (1994b), who used approximations to the required posterior distributions. Rather than follow this approach here, we will extend the WinBUGS analysis described earlier. The appropriate code is given in the following box.

WinBUGS code for 2×2 cross-over trial with baselines:

```
model {
 for (j in 1:N) {
   s[j] ~ dnorm(0,prec.s);
   for (k in 1:P) {
   Y[j,k] ~ dnorm(m[j,k],prec.e);
```

WinBUGS code for 2×2 *cross-over trial with baselines (Continued):*

```
   m[j,k] <- mu + seq[j]*gamma
   + equals(k,1)*(pi1)
   + equals(k,2)*(pi2+seq[j]*tau)
   + equals(k,3)*(pi3+seq[j]*theta)
   + equals(k,4)*(-pi1-pi2-pi3+seq[j]
   *(-tau+lambda))
   + s[j]; }}
   mu ~ dnorm(0,1.0E-3);
   gamma ~ dnorm(0,1.0E-3);
   tau ~ dnorm(0,1.0E-3);
   pi1 ~ dnorm(0,1.0E-3);
   pi2 ~ dnorm(0,1.0E-3);
   pi3 ~ dnorm(0,1.0E-3);
   theta ~ dnorm(0,1.0E-3);
        #use for model with theta included
#  theta <- 0; #use for model with theta=0
   lambda ~ dnorm(0,1.0E-3);
#use for model with lambda included
#  lambda <- 0; #use for model with lambda=0
   prec.e ~ dgamma(1.0E-3,1.0E-3);
   prec.s ~ dgamma(1.0E-3,1.0E-3);}
list(N=16,P=4, seq = c(1, 1,
1,1,1,1,1,1,-1,-1,-1,-1,-1,-1,-1,-1,-1),
Y = structure(.Data =c(1.09, 1.28, 1.24,
1.33, 1.38, 1.60, 1.90, 2.21, 2.27, 2.46,
2.19, 2.43, ..., 0.96, 1.16, 1.01, 1.25 ),
.Dim = c(16, 4)  ) )
list(mu=0, gamma=0, tau=0, pi1=0, pi2=0,
pi3=0,prec.s=0.1,prec.e=1)
```

Fitting the complete model, we obtain $\hat{\theta} = -0.046$ with a 90% credible interval for θ of $(-0.36, 0.26)$. We have no reason to reject the null hypothesis that $\theta = 0$. If θ is removed and the model refitted, we obtain $\hat{\lambda} = -0.12$, with a 90% credible interval for λ of $(-0.37, 0.13)$. Again we have no reason to reject the null hypothesis that $\lambda = 0$. We are therefore left with the estimator of the treatment effect that does not make use of the baselines at all and the Bayesian model we fitted earlier.

2.11 Use of covariates

It often happens in clinical trials that additional information is available about each subject, for example, age, weight or disease state. These additional data are usually called **covariates** and they can be put to two important uses. It may be that we wish to know if a treatment effect is related to the values taken by a covariate. Or, if a covariate does not seem to be related to any treatment effect, it may be that it is still related to a subject's response and then the possibility exists that some of the between-subject variation can be accounted for by the covariate values. In this way the between-subject residual variance might be reduced. We can only use a covariate for this purpose if it is first established that the covariate is indeed unrelated to the treatment effect. In the 2×2 trial this second use of the covariate is relevant only for the investigation of the direct-by-period interaction because other comparisons are based on within-subject differences from which between-subject variation is eliminated. In this section we shall only outline the ways in which covariates are used. The computation required by the analyses is standard, although more involved than that described previously, and can be done by most statistical computer packages. For further details of the computation involved we refer to Armitage and Berry (1987), Chapters 8 and 9.

A covariate may be categorical, like sex, or continuous, like weight. We shall begin by looking at the use of the former. The introduction of a categorical covariate is equivalent to introducing a further factor into the trial and we simply need to generalize the analysis of variance, as given in Table 2.5. Quite often the trial is run at a number of different treatment centers. The variable which identifies center is then a categorical covariate. Suppose, for example, that we have a single additional factor A (e.g., center) with a levels. If the trial has a total of n subjects, the corresponding analysis of variance has the skeleton form given in Table 2.16.

Table 2.16: Skeleton analysis of variance for a 2×2 cross-over trial with an additional categorical covariate.

Source	d.f.
Between-subjects:	
A main effect	$a-1$
Direct treatment $\times$ Period interaction	1
$A\times$ Direct treatment $\times$ Period interaction	$a-1$
Between-subjects residual	$n-2a$
Within-subjects:	
Period main effect	1
Direct treatment main effect	1
$A\times$ Period interaction	$a-1$
$A\times$ Direct treatment interaction	$a-1$
Within-subjects residual	$n-2a$
Total	$2n-1$

An association between the covariate and the direct treatment effect is indicated by a large A-by-direct interaction. In the presence of such an interaction it is necessary to examine the direct treatment effect at each of the levels of A. This does not preclude the possibility of there being a clear overall direct treatment effect, but any such conclusion will depend on the differences in direction of the direct treatment effect among the levels of A and on the relative sizes of the direct treatment main effect and A-by-direct interaction. It is possible to examine in a similar way the interaction between A and the direct-by-period interaction. The A-by-period interaction is included in the analysis of variance table for completeness but is unlikely to be of great interest. The generalization of this procedure to more covariate factors should be clear at this point. Should there be no interaction between A and the direct treatments, then the incorporation of A into the analysis with the aim of reducing the between-subject error amounts to its use as a blocking factor. Its effectiveness will then depend on the size of the A main effect mean square relative to the between-subjects residual mean square. If it was known before the trial that A was to be used in this way, then subjects should be randomized within each level of A and it would then be essential that A be included in the analysis.

Suppose that we now have a continuous covariate. We take as an example a 2×2 trial from an investigation of the relationship between plasma estradiol levels in women and visuo-spatial ability. The study was carried out by Dr. Robert Woodfield at King's College Hospital, London. Populations of women were chosen to reflect the widest possible range of plasma estradiol concentration and our example is taken from one such population: women undergoing in vitro fertilization (IVF). These were evaluated in the proliferative phase and at the end of ovarian hyperstimulation. These two conditions, corresponding to low (treatment A) and high (treatment B) estradiol concentrations, respectively, define the two treatments in the trial. By selecting the times of the first test period, it was possible to determine which condition a subject would have first. Hence it was possible to randomize the allocation to the two sequence groups. After allowing for exclusions, there were, respectively, 12 and 11 women in the two groups (low-to-high and high-to-low). Visuo-spatial ability was assessed using several tests. We use the results from one, the Embedded Figures Test (EFT). This response is the time taken to complete a task and therefore lower values correspond to a higher measured ability. The distribution of these times is highly skewed, and, following the investigator's approach, we use a log transformation. The log-transformed EFT scores are given in Table 2.17 along with an IQ score for each subject. It is known that EFT score and IQ are strongly associated and we therefore introduce as our covariate the IQ score obtained at the time of the first period test. The IQ score is obtained as a series of tests and is considered to be quite stable to changes in the conditions being compared. As well as accounting for some of the between-subject variation in log EFT scores, the inclusion of the IQ as a covariate allows us to investigate

Table 2.17: Log(EFT) and IQ values.

Group 1 (AB)			
Subject	Covariate (IQ)	Period 1	Period 2
1	98.8	4.399	3.779
2	75.0	4.748	4.524
3	92.5	4.202	3.185
4	82.5	4.487	4.154
5	100.0	4.614	3.724
6	117.5	2.376	1.297
7	90.0	4.123	3.656
8	103.8	3.463	2.452
9	106.3	3.123	1.258
10	108.8	3.455	3.089
11	106.3	4.132	2.734
12	103.8	3.539	2.742
Group 2 (BA)			
Subject	Covariate (IQ)	Period 1	Period 2
1	117.5	3.166	3.625
2	118.8	3.714	3.273
3	88.8	3.209	2.667
4	112.5	2.692	3.175
5	91.3	4.406	4.638
6	87.5	4.890	4.971
7	101.3	3.470	2.141
8	101.3	3.732	4.008
9	101.3	4.644	4.307
10	107.5	3.792	3.646
11	103.8	3.605	2.452

a possible association between IQ and the effect of condition on EFT score, should such an effect be found to exist.

We start by plotting the data. A scatter plot of log EFT times against IQ is given for each group in Figure 2.16. In these plots a different symbol is used for each period. As expected, there is a strong negative association between IQ and log EFT time, although this is much more apparent in Group 1 and the relationship appears to be roughly linear. If the slope of this relationship was not the same for the two conditions (the treatments), this would indicate a relationship between IQ and the condition effect. However, it is difficult to detect this from the plots in the presence of possible period effects, and, given the strong association, it is difficult to judge whether there is an overall effect associated with the conditions. As before, we get a clearer picture by looking separately at the totals and differences.

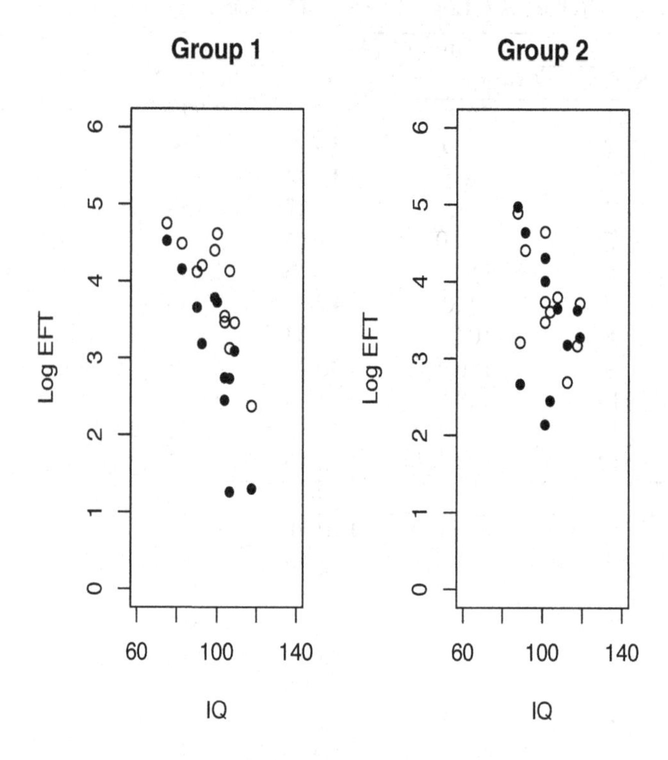

Figure 2.16: Scatter plots of log EFT time against IQ for each group/period category.

We first look at the subject totals. The plots of these are given in Figure 2.17 for each of the two groups. The strong negative trend is clear from this. As before, we use the subject totals to investigate the direct-by-period interaction, in this case the condition-by-period interaction, and a difference in the trend between the two groups would indicate that there is a condition-by-period interaction that changes with IQ, that is, a condition-by-period-by-IQ interaction. If the trend lines have the same slope in each group but are at different heights, this indicates the presence of a condition-by-period interaction that is independent of IQ. In keeping with conventional analysis of covariance, we are assuming that relationships with covariates are linear. This need not be true, of course, although it appears to be a reasonable assumption in this case, and the arguments used here can be extended to allow for nonlinear relationships. We test formally for these effects using the analysis of covariance of the totals. We have here the simplest example of such an analysis, with one factor (Groups)

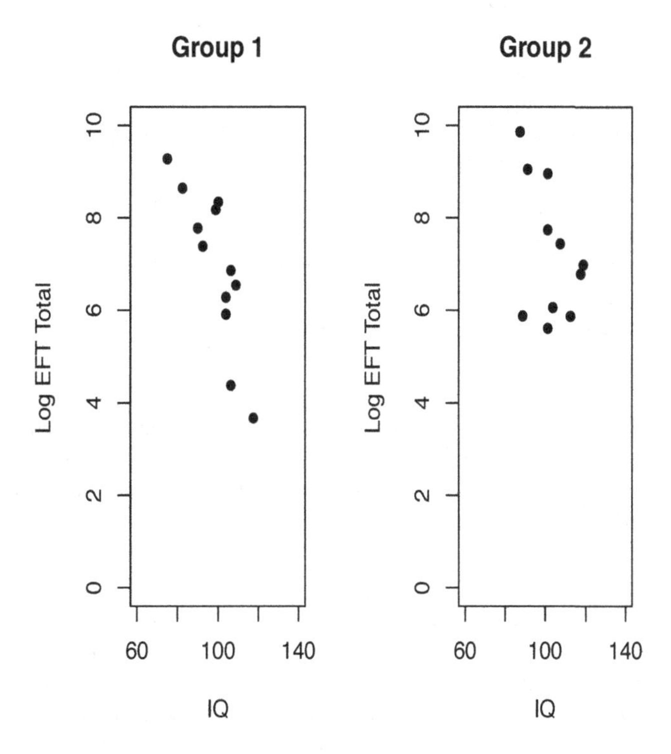

Figure 2.17: Scatter plots of the subject totals of log EFT time against IQ for each group.

with two levels and one covariate (IQ). The analysis of covariance table is presented in Table 2.18.

The large F-ratio for IQ confirms the strong association observed in the plots. The remaining effects are negligible. Although there is no evidence of an interaction with IQ, this does not mean that the inclusion of the covariate

Table 2.18: Log(EFT) and IQ values.

Source	d.f.	SS	MS	F
Covariate (IQ)	1	21.030	21.030	14.68
Groups (Condition × Period)	1	2.982	2.982	2.08
Group × Covariate (Condition × Period × IQ)	1	2.463	2.463	1.72
Residual	19	27.214	1.432	

Table 2.19: Log(EFT) and IQ values.

Source	d.f.	SS	MS	F
Correction factor (Period main effect)	1	6.775	6.775	24.11
Covariate (Condition × Period)	1	0.072	0.072	0.26
Groups (Condition main effect)	1	2.434	2.434	8.65
Group × Covariate (Condition × IQ)	1	0.654	0.654	2.32
Residual	19	5.344	0.281	

has served no purpose. Its use has led to a reduction in the residual mean square from 2.522 to the observed value of 1.43. It can be seen from this how the use of a suitably chosen covariate is one method for increasing the sensitivity of the test for direct-by-period interaction.

We now consider the analysis of the within-subject differences. First we plot the differences in log EFT times against IQ for each of the two groups (Figure 2.18). The first thing to note is the preponderance of negative values, particularly in the first group. The Period 1–Period 2 differences are being used in the analysis and this therefore suggests a large period effect, with the second period scores being the higher. This is in fact expected from the nature of the test, for which there is likely to be a marked learning effect. There is a hint of a slope in the scatter plot for Group 1 but not for Group 2, which suggests at most a small interaction between IQ and the difference between the conditions. The analysis of covariance table for the differences is given in Table 2.19. Note the inclusion of the correction factor as a line in the table: in this analysis this corresponds to the period main effect and, as expected, the effect is very large. There are no effects associated with IQ but there is a large condition effect. Ignoring the covariate, the mean difference in log EFT times between the conditions (high-low) is 0.619 with a standard error of 0.229.

2.12 Nonparametric analysis

If the data from a cross-over trial are such that it would be unreasonable to assume that they are normally distributed, then the usual t-tests, as described in Section 2.3, can be replaced by Wilcoxon rank-sum tests, or equivalently by Mann–Whitney U-tests. As with normal data, these nonparametric tests are based on subject totals and differences.

A nonparametric test would be required, for example, if the data could not be transformed to satisfy the usual assumptions or the observed response was categorical with more than four or five categories. The analysis of binary data

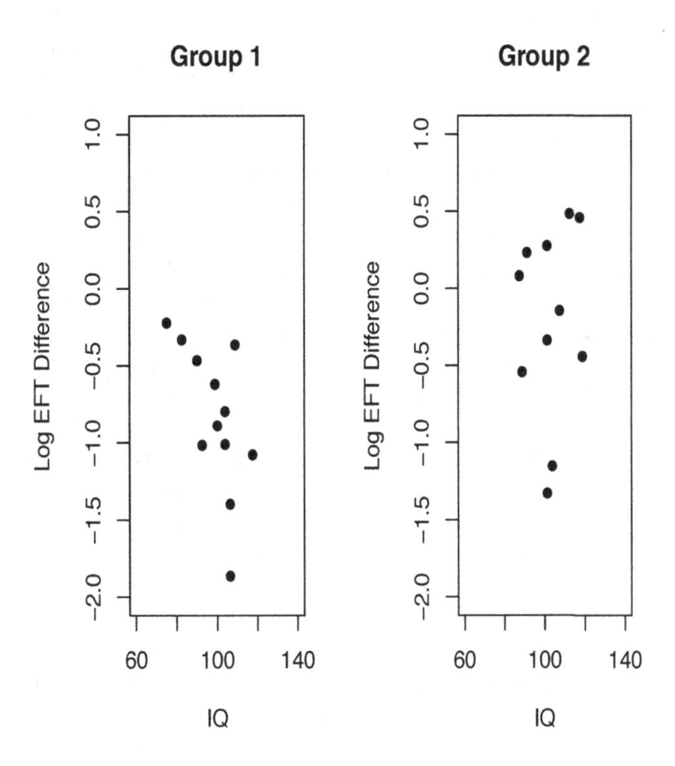

Figure 2.18: Scatter plots of within-subject log EFT differences against IQ for each group.

and categorical data with a small number of categories will be covered more fully in Chapter 6.

The nonparametric analysis for the 2×2 cross-over was first described by Koch (1972) and later illustrated by Cornell (1980) in the context of evaluating bioavailability data. An excellent review of nonparametric methods for the analysis of cross-over trials is given by Tudor and Koch (1994). For a more extensive coverage of the methods covered in this section, see Stokes et al. (2012).

To illustrate the nonparametric tests, we will use the data described in Example 2.2 and presented in Table 2.20. When analyzed under the usual assumptions of normality, equal variance, etc., the residuals from the fitted model indicate that not all these assumptions hold. Transforming the data (using the log and square-root transformation) was not totally successful and so a nonparametric analysis is used. A further reason for a nonparametric analysis is that, even if a transformation could be found to make the analysis more compatible with normality assumptions, the differences on the transformed scale might not be interpretable. Of course, for large trials the central limit theorem can be used to support the assumption of normality of means and then a parametric analysis might be used.

Example 2.2 In this 2×2 trial an oral mouthwash (treatment A) was compared with a placebo mouthwash (treatment B). The trial was double-blind and lasted fifteen weeks. This period was divided into two six-week treatment periods and a three-week wash-out period. One variable of interest was the average plaque score. This was obtained for each subject by allocating a score of 0, 1, 2 or 3 to each tooth and averaging over all teeth present in the mouth. The scores of 0, 1, 2 and 3 for each tooth corresponded, respectively, to (i) no plaque, (ii) a film of plaque visible only by disclosing and (iii) a moderate accumulation of deposit visible to the naked eye or an abundance of soft matter. Of the 41 subjects who entered the trial, only 38 completed it. The reasons for the withdrawals were unrelated to the treatments. Of these 38, complete records were obtained for only 34. The reasons for the missing data were again unrelated to the treatments. The complete records are given in Table 2.20. □□□

The analysis proceeds in exactly the same way as described in Section 2.3, except that the significance test we use is the Wilcoxon rank-sum test rather than the t-test. The Wilcoxon rank-sum test assumes that the subject totals, period differences and cross-over differences are expressed on an interval (or metric) scale, so that the same shift on the scale has the same interpretation regardless of its location. Further assumptions made in using this test include randomization of patients to the groups with random sampling from the same family of distributions with differences between groups only being for location.

The subject totals, period differences and cross-over differences are given in Table 2.21, along with their corresponding ranks. The ranking is done in terms of the total number of subjects, not separately for each group.

2.12.1 Testing $\lambda_1 = \lambda_2$

Although it has not happened with our subject totals, it is possible that some of them will be the same, i.e., there may be ties in the data. If this happens, we assign to the tied observations the average of the ranks they would have gotten if they had been slightly different from each other. This can be seen in the columns of Table 2.21 which refer to the period and cross-over differences. There are, for example, two period differences which take the value 0.000. They have both been assigned the average of the ranks 18 and 19, i.e., a rank of 18.5.

Let $R_i =$ [the sum of the ranks of group i], $i = 1,2$. Under the null hypothesis that $\lambda_1 = \lambda_2$,

$$E[R_1] = n_1(n_1 + n_2 + 1)/2,$$

Table 2.20: Data from mouthwash trial.

Group 1 (AB)		
Subject	Period 1	Period 2
1	0.796	0.709
2	0.411	0.339
3	0.385	0.596
4	0.333	0.333
5	0.550	0.550
6	0.217	0.800
7	0.086	0.569
8	0.250	0.589
9	0.062	0.458
10	0.429	1.339
11	0.036	0.143
12	0.036	0.661
13	0.200	0.275
14	0.065	0.226
15	0.117	0.435
16	0.121	0.224
17	0.250	1.271
18	0.180	0.460
Group 2 (BA)		
Subject	Period 1	Period 2
1	0.062	0.000
2	0.143	0.000
3	0.453	0.344
4	0.235	0.059
5	0.792	0.937
6	0.852	0.024
7	1.200	0.033
8	0.080	0.000
9	0.241	0.019
10	0.271	0.687
11	0.304	0.000
12	0.341	0.136
13	0.462	0.000
14	0.421	0.395
15	0.187	0.167
16	0.792	0.917

Table 2.21: Subject totals and differences and their ranks.

Group 1 (AB)						
Subject	Total	Rank	Period Difference	Rank	Cross-over Difference	Rank
1	1.505	30	0.087	25.0	0.087	31.0
2	0.750	20	0.072	23.0	0.072	30.0
3	0.981	26	−0.211	11.0	−0.211	15.0
4	0.666	18	0.000	18.5	0.000	28.5
5	1.100	28	0.000	18.5	0.000	28.5
6	1.017	27	−0.583	4.0	−0.583	6.0
7	0.655	17	−0.483	5.0	−0.483	7.0
8	0.839	23	−0.339	8.0	−0.339	10.0
9	0.520	14	−0.396	7.0	−0.396	9.0
10	1.768	34	−0.910	2.0	−0.910	3.0
11	0.179	4	−0.107	15.0	−0.107	21.0
12	0.697	19	−0.625	3.0	−0.625	5.0
13	0.475	12	−0.075	17.0	−0.075	24.0
14	0.291	6	−0.161	12.0	−0.161	18.0
15	0.552	15	−0.318	9.0	−0.318	11.0
16	0.345	9	−0.103	16.0	−0.103	22.0
17	1.521	31	−1.021	1.0	−1.021	2.0
18	0.640	16	−0.280	10.0	−0.280	13.0
Mean	0.806	19.4	−0.303	11.4	−0.303	15.8
Group 2 (BA)						
Subject	Total	Rank	Period Difference	Rank	Cross-over Difference	Rank
1	0.062	1	0.062	22.0	−0.062	25.0
2	0.143	3	0.143	27.0	−0.143	19.0
3	0.797	21	0.109	26.0	−0.109	20.0
4	0.294	7	0.176	28.0	−0.176	17.0
5	1.729	33	−0.145	13.0	0.145	33.0
6	0.876	24	0.828	33.0	−0.828	4.0
7	1.233	29	1.167	34.0	−1.167	1.0
8	0.080	2	0.080	24.0	−0.080	23.0
9	0.260	5	0.222	30.0	−0.222	14.0
10	0.958	25	−0.416	6.0	0.416	34.0
11	0.304	8	0.304	31.0	−0.304	12.0
12	0.477	13	0.205	29.0	−0.205	16.0
13	0.462	11	0.462	32.0	−0.462	8.0
14	0.816	22	0.026	21.0	−0.026	26.0
15	0.354	10	0.020	20.0	−0.020	27.0
16	1.709	32	−0.125	14.0	0.125	32.0
Mean	0.660	15.4	0.195	24.4	−0.195	19.4

$$E[R_2] = n_2(n_1 + n_2 + 1)/2$$

and

$$\text{Var}[R_1] = \text{Var}[R_2] = n_1 n_2 (n_1 + n_2 + 1 - T)/12,$$

where T is a correction for ties.

If there are no ties, then $T = 0$. If there are v tied sets, with t_s ties in the sth set, where $s = 1, 2, \ldots, v$, then

$$T = \frac{\sum_{s=1}^{v} t_s(t_s^2 - 1)}{[(n_1 + n_2)(n_1 + n_2 - 1)]}.$$

For our subject totals, $n_1 = 18$, $n_2 = 16$ and

$$E[R_1] = 315,$$

$$E[R_2] = 280,$$

$$T = 0$$

and

$$\text{Var}[R_1] = \text{Var}[R_2] = 840.$$

An asymptotic test of the null hypothesis can be based on either R_1 or R_2. For R_1 we calculate

$$z = \frac{R_1 - E[R_1]}{(\text{Var}[R_1])^{\frac{1}{2}}}$$

and compare it with the standard normal distribution.

The two-sided hypothesis would be rejected at the 5% significance level if $|z| \geq 1.96$. A similar test can be based on R_2. For our data $R_1 = 349$ and

$$z = \frac{349 - 315}{(840)^{\frac{1}{2}}} = 1.173.$$

Therefore, there is insufficient evidence to reject the null hypothesis.

Of course, this test can be done using software such as the `proc npar1way` procedure in SAS. The necessary commands to run this procedure on the subject totals, and the resulting output, are given in the following two boxes. It will be seen that we have used the `exact` option, which ensures that the exact, in addition to the asymptotic, version of the hypothesis test is done. The exact version of the test uses the full permutation distribution of the observed ranks to obtain the probability of obtaining a result equal to or more extreme than that observed in the data. This approach also ensures that ties are dealt with appropriately.

The `npar1way` procedure calculates a continuity corrected asymptotic test statistic and so the result is slightly different from that obtained in the above hand calculations. The P-value for the asymptotic and exact tests are almost the same for this example, but often that is not the case, especially for small data sets. There is no evidence of a difference in carry-over effects.

SAS commands to run `proc npar1way` *to test for a difference in carry-over effects:*

```
proc npar1way wilcoxon data=mouthwash;
var sum;
class seq;
exact wilcoxon;
run;
```

NPAR1WAY output for the test for a difference in carry-over effects:

```
N P A R 1 W A Y  P R O C E D U R E
Wilcoxon Scores (Rank Sums) for Variable SUM

           Sum of   Expected  Std Dev    Mean
SEQ  N     Scores   Under H0  Under H0   Score
1    18    349.0    315.0     28.9828   19.3889
2    16    246.0    280.0     28.9828   15.3750

Wilcoxon 2-Sample Test       S =  246.000

Exact P-Values
(One-sided)    Prob <= S            = 0.1257
(Two-sided)   Prob >= |S - Mean| = 0.2514

Normal Approximation
(with Continuity Correction of .5)
Z = -1.15586        Prob > |Z| = 0.2477

T-Test Approx. Significance = 0.2560

Kruskal-Wallis Test (Chi-Square Approximation)
CHISQ =  1.3762  DF =  1 Prob > CHISQ = 0.2408
```

2.12.2 *Testing $\tau_1 = \tau_2$, given that $\lambda_1 = \lambda_2$*

The period differences and their ranks are given in Table 2.21. Letting R_1 now refer to the sum of the ranks of the period differences for Group 1, our test statistic is $z = \frac{205-315}{(840)^{\frac{1}{2}}} = -3.795$. Clearly there is strong evidence of a direct treatment difference (P = 0.000147). In the above test, $R_1 = 205$ and $E[R_1]$ and $\text{Var}[R_1]$ are as before. In fact, as there are ties in the period differences, $\text{Var}[R_1]$ should have been adjusted by using the value of T as defined above. However, as $T = 0.00535$ here, we did not bother to include it in the test statistic, as it would have made little difference to the result. Using the `npar1way` procedure with the `exact` option gives a similar and highly significant result.

2.12.3 *Testing $\pi_1 = \pi_2$, given that $\lambda_1 = \lambda_2$*

Using the ranks of the cross-over differences, we obtain $R_1 = 284$ and the test statistic is -1.07. There is no evidence therefore to suggest a period difference.

Although using software to calculate exact significance tests is the preferred option, it is possible to calculate exact tests using published tables. We illustrate the use of tables in the following example.

2.12.4 *Obtaining the exact version of the Wilcoxon rank-sum test using tables*

If $n_1 = n_2$ is small (less than 12 according to Gibbons (1985), p. 166), then the asymptotic test should be replaced by its exact version. To conduct this test we need the null distribution of the rank-sum statistic. The upper tail of this distribution has been tabulated by, for example, Hollander and Wolfe (1999) in their Table A.6. This table is in terms of m and n, where n is the size of the smaller group and m is the size of the larger. The table covers the following values of m and n: $m = 3, 4, ..., 10$ and $n = 1, 2, ..., m$ and $m = 11, 12, ..., 20$ and $n = 1, 2, 3$ and 4. We note that the tables for the exact distribution are based on no ties being present.

As we require $n = 16$ and $m = 18$, the tables are of no use. Indeed, for these group sizes, the asymptotic test was quite suitable. To provide an illustration of the exact test we will use the data from the subjects in the first half of each group. The resulting table obtained from these data is given as Table 2.22. We must emphasize that we are using this smaller set of data for the purposes of illustration only, and do not recommend basing inferences on fewer than the observed number of subjects!

To test each of our null hypotheses we compare the value of the rank-sum statistic for the group with the smaller number of subjects with the appropriate lower- and upper-tail values of the null distribution. As the distribution is discrete, we may not be able to achieve exactly the significance level we would like. For example, for $n = 8$ and $m = 9$, the closest we can get to a probability of 0.025 in each tail is to use the values of 51 and 93 obtained from Table A.6 of Hollander and Wolfe (1999). These values correspond to a probability of 0.023 in each tail. If our observed statistic is 51 or smaller or is 93 or larger, we would reject the null hypothesis at the 4.6% significance level.

The observed rank-sum for testing $\lambda_1 = \lambda_2$ is 62, and so we have no reason to reject the null hypothesis. For testing $\tau_1 = \tau_2$ the rank-sum is 101, and so there is evidence of a direct treatment difference. For testing $\pi_1 = \pi_2$ the rank-sum is 70, and there is, therefore, no evidence of a period difference.

Table 2.22: Subject totals and differences and their ranks (first-half data).

Group 1 (AB)						
			Period		Cross-over	
Subject	Total	Rank	Difference	Rank	Difference	Rank
1	1.505	16	0.087	12.0	0.087	16.0
2	0.750	8	0.072	10.0	0.072	15.0
3	0.981	12	−0.211	5.0	−0.211	7.0
4	0.666	7	0.000	7.5	0.000	13.5
5	1.100	14	0.000	7.5	0.000	13.5
6	1.017	13	−0.583	1.0	−0.583	3.0
7	0.655	6	−0.483	2.0	−0.483	4.0
8	0.839	10	−0.339	4.0	−0.339	6.0
9	0.520	5	−0.396	3.0	−0.396	5.0
Mean	0.893	10.1	−0.206	5.8	−0.206	9.2
Group 2 (BA)						
			Period		Cross-over	
Subject	Total	Rank	Difference	Rank	Difference	Rank
1	0.062	1	0.062	9.0	−0.062	12.0
2	0.143	3	0.143	14.0	−0.143	9.0
3	0.797	9	0.109	13.0	−0.109	10.0
4	0.294	4	0.176	15.0	−0.176	8.0
5	1.729	17	−0.145	6.0	0.145	17.0
6	0.876	11	0.828	16.0	−0.828	2.0
7	1.233	15	1.167	17.0	−1.167	1.0
8	0.080	2	0.080	11.0	−0.080	11.0
Mean	0.652	7.8	0.302	12.6	−0.303	8.8

2.12.5 *Point estimate and confidence interval for* $\delta = \tau_1 - \tau_2$

Point estimates and confidence intervals (Hodges and Lehman, 1963) for the direct treatment difference can be obtained using tables or from software for exact testing such as StatXact (Cytel, 1995). Here we will illustrate both approaches, beginning with the use of tables.

Let us label the data in Group 1 as X_i, $i = 1,2,\ldots,m$ and the data in Group 2 as Y_j, $j = 1,2,\ldots,n$, where n is the size of the smaller group. That is, $n_1 = m$ and $n_2 = n$.

Before we can calculate the point estimate we must first form the $m \times n$ differences $Y_j - X_i$, for $i = 1,2,\ldots,m$ and $j = 1,2,\ldots,n$. The point estimate $\hat{\delta}$ is then the median of these differences.

To obtain the median we first order the differences from smallest to largest. If $m \times n$ is odd and equals $2p+1$, say, then the median is the $(p+1)$th ordered difference. If $m \times n$ is even and equals $2p$, say, then the median is the average of the pth and $(p+1)$th ordered differences.

For the smaller of our example data sets, $m = 9$ and $n = 8$. Therefore, $m \times n = 72$ and the median is the average of the 36th and 37th ordered differences.

The ordered differences for the smaller data set are

−1.750 −1.650 −1.563 −1.506 −1.411 −1.378 −1.311 −1.224 −1.167
−1.167 −1.167 −1.095 −1.080 −1.039 −0.828 −0.828 −0.759 −0.756
−0.741 −0.726 −0.692 −0.663 −0.659 −0.645 −0.626 −0.592 −0.572
−0.563 −0.545 −0.539 −0.515 −0.505 −0.482 −0.476 −0.458 −0.448
−0.438 −0.419 −0.401 −0.387 −0.354 −0.338 −0.320 −0.291 −0.273
−0.251 −0.194 −0.176 −0.176 −0.143 −0.143 −0.109 −0.109 −0.104
−0.089 −0.080 −0.080 −0.071 −0.066 −0.062 −0.062 −0.056 −0.037
−0.022 −0.008 0.007 0.010 0.025 0.145 0.145 0.217 0.232

The point estimate is $\hat{\delta} = (-0.448 + -0.438)/2 = -0.443$, so the point estimate for the direct treatment difference is −0.22.

Using the larger data set, the point estimate is $\hat{\delta} = -0.4135$, so the point estimate for the direct treatment difference is −0.20.

To obtain a symmetric two-sided confidence interval for δ, with confidence coefficient $1 - \alpha$, we first obtain an integer C_α using Table A.6 of Hollander and Wolfe (1999). To obtain this integer for our particular values of m, n and α we first obtain the value $w(\alpha/2, m, n)$ from Table A.6. This value is such that, on the null hypothesis, $P[W \geq w(\alpha/2, m, n)] = \alpha/2$, where W is the rank-sum statistic. The value of C_α is then obtained by noting that $[n(2m+n+1)/2] - C_\alpha + 1 = w(\alpha/2, m, n)$.

On the null hypothesis, the integer C_α is, in fact, the largest integer such that

$$P\left[\left(\frac{n(n+1)}{2} + C_\alpha\right) \leq W \leq \left(\frac{n(2m+n+1)}{2} - C_\alpha\right)\right] \geq 1 - \alpha.$$

We then order the differences $Y_j - X_i$ as done in the previous sub-section.

The $(1 - \alpha)$ confidence interval is the $\frac{1}{2}(\delta_L, \delta_U)$, where δ_L is the C_αth ordered difference and δ_U is the $(mn + 1 - C_\alpha)$th ordered difference.

For our smaller data set $w(0.023, 9, 8) = 93$ and hence $C_\alpha = 16$. The confidence interval is then obtained as the 16th and 57th ordered differences. That is, a 95.4% confidence interval for δ is (−0.828/2, −0.080/2), i.e., (−0.41,−0.04) for the direct treatment difference. We note that the required positions of the ordered differences can be obtained from the critical values, 51 and 93, of the test statistic. Noting that $n_1(n_1 + 1)/2 = 8(9)/2 = 36$, the positions in the ranking for the lower and upper limits of the confidence interval are $51 - 36 + 1 = 16$ and $93 - 36 = 57$.

For large m and n, the integer C_α may, according to Hollander and Wolfe, be approximated by

$$C_\alpha = \frac{mn}{2} - z_{\alpha/2}\left[\frac{mn(m+n+1)}{12}\right]^{\frac{1}{2}}$$

where $z_{\alpha/2}$ is the upper $(1-\alpha/2)$ point of the standard normal distribution. To account for ties we can replace $\frac{mn(m+n+1)}{12}$ by $\text{Var}[R_1]$. Ignoring ties is a conservative approach which will provide a wider interval as compared to allowing for ties.

For our larger data set, and taking $z_{0.025} = 1.96$, we get $C_\alpha = 87$. That is, the 95% confidence interval is obtained by taking δ_L as the 87th ordered difference and δ_U as the 202nd ordered difference. The resulting 95% confidence interval for δ is (−0.687, −0.205)/2, i.e., (−0.34, −0.10) for the direct treatment difference.

We also note that for the smaller data set the asymptotic approximation gives 16, as we obtained from the exact formula.

Of course, the exact point estimate and confidence interval can also be obtained using StatXact, without any approximation needed for the larger dataset. The results of doing this are that the confidence interval for the direct treatment difference is (−0.41, −0.04), using the smaller data set and (−0.34, −0.10) if the full dataset is used.

For the above Wilcoxon rank-sum tests to be valid, the data in each group must have the same variability. As our groups of subjects are (or should be) a random division of those available for the trial, this assumption will usually hold for cross-over data. However, if we are worried about this, there are non-parametric tests we can use (see Hollander and Wolfe (1999), Chapter 5). See also Cornell (1991) for a particular test for cross-over data.

2.12.6 A more general approach to nonparametric testing

It will be recalled that in Section 2.3 we defined the period differences

$$d_{1k} = y_{11k} - y_{12k} \quad \text{for the } k\text{th subject in Group 1}$$

and

$$d_{2k'} = y_{21k'} - y_{22k'} \quad \text{for the } k'\text{th subject in Group 2}$$

and corresponding mean period differences $\bar{d}_{1.}$ and $\bar{d}_{2.}$, respectively.

As already noted in Section 2.7, if we do not make the assumption that $\lambda_1 = \lambda_2$, a comparison of the mean differences $\bar{d}_{1.}$ and $\bar{d}_{2.}$ provides a test of the null hypothesis

$$H_0 : 2(\tau_1 - \tau_2) - (\lambda_1 - \lambda_1) = 0. \tag{2.10}$$

In order to provide a test of H_0, Tudor and Koch (1994) considered the statistic

$$Q = \frac{(\bar{d}_{1.} - \bar{d}_{2.})^2}{v_d} \tag{2.11}$$

where

$$v_d = \frac{n_1 + n_2}{n_1 n_2 (n_1 + n_2 - 1)} \sum_{i=1}^{2} \sum_{k=1}^{n_i} (d_{ik} - \bar{d})^2$$

and

$$\bar{d} = \frac{(n_1\bar{d}_{1.} + n_2\bar{d}_{2.})}{(n_1 + n_2)}.$$

We note that v_d incorporates an adjustment for ties when the ranks are midranks for the ties.

When sample sizes are large (e.g., $n_i > 15$), Q has approximately the χ^2 distribution with 1 degree of freedom. For small (or large) sample sizes the randomization of subjects to groups implies that an hypothesis test can be based on the randomization distribution of Q over its $\frac{(n_1+n_2)!}{n_1!n_2!}$ possible realizations.

Tudor and Koch (1994) note that Q has a unifying role in that it can be used for a variety of forms of response y_{ijk}. When the response is binary (0 or 1), then Q is same as the Mantel (1963) counterpart to the trend test of Armitage (1955) for a 2×3 contingency table with integer-valued outcomes in its columns: this is equivalent to the Prescott (1981) test we will briefly describe in Section 2.13.5. If the responses are replaced by ranks, then Q corresponds to the Wilcoxon rank-sum test described in some detail earlier in this section. A particular advantage in using Q from our point of view is that it can be extended to allow for stratification among the subjects, e.g., by centers in a multicenter trial or by a categorical covariate. We will illustrate this extension later in this sub-section. Before doing this we review Tudor and Koch's approach to the analysis of the 2×2 trial, as this offers an alternative that does not suffer from the disadvantages of preliminary testing, as discussed in Section 2.7.

The null hypothesis (2.10) can be thought of as being made up of the sum of two sub-hypotheses: $\tau_1 - \tau_2 = 0$ and $\tau_1 - \tau_2 - (\lambda_1 - \lambda_2) = 0$. The first of these can be tested using only the data from Period 1 and the second can be tested using only the Period 2 data. The combined null hypothesis (2.10) is then a test for a prevailing treatment difference across the two periods. Clarification of whether it is a direct treatment difference or a carry-over difference that is the principal reason for any rejection of (2.10) would then come from supportive evaluation of hypothesis tests on the carry-over effects and on the direct treatment difference in Period 1 (as described in Section 2.3). These supportive hypothesis tests would only be done as a second step following a significant rejection of (2.10). In addition, supportive evidence such as the length of any wash-out periods and the pharmacological properties of the treatments will also be needed to make any decisions as to whether rejection of (2.10) is due to direct treatment and/or carry-over differences. This approach to testing potentially has three stages: (1) test hypothesis (2.10), (2) test $H_{0\lambda} : \lambda_1 = \lambda_2$ and (3) test $H_{0\tau} : \tau_1 = \tau_2$ (using Period 1 data). However, as significance at a prior stage is required before proceeding to the next stage, the Type I error rate is not inflated. See Tudor and Koch (1994), pages 352–354, for further discussion of the implications for the Type I error rate of this three-stage strategy and their use of a weighted difference of the Period 1 and Period 2 responses to address a possibly unclear result of the test for $H_{0\tau} : \tau_1 = \tau_2$ when (2.10) and

$H_{0\lambda}$ are contradicted. These authors also give an extended Mantel–Haenszel statistic for testing if the variances of the responses under each treatment are the same.

As an illustration, we give, in the following two boxes, the `proc freq` input and output for testing for a carry-over difference and a direct treatment difference. The period differences are stored in the variate `difftrt`. The P-values for the 1 degree of freedom tests are the ones we need.

`proc freq` *code to use Q statistic to test for a difference in carry-over and direct treatment effects:*

```
proc freq data=mouthwash;
tables seq*sum/noprint cmh2
score=modridit;
tables seq*difftrt/noprint cmh score=modridit;
```

Use of the Q statistic to test for a difference in carry-over and treatment effects:

```
SUMMARY STATISTICS FOR SEQ BY SUM
Cochran-Mantel-Haenszel Statistics
(Modified Ridit Scores)

Statistic Alternative Hypothesis    DF  Value   Prob
-----------------------------------------------------
Nonzero Correlation                  1   1.376  0.241
Row Mean Scores Differ               1   1.376  0.241
General Association                 33  33.000  0.467

SUMMARY STATISTICS FOR SEQ BY DIFFTRT
Cochran-Mantel-Haenszel Statistics
(Modified Ridit Scores)
Statistic Alternative Hypothesis    DF  Value   Prob
-----------------------------------------------------
Nonzero Correlation                  1  14.407  0.001
Row Mean Scores Differ               1  14.407  0.001
General Association                 32  33.000  0.418
```

If the subjects in the trial can be stratified in some way, e.g., by centers in a multicenter trial or by some demographic variable such as age or sex or by some baseline characteristic such as severity of condition, then Tudor and Koch define an extended Mantel–Haenszel counterpart of the statistic Q:

$$Q_{EMH} = \frac{\left\{\sum_{h=1}^{q}\left(\frac{n_{h,1}n_{h,2}}{n_h}\right)\left(\bar{d}_{h,1.} - \bar{d}_{h,2.}\right)\right\}^2}{\left\{\sum_{h=1}^{q}\left(\frac{n_{h,1}n_{h,2}}{n_h}\right)^2 v_{d,h}\right\}} \tag{2.12}$$

where h defines the stratum and the other quantities are the within stratum counterparts of the quantities used to define Q. Tudor and Koch note that for sufficiently large sample size ($\sum_{h=1}^{q} n_h \geq 40$) Q_{EMH} should have approximately a χ^2 distribution with 1 degree of freedom. The computation of Q_{EMH} is conveniently done using the `proc freq` procedure in SAS. For small samples, exact P-values based on the permutation distribution of Q_{EMH} can be calculated.

As an example of using the stratified test, we analyse the data given in Tables 2.23 and 2.24, which are taken from the results of the trial described in Example 2.1. These data refer to a secondary endpoint, the percentage number of nights when no additional bronchodilator medication was taken. For each patient, three values are obtained: a baseline derived from the diary data recorded in the run-in period, a corresponding value for Period 1 and a corresponding value for Period 2. In addition, a new binary variable has been derived from the baseline, and takes the value 1 if the baseline percentage is 100 and is 0 otherwise. This divides the patients into two groups: those that needed no additional medication and those that needed some.

The results of using the unstratified Q statistic to test for a direct treatment difference (based on the within-patient period differences) are given in the following box. We see that the P-value is 0.059, which is marginally non-significant.

Use of the Q statistic to test for a direct treatment difference: no additional medication at night:

```
SUMMARY STATISTICS FOR SEQ BY DIFFTRT
Cochran-Mantel-Haenszel Statistics
(Modified Ridit Scores)
Statistic Alternative Hypothesis    DF  Value  Prob
---------------------------------------------------
Nonzero Correlation                  1   3.574  0.059
Row Mean Scores Differ               1   3.574  0.059
General Association                 27  25.670  0.537
Total Sample Size = 54
```

To apply the stratified Q test, we used the SAS code given in the next box. The output it produces is given in the following box. Stratifying on the binary covariate (no medication vs the rest) has improved the power of the test (based on Q_{EMH}) and a significant P-value of 0.038, obtained from the chi-squared approximation, has been obtained.

SAS code for stratified Q test for a direct treatment difference:

```
proc freq data=newbase;
tables nbase*seq*difftrt/noprint cmh2
score=modridit;
run;
```

Table 2.23: Group 1 (AB) percentage of nights with no additional medication.

Subject Number	Subject Label	Baseline	Period 1	Period 2	Coded Baseline
1	7	100	100	100	1
2	8	80	100	100	0
3	09	0	55	38.095	0
4	13	100	90.476	71.429	1
5	14	100	90.476	100	1
6	15	100	100	0	1
7	17	85.714	100	100	0
8	21	0	47.368	7.692	0
9	22	100	100	36.842	1
10	28	100	100	100	1
11	35	100	90	30	1
12	36	0	0	0	0
13	37	33.333	100	25	0
14	38	100	100	100	1
15	41	100	100	100	1
16	44	0	0	0	0
17	58	100	100	100	1
18	66	71.429	100	100	0
19	71	0	71.429	33.333	0
20	76	100	100	100	1
21	79	100	37.5	5	1
22	80	100	100	72.222	1
23	81	28.571	57.143	100	0
24	82	16.667	16.667	0	0
25	86	66.667	76.923	85	0
26	89	57.143	42.105	52.632	0
27	90	100	0	0	1

Use of the stratified Q statistic to test for a direct treatment difference: no additional medication at night:

```
SUMMARY STATISTICS FOR SEQ BY DIFFTRT
CONTROLLING FOR NBASE
Cochran-Mantel-Haenszel Statistics
(Modified Ridit Scores)
Statistic Alternative Hypothesis     DF  Value   Prob
-------------------------------------------------------
Nonzero Correlation                   1   4.288  0.038
Row Mean Scores Differ                1   4.291  0.038
General Association                  27  26.987  0.464
Total Sample Size = 54
```

Table 2.24: Group 2 (BA) percentage of nights with no additional medication.

Subject Number	Subject Label	Baseline	Period 1	Period 2	Coded Baseline
1	3	100	100	100	1
2	10	100	100	100	1
3	11	100	100	100	1
4	16	0	52.381	27.778	0
5	18	100	80.952	80	1
6	23	100	100	100	1
7	27	28.571	90	100	0
8	29	16.667	5	33.333	0
9	30	71.429	100	68.75	0
10	32	100	100	0	1
11	33	100	95	95	1
12	39	100	87.5	84.211	1
13	43	85.714	5.263	14.286	0
14	47	100	100	100	1
15	51	100	11.111	85.714	1
16	52	100	100	100	1
17	55	66.667	6.25	23.81	0
18	59	100	100	100	1
19	68	71.429	42.857	100	0
20	70	100	100	100	1
21	74	100	100	100	1
22	77	71.429	100	100	0
23	78	100	100	100	1
24	83	100	100	95.238	1
25	84	100	100	100	1
26	85	100	88.889	100	1
27	99	0	0	0	0

2.12.7 Nonparametric analysis of ordinal data

Tudor and Koch (1994) describe a bivariate Wilcoxon rank-sum statistic for testing the combined null hypothesis that there is no carry-over difference and no direct treatment difference.

Let R_{ijk} denote the rank of the response from patient j in sequence i in period k among the responses in the kth period from the $n = n_1 + n_2$ patients in the pooled sequence groups (note that here the ordering of the subscripts is different from that used earlier in this chapter). We define $\mathbf{R}_{ij} = (R_{ij1}, R_{ij2})^\top$ and $\bar{\mathbf{R}}_i = (\bar{R}_{i1}, \bar{R}_{i2})^\top$, where $\bar{R}_{ik} = \sum_{j=1}^{n_i} R_{ijk}/n_i$. Then the bivariate Wilcoxon rank-sum statistic is

$$Q_R = (\bar{\mathbf{R}}_1 - \bar{\mathbf{R}}_2)^\top \mathbf{V}_R^{-1} (\bar{\mathbf{R}}_1 - \bar{\mathbf{R}}_2) \tag{2.13}$$

where

$$\mathbf{V}_R = \frac{n}{n_1 n_2 (n-1)} \sum_{i=1}^{2} \sum_{j=1}^{n_i} (\mathbf{R}_{ij} - \bar{\mathbf{R}})(\mathbf{R}_{ij} - \bar{\mathbf{R}})^\top \tag{2.14}$$

and $\bar{\mathbf{R}} = (n_1 \bar{\mathbf{R}}_1 + n_2 \bar{\mathbf{R}}_2)/n$. Tudor and Koch note that for sufficiently large sample sizes Q_R approximately has the χ^2 distribution with 2 degrees of freedom.

To illustrate the analysis of a categorical response, we consider the data given in Tables 2.25 and 2.26, which are taken from the trial described in Example 2.1. These are data on a secondary variable, the severity of symptoms that occurred during the night. For each of the periods of the trial, each patient kept a diary of the severity of the symptoms using a five-point scale, where 0 = no symptoms, 1 = symptoms which caused the patient to wake once or wake early, 2 = symptoms which caused the patient to wake twice or more (including waking early), 3 = symptoms causing the patient to be awake for most of the night and 4 = symptoms so severe that the patient did not sleep at all. The symptom scores given in Tables 2.25 and 2.26 are the median values over a three-week period. The median for patient 82 in Period 2 was 1.5, and this was rounded up to 2. The decision to round up or down was taken on the result of a coin toss. The last two columns in these tables are the ranks (midranks for ties) over both sequences for the symptom scores within a period. There are 27 patients in the AB group and 31 patients in the BA group.

For these data

$$\bar{\mathbf{R}}_1 = \begin{bmatrix} 32.259 \\ 32.815 \end{bmatrix}, \; \bar{\mathbf{R}}_2 = \begin{bmatrix} 27.097 \\ 26.613 \end{bmatrix} \text{ and } \bar{\mathbf{R}} = \begin{bmatrix} 29.5 \\ 29.5 \end{bmatrix}$$

and

$$\mathbf{V}_R = \begin{bmatrix} 15.181 & 11.154 \\ 11.154 & 15.424 \end{bmatrix}.$$

Then $Q_R = 2.56$ on 2 d.f. Obviously, from this value and by looking at the raw data, there is no evidence of any difference between the two groups. With so many tied observations, the appropriateness of the asymptotic approximation must be in some doubt, and in this case an exact permutation test would be more appropriate. However, we do not pursue this here.

If the test had been significant, then similar tests with one degree of freedom can be calculated to test for a direct-by-period interaction, and for carry-over and direct treatment differences, respectively (see Tudor and Koch (1994)).

Table 2.25: Group 1 (AB) night-time symptom score.

Subject Label	Period 1	Period 2	Period 1 Rank	Period 2 Rank
7	1	0	43.5	17.5
8	2	0	55.0	17.5
9	1	1	43.5	42.0
13	0	1	17.5	42.0
14	0	0	17.5	17.5
15	3	3	58.0	56.0
17	1	1	43.5	42.0
21	0	0	17.5	17.5
22	0	0	17.5	17.5
28	0	0	17.5	17.5
35	0	1	17.5	42.0
36	2	2	55.0	51.5
37	0	2	17.5	51.5
38	0	0	17.5	17.5
41	1	1	43.5	42.0
44	2	3	55.0	56.0
58	0	0	17.5	17.5
66	0	0	17.5	17.5
71	1	1	43.5	42.0
76	0	0	17.5	17.5
79	0	0	17.5	17.5
80	2	3	55.0	56.0
81	0	0	17.5	17.5
82	1	2	43.5	51.5
86	0	0	17.5	17.5
89	1	1	43.5	42.0
90	1	1	43.5	42.0

2.12.8 Analysis of a multicenter trial

Here we will illustrate the analysis of a multicenter trial using the methods described in Section 2.12.6.

Example 2.3 This example is taken from a trial described by Koch et al. (1983) to compare an active treatment (A) against a placebo treatment (P) for the relief of heartburn. At each of two centers, 30 patients attended on two separate occasions and ate a symptom-provoking meal. Half the patients at each center received the treatments in the order AP (Sequence 1) and the other half at each center received the treatments in the order PA (Sequence 2). The response recorded was the time in minutes to relief of symptoms after taking one dose of treatment. If no relief was obtained after 15 minutes, a second dose could be taken. The variables MD1 and MD2 (for Period 1 and Period 2,

Table 2.26: Group 2 (BA) night-time symptom score.

Subject Label	Period 1	Period 2	Period 1 Rank	Period 2 Rank
3	0	0	17.5	17.5
4	1	1	43.5	42.0
10	0	0	17.5	17.5
11	0	0	17.5	17.5
16	0	0	17.5	17.5
18	1	0	43.5	17.5
23	0	0	17.5	17.5
24	1	3	43.5	56.0
26	0	0	17.5	17.5
27	1	3	43.5	56.0
29	1	1	43.5	42.0
30	0	0	17.5	17.5
32	1	1	43.5	42.0
33	0	0	17.5	17.5
39	0	0	17.5	17.5
43	1	1	43.5	42.0
47	0	0	17.5	17.5
51	1	0	43.5	17.5
52	0	0	17.5	17.5
55	0	1	17.5	42.0
59	0	0	17.5	17.5
68	1	1	43.5	42.0
70	2	2	55.0	51.5
73	0	0	17.5	17.5
74	0	0	17.5	17.5
77	0	0	17.5	17.5
78	0	0	17.5	17.5
83	0	0	17.5	17.5
84	0	0	17.5	17.5
85	0	0	17.5	17.5
99	1	1	43.5	42.0

respectively) are defined in Tables 2.27 and 2.28 as follows. For Period 1: MD1 = time to relief from first dose during Period 1 if time is less than 20; MD1 = (20 + time to relief from second dose during Period 1) if time is between 20 and 40; MD1 = 60 if no relief from either first or second dose during Period 1. A similar definition applies to MD2 with Period 1 replaced by Period 2. In addition, a categorical score was created: 1 if relief from first dose is within 15 minutes; 2 if relief from second dose is within 15 minutes after that dose (given no relief from first dose within 15 minutes); 3 if no relief from first dose

Table 2.27: Center 1 data from clinical trial for relief of heartburn.

Site	Sequence	ID	Age	Sex	Freq	MD1	MD2	CAT1	CAT2
1	1	2	55	2	7	7	35	1	2
1	1	3	35	2	3	5	60	1	4
1	1	6	36	2	4	10	28	1	2
1	1	7	44	2	4	14	36	1	4
1	1	9	38	2	7	60	35	4	2
1	1	11	46	2	4	5	15	1	1
1	1	13	56	1	5	2	13	1	1
1	1	15	30	2	3	32	60	2	4
1	1	18	42	2	2	60	35	4	2
1	1	19	39	2	2	25	14	2	1
1	1	22	30	2	4	15	15	1	1
1	1	23	34	2	3	26	60	2	4
1	1	26	29	2	3	60	60	4	4
1	1	27	37	2	3	60	60	4	4
1	1	30	35	2	3	15	35	1	2
1	2	1	27	2	5	11	35	1	2
1	2	4	33	2	4	6	13	1	1
1	2	5	29	2	2	4	60	1	4
1	2	8	32	2	4	9	60	1	4
1	2	10	38	2	3	6	18	1	3
1	2	12	52	2	6	60	60	4	4
1	2	14	25	2	3	60	10	4	1
1	2	16	65	2	3	3	15	1	1
1	2	17	50	2	4	60	10	4	1
1	2	20	28	2	2	10	10	1	1
1	2	21	39	2	3	10	15	1	1
1	2	24	50	2	2	60	12	4	1
1	2	25	52	1	4	6	15	1	1
1	2	28	38	2	3	60	15	4	1
1	2	29	31	2	3	15	35	1	2

Note: From Koch et al. (1983). Reproduced by permission of John Wiley and Sons Limited.

within 15 minutes, but some relief between 15 and 20 minutes and no second dose given; 4 if no relief from both first and second doses within 15 minutes of either. □□□

The following panel gives the `proc freq` instructions to analyze each center (labeled site here) separately and both centers combined using the extended Cochran–Mantel–Haenszel statistic. For each dataset, four analyses are done: Period 1 only, Period 2 only, carry-over (using period sums) and direct treat-

Table 2.28: Center 2 data from clinical trial for relief of heartburn.

Site	Sequence	ID	Age	Sex	Freq	MD1	MD2	CAT1	CAT2
2	1	1	31	2	4	8	60	1	4
2	1	4	30	2	3	60	60	4	4
2	1	6	28	2	4	60	60	4	4
2	1	8	48	1	5	4	60	1	4
2	1	9	27	1	2	7	60	1	4
2	1	11	54	2	3	7	60	1	4
2	1	14	30	1	2	60	12	4	1
2	1	15	30	1	2	60	60	4	4
2	1	18	31	2	2	9	60	1	4
2	1	19	27	2	3	18	60	3	4
2	1	21	30	2	3	28	60	2	4
2	1	23	29	1	5	32	25	2	2
2	1	26	34	2	2	15	60	1	4
2	1	27	.	1	4	11	60	1	4
2	1	29	48	2	5	32	60	2	4
2	2	2	32	2	3	60	7	4	1
2	2	3	22	1	2	60	7	4	1
2	2	5	29	2	5	60	8	4	1
2	2	7	29	1	5	32	10	2	1
2	2	10	26	2	4	60	8	4	1
2	2	12	30	1	2	60	8	4	1
2	2	13	47	1	3	60	4	4	1
2	2	16	33	2	3	25	60	2	4
2	2	17	38	1	4	32	60	2	4
2	2	20	29	2	5	60	4	4	1
2	2	22	28	2	3	12	60	1	4
2	2	24	26	1	2	9	35	1	2
2	2	25	34	2	2	10	26	1	2
2	2	28	32	2	3	60	13	4	1
2	2	30	31	2	2	30	15	2	1

Note: From Koch et al. (1983). Reproduced by permission of John Wiley and Sons Limited.

ment (using period differences). Table 2.29 gives the results. For each site, separately, is quite different, as are the results for Periods 1 and 2 in Center 2. For Center 1, none of the four test results is significant at the 5% level for either Pattern of relief or Time to relief. However, for Center 2 there is strong evidence of a difference between the groups at Period 2, of a carry-over difference and of a direct treatment difference. This all points to the presence of a direct-by-period interaction in Center 2. As the effects present in the two centers are quite different, the results from combining the centers are not so useful. However, we note that the Center 2 results seem to be dominating the combined results. Koch et al. (1983) discuss the interpretation of the results in the presence of such a significant direct-by-period interaction and focus on the nature of the Placebo treatment. See Koch et al. (1983) for further information.

2.12.9 Tests based on nonparametric measures of association

Here we will use a nonparametric measure of association between the groups as the metric of comparison. Details of the methodology are given by Jung and Koch (1999). We will illustrate this approach using the following example.

SAS commands to run `proc freq` *for multicenter heartburn trial:*

```
** site 1 only **; proc freq data=site1;
tables sequence*md1/noprint cmh score=modridit;
tables sequence*md2/noprint cmh score=modridit;
tables sequence*sum/noprint cmh score=modridit;
tables sequence*difftrt/noprint cmh score=modridit;
tables sequence*cat1/noprint cmh score=modridit;
tables sequence*cat2/noprint cmh score=modridit;
tables sequence*csum/noprint cmh score=modridit;
tables sequence*cdifftrt/noprint cmh score=modridit;
run;
** site 2 only
**; proc freq data=site2;
... repeat of above code for site 1
...
run;
** both sites combined **;
proc freq data=original;
...
repeat of above code for site 1
...
run;
```

Example 2.4. The data in Table 2.30 were given by Tudor and Koch (1994) and were obtained in a trial to investigate the effect of exposure to low levels of carbon monoxide on exercise capacity of patients suffering from ischemic heart disease. The responses given in Table 2.30 are the exercise times in seconds of the patients. The two treatments in this case are exposure to regular air (A) and exposure to carbon monoxide (B).□□□

Let us now consider analyses based on rank measures of association. To get started, let us consider just the data from Period 1. Let

$$\xi_1 = P(Y_{11k} > Y_{21k'}),$$

Table 2.29: `proc freq` results for each center and combined data for heartburn trial.

Pattern of Relief				
Center	Period 1	Period 2	Carry-over	Treatment
1	0.128(0.721)	2.605(0.107)	1.222(0.269)	0.768(0.381)
2	2.513(0.113)	13.440(0.001)	4.774(0.029)	8.883(0.003)
Combined	0.850(0.357)	13.671(0.001)	5.266(0.022)	7.455(0.006)
Time to Relief				
Center	Period 1	Period 2	Carry-over	Treatment
1	0.234(0.628)	3.532(0.0.060)	0.912(0.339)	0.692(0.405)
2	3.567(0.059)	13.321(0.001)	4.865(0.027)	10.495(0.001)
Combined	0.954(0.329)	14.954(0.001)	4.991(0.025)	8.296(0.004)

where Y_{11k} is the observation from a randomly chosen subject k in Group 1 and $Y_{21k'}$ is the observation from a randomly chosen subject k' in Group 2. A possible linear model that explains ξ_1 can be written as

$$\text{logit}(\xi_1) = \text{logit}\{P(Y_{11k} > Y_{21k'})\} = \tau_1 - \tau_2,$$

where $\text{logit}(p) = \log(\frac{p}{1-p})$.

Fitting the above logit model would determine if the chance of getting a larger response in one treatment group depended on the direct treatment difference. This idea can be extended to give three more comparisons between groups: Period 2 in Group 1 vs Period 2 in Group 2, Period 1 in Group 1 vs Period 2 in Group 2 and finally Period 2 in Group 1 vs Period 1 in Group 2. The corresponding logits can be written as

$$\text{logit}(\xi_2) = \text{logit}\{P(Y_{12k} > Y_{22k'})\} = -(\tau_1 - \tau_2) + (\lambda_1 - \lambda_2),$$

$$\text{logit}(\xi_3) = \text{logit}\{P(Y_{11k} > Y_{22k'})\} = \pi_1 - \pi_2 - \lambda_2,$$

$$\text{logit}(\xi_4) = \text{logit}\{P(Y_{12k} > Y_{21k'})\} = -(\pi_1 - \pi_2 - \lambda_2) + (\lambda_1 - \lambda_2).$$

If estimates of ξ_m, $m = 1,2,\ldots,4$ can be obtained and are denoted by $\hat{\xi} = (\hat{\xi}_1, \hat{\xi}_2, \hat{\xi}_3, \hat{\xi}_4)^\top$, then Jung and Koch propose the model

$$\text{logit}(\hat{\xi}) = \begin{bmatrix} 1 & 0 & 0 \\ -1 & 0 & 1 \\ 0 & 1 & 0 \\ 0 & -1 & 1 \end{bmatrix} \begin{bmatrix} \tau_1 - \tau_2 \\ \pi_1 - \pi_2 - \lambda_2 \\ \lambda_1 - \lambda_2 \end{bmatrix} = \mathbf{X}\beta. \qquad (2.15)$$

To estimate the ξ_m, Jung and Koch use Mann–Whitney statistics for comparing two groups:

Table 2.30: Duration of exercise in seconds from patients suffering ischemic heart disease.

Patient	Baseline	Period 1	Period 2
		Group 1 (AB)	
1	540	720	759
2	1200	840	840
3	855	614	750
4	395	1020	780
5	540	510	550
6	510	780	780
7	780	740	720
8	840	720	490
9	1100	1280	1170
10	400	345	320
11	640	795	720
12	285	280	280
13	405	325	300
14	390	370	300
		Group 2 (BA)	
15	900	720	798
16	475	540	462
17	1002	1020	1020
18	360	322	510
19	190	360	540
20	300	330	505
21	750	840	868
22	780	780	780
23	810	780	780
24	240	180	180
25	560	540	540
26	1020	1020	1020
27	540	480	540
28	450	370	406
29	270	220	220
30	240	285	270

Note: Reproduced with permission from Tudor and Koch (1994).

$$\hat{\xi}_m = \frac{\hat{\theta}_{m1}}{\hat{\theta}_{m2}}$$

where

$$\hat{\theta}_{m1} = \sum_{q=1}^{n} \sum_{q' \neq q}^{n} U_{mqq'} / (n(n-1))$$

and

$$\hat{\theta}_{m2} = \sum_{q=1}^{n} \sum_{q' \neq q}^{n} M_{mqq'}/(n(n-1))$$

where $n = n_1 + n_2$.

To define $U_{mqq'}$ and $M_{mqq'}$, let $\tilde{Y}_m$ denote the data for both groups combined that are used in the mth comparison. So, for example, $\tilde{Y}_1$ denotes the data from Period 1 for both groups combined and $\tilde{Y}_4$ denotes the combination of the data from Period 2 of Group 1 and Period 1 of Group 2 (see Table 2.31). In addition, we define $X_q = 1$ if subject q is in Group 1 and $X_q = -1$ if subject q is in Group 2, $q = 1, 2, \ldots, n$. Then

$$U_{mqq'} = \begin{cases} 1 & (X_q - X_{q'})(\tilde{Y}_{1q} - \tilde{Y}_{1q'}) > 0 \\ 0.5 & (X_q - X_{q'})^2 > 0 \text{ and } (\tilde{Y}_{1q} - \tilde{Y}_{1q'}) = 0 \\ 0 & \text{otherwise} \end{cases}$$

and

$$M_{mqq'} = \begin{cases} 1 & (X_q - X_{q'})^2 > 0 \\ 0 & \text{otherwise.} \end{cases}$$

Note that $U_{mqq'}$ can equal 0.5 if $(X_q - X_{q'})^2 > 0$ and $(\tilde{Y}_{1q} - \tilde{Y}_{1q'})$ is missing. Let

$$\mathbf{F}_q = (U_{1q}, U_{2q}, U_{3q}, U_{4q}, M_{1q}, M_{2q}, M_{3q}, M_{4q})^\top,$$

where $U_{mq} = \sum_{q' \neq q}^{n} U_{mqq'}/(n-1)$ and $M_{mq} = \sum_{q' \neq q}^{n} M_{mqq'}/(n-1)$. Then

$$\bar{\mathbf{F}} = \sum_{q=1}^{n} \mathbf{F}_q/n = (\hat{\theta}_{11}, \hat{\theta}_{21}, \hat{\theta}_{31}, \hat{\theta}_{41}, \hat{\theta}_{12}, \hat{\theta}_{22}, \hat{\theta}_{32}, \hat{\theta}_{42})^\top = (\hat{\theta}_1^\top, \hat{\theta}_2^\top)^\top.$$

The covariance matrix for $\bar{\mathbf{F}}$ can be consistently estimated by

$$\mathbf{V}_{\bar{\mathbf{F}}} = \frac{4}{n(n-1)} \sum_{q=1}^{n} (\mathbf{F}_q - \bar{\mathbf{F}})(\mathbf{F}_q - \bar{\mathbf{F}})^\top.$$

Asymptotically (see Jung and Koch), the vector of Mann–Whitney statistics

$$\hat{\xi} = \mathbf{D}_{\hat{\theta}_2}^{-1} \hat{\theta}_1^\top,$$

where $\mathbf{D}_g$ is the diagonal matrix with the elements of vector $\mathbf{g}$ on the diagonal, has the multivariate normal distribution with mean vector ξ and a covariance matrix which can be consistently estimated by

$$\mathbf{V}_{\hat{\xi}} = \mathbf{D}_{\hat{\xi}} [\mathbf{D}_{\hat{\theta}_1}^{-1}, -\mathbf{D}_{\hat{\theta}_2}^{-1}] \mathbf{V}_{\bar{\mathbf{F}}} [\mathbf{D}_{\hat{\theta}_1}^{-1}, -\mathbf{D}_{\hat{\theta}_2}^{-1}]^\top \mathbf{D}_{\hat{\xi}}.$$

To link the Mann–Whitney statistics to the period, direct treatment and carry-over effects, we assume the model

$$\text{logit}(\hat{\xi}) = \mathbf{X}\beta$$

where logit(ξ) is the vector of parameters $\ln(\xi_m/(1-\xi_m))$, $m = 1,2,3,4$, $\mathbf{X}$ is a full rank 4×3 design matrix and β is the corresponding 3×1 vector of parameters: $(\tau_1 - \tau_2, \pi_1 - \pi_2 - \lambda_2, \lambda_1 - \lambda_2)^\top$.

If $\mathbf{f} = \text{logit}(\hat{\xi})$, then a consistent estimate of the covariance matrix of $\mathbf{f}$ is $\mathbf{V_f}$, where

$$\mathbf{V_f} = \mathbf{D}_{\hat{\eta}}^{-1}\mathbf{V}_{\hat{\xi}}\mathbf{D}_{\hat{\eta}}^{-1}$$

and $\hat{\eta}$ is the vector with elements $\hat{\eta}_m = \hat{\xi}_m(1-\hat{\xi}_m)$, $m = 1,2,3,4$.

The modified weighted least squares estimate of β is

$$\hat{\beta} = (\mathbf{X}^\top\mathbf{A}^\top(\mathbf{A}\mathbf{V_f}\mathbf{A}^\top)^{-1}\mathbf{A}\mathbf{X})^{-1}\mathbf{X}^\top\mathbf{A}^\top(\mathbf{A}\mathbf{V_f}\mathbf{A}^\top)^{-1}\mathbf{A}\mathbf{f}$$

where

$$\mathbf{A} = \begin{bmatrix} 1 & 1 & 1 & 1 \\ 1 & -1 & 1 & -1 \\ 1 & -1 & -1 & 1 \end{bmatrix}.$$

Modified weighted least squares is used to address near singularities in $\mathbf{V}_{\bar{\mathbf{F}}}$ that are not in $(\mathbf{A}\mathbf{V_f}\mathbf{A}^\top)$.

From Table 2.32 and using the values of the M-statistics, which are either 14 or 16, we obtain $\bar{\mathbf{F}}^\top = (\hat{\theta}_1^\top, \hat{\theta}_2^\top)^\top$, where $\hat{\theta}_1^\top = (0.315, 0.271, 0.289, 0.289)$ and $\hat{\theta}_2^\top = (0.515, 0.515, 0.515, 0.515)$, leading to $\hat{\xi}^\top = (0.611, 0.527, 0.560, 0.550)$.

The asymptotic covariance matrix of $\hat{\xi}$ is

$$\mathbf{V}_{\hat{\xi}} = \begin{bmatrix} 0.0108 & 0.0104 & 0.0107 & 0.0108 \\ 0.0104 & 0.0120 & 0.0112 & 0.0115 \\ 0.0107 & 0.0112 & 0.0116 & 0.0111 \\ 0.0108 & 0.0115 & 0.0111 & 0.0117 \end{bmatrix}.$$

The parameter estimates, their corresponding standard errors and asymptotic P-values are given in Table 2.33.

When the carry-over parameter was dropped from the model, the results given in Table 2.34 were obtained. The P-value for the test of $\tau_1 - \tau_2 = 0$ is 0.055, giving some evidence of a (significant) direct treatment difference.

The baseline values can also be included in the model. The Mann–Whitney estimator for these is $\hat{\xi}_5 = 0.592$. By including baselines in the model, and forcing their parameter estimate to zero, we can allow for any baseline imbalance between the two groups. This imbalance, if present, is due only to randomization: we assume that the two groups of patients are randomly sampled from a common population and so the true mean baseline difference between the groups is zero. By setting the baseline parameter in the model to zero, we force the model to take account of this. In our example the conclusions were not altered when the baseline values were taken into account (there

Table 2.31: Columns of combined data for exercise duration trial.

Group	Subject	$\tilde{Y}_1$	$\tilde{Y}_2$	$\tilde{Y}_3$	$\tilde{Y}_4$
1	1	720	759	720	759
1	2	840	840	840	840
1	3	614	750	614	750
1	4	1020	780	1020	780
1	5	510	550	510	550
1	6	780	780	780	780
1	7	740	720	740	720
1	8	720	490	720	490
1	9	1280	1170	1280	1170
1	10	345	320	345	320
1	11	795	720	795	720
1	12	280	280	280	280
1	13	325	300	325	300
1	14	370	300	370	300
2	15	720	798	798	720
2	16	540	462	462	540
2	17	1020	1020	1020	1020
2	18	322	510	510	322
2	19	360	540	540	360
2	20	330	505	505	330
2	21	840	868	868	840
2	22	780	780	780	780
2	23	780	780	780	780
2	24	180	180	180	180
2	25	540	540	540	540
2	26	1020	1020	1020	1020
2	27	480	540	540	480
2	28	370	406	406	370
2	29	220	220	220	220
2	30	285	270	270	285

was no evidence of a significant mean baseline difference between the groups, P = 0.4).

A simple analysis that can be used to obtain a P-value to compare with the one obtained above (P = 0.055) is to (1) combine the sequence groups and rank the responses in each period, (2) take the difference in these ranks between the periods and (3) compare the groups in terms of this difference using SAS `proc freq`. The SAS code and output for doing this are given below. We see

Table 2.32: Values of U-statistics for exercise duration trial.

Group	Index	$\tilde{Y}_1$	$\tilde{Y}_2$	$\tilde{Y}_3$	$\tilde{Y}_4$
1	1	10.5	10	10	11
1	2	13.5	13	13	13.5
1	3	10	10	10	11
1	4	15	11	15	12
1	5	8	10	6.5	10
1	6	12	11	11	12
1	7	11	10	10	10.5
1	8	10.5	5	10	8
1	9	16	16	16	16
1	10	5	3	3	3
1	11	13	10	12	10.5
1	12	2	3	3	2
1	13	4	3	3	3
1	14	6.5	3	3	3
2	15	7	2	3	7
2	16	9	10	10	9
2	17	1.5	1	1.5	1
2	18	13	9	9.5	10
2	19	11	9	9	10
2	20	12	9	10	10
2	21	2.5	1	2	1.5
2	22	4.5	3	4.5	3
2	23	4.5	3	4.5	3
2	24	14	14	14	14
2	25	9	9	9	9
2	26	1.5	1	1.5	1
2	27	10	9	9	10
2	28	10.5	10	10	10
2	29	14	14	14	14
2	30	13	14	14	13

Table 2.33: Parameter estimates for exercise duration trial (with carry-over).

Parameter	Estimate	Std error	χ^2	P-value
$\tau_1 - \tau_2$	0.435	0.438	0.984	0.321
$\pi_1 - \pi_2 - \lambda_2$	0.261	0.434	0.364	0.546
$\lambda_1 - \lambda_2$	0.523	0.860	0.370	0.543

Table 2.34: Parameter estimates for exercise duration trial (no carry-over).

Parameter	Estimate	Std error	χ^2	P-value
$\tau_1 - \tau_2$	0.174	0.091	3.678	0.055
$\pi_1 - \pi_2$	0.001	0.070	0.000	0.986

that the P-value is 0.054, which is very similar to that obtained from the more sophisticated analysis.

`proc freq` *code for simple analysis of exercise duration data:*

```
data diff;
input group rankper1 rankper2 diffranks;
datalines;
1 10.5  5.5  5.0
1  6.0  5.5  0.5
.    .    .    .
.    .    .    .
.    .    .    .
2 14.5  9.0  5.5
2 18.0 25.0 -7.0 ;
run; proc freq data=diff;
tables group*diffranks/ cmh2 noprint;
run;
```

`proc freq` *output for simple analysis of exercise duration data:*

```
The FREQ Procedure Summary Statistics
for GROUP by DIFFRANKS
Cochran-Mantel-Haenszel Statistics
(Based on Table Scores)
Statistic Alternative Hypothesis DF  Value   Prob
--------------------------------------------------
Nonzero Correlation               1   3.7240  0.0536
Row Mean Scores Differ            1   3.7240  0.0536
```

2.13 Binary data

2.13.1 Introduction

A binary observation can take only two values, traditionally labeled 0 and 1; examples are no/yes, failure/success and no effect/effect. In keeping with standard practice, we shall refer to the responses 1 and 0 as a success and a failure, respectively, and we shall refer to a 2 × 2 cross-over with binary data as a binary 2 × 2 cross-over. The design of the trial will take exactly the same form as before: the subjects are divided into Groups 1 and 2 (treatment orders AB and BA, respectively) and we assume that we have a single observation that takes the value 0 or 1 from each subject in each period.

Example 2.5 This example consists of safety data from a trial on the disease cerebrovascular deficiency in which a placebo (A) and an active drug (B) were compared. A 2 × 2 design was used at each of two centers, with 33 and 67 subjects, respectively, at each center. The response measured was binary and was defined according to whether an electrocardiogram was considered by a

Table 2.35: 2×2 Binary cross-over trial.

Group	(0,0)	(0,1)	(1,0)	(1,1)	Total
1 (AB)	n_{11}	n_{12}	n_{13}	n_{14}	$n_{1.}$
2 (BA)	n_{21}	n_{22}	n_{23}	n_{24}	$n_{2.}$
Total	$n_{.1}$	$n_{.2}$	$n_{.3}$	$n_{.4}$	$n_{..}$

cardiologist to be normal (1) or abnormal (0). In such a trial each subject supplies a pair of observations (0,0), (0,1), (1,0) or (1,1) where (a,b) indicates a response a in Period 1 and b in Period 2. We can therefore summarize the data from one 2×2 trial in the form of a 2×4 contingency table as given in Table 2.35.

In this table, the entry n_{11}, for example, is the number of subjects in Group 1 who gave a (0,0) response. The other entries in the body of the table are defined in a similar way and the sizes of the two groups are given by the marginal totals $n_{1.}$ and $n_{2.}$. The tables of data from the two centers are given in Table 2.36.□□□

Table 2.36: Data from a two-center 2×2 trial on cerebrovascular deficiency. Outcomes 0 and 1 correspond to abnormal and normal electrocardiogram readings.

			Center 1		
Group	(0,0)	(0,1)	(1,0)	(1,1)	Total
1 (AB)	6	2	1	7	16
2 (BA)	4	2	3	8	17
Total	10	4	4	15	33
			Center 2		
1 (AB)	6	0	6	22	34
2 (BA)	9	4	2	18	33
Total	15	4	8	40	67

Here we describe a series of tests that can be used to investigate effects in the 2×4 contingency table described earlier. The tests we shall be using are based on standard contingency table methods, and those not already familiar with these are referred to Stokes et al. (2012). We will make the assumption that there is no direct-by-period interaction or differential carry-over effect. This is to avoid the issues of preliminary testing we discussed earlier for continuous data. We describe three tests for a direct treatment effect that are valid under these conditions and it will be seen that corresponding to each of these is a test for a period effect. The emphasis in this section is on hypothesis testing and this is a consequence of using contingency table methods and of avoiding explicit statistical models.

2.13.2 McNemar's test

In the absence of a period effect and under the null hypothesis of no direct treatment effect, then, given that a subject has shown a preference (i.e., a 1), the choice is equally likely to have been for either treatment. There is a total of $n_p = n_{.2} + n_{.3}$ subjects who show a preference and out of these $n_A = n_{13} + n_{22}$ show a preference for A. Hence, under the null hypothesis, n_A has a binomial distribution with parameters $\frac{1}{2}$ and n_P. That is, $n_A \sim Binomial(\frac{1}{2}, n_p)$.

To obtain the probability of a result as extreme as this under the null hypothesis, we sum the appropriate binomial probabilities. This gives, for a one-sided test, for $n_A/n_P > \frac{1}{2}$,

$$P = \sum_{r=n_A}^{n_p} \binom{n_p}{r} \left(\frac{1}{2}\right)^r \left(\frac{1}{2}\right)^{n_p - r} = \left(\frac{1}{2}\right)^{n_p} \sum_{r=n_A}^{n_p} \binom{n_p}{r}.$$

For $n_A/n_p < \frac{1}{2}$, n_A is replaced by $n_B = n_p - n_A$ in this expression. For a two-sided test, P is doubled. This is known as McNemar's test (McNemar, 1947) and is just an example of the well-known sign test. We can also construct an approximate two-sided version of the test which is easier to calculate. Under the null hypothesis, $\text{Var}(n_A) = n_p/4$ and hence the ratio

$$\frac{(n_A - \frac{1}{2}n_p)^2}{\text{Var}(n_A)} = \frac{(n_A - n_B)^2}{n_p}$$

has an asymptotic χ_1^2 distribution.

In Example 2.5, for Center 2, $n_A = 10$ and $n_B = 2$, giving $n_p = 12$. We then have $P = 0.019$ and doubling this for a two-sided test we get a probability of 0.038. For the approximate version we compare

$$\frac{(10-2)^2}{12} = 5.33$$

with the χ_1^2 distribution to get a two-sided probability of 0.021. This is rather more extreme than the exact probability above.

The SAS `proc freq` commands to apply McNemar's test are given in the following box. Note that we have asked for the exact version of the test.

`proc freq` *code for McNemar's test:*

```
data center2;
input A_pref$  B_pref$ count;
datalines;
no   no  15
no   yes  2
yes  no  10
yes  yes 40 ;
proc freq order=data;
weight count;
tables A_pref*B_pref/norow ncol nopct agree;
exact mcnemar;
run;
```

The results of applying McNemar's test are given in the following box.

`proc freq` *output for McNemar's test:*

```
McNemar test for 2x2 trial - Center 2
The FREQ Procedure
Table of A_PREF by B_PREF
A_PREF     B_PREF
Frequency|no      |yes     |  Total
---------+--------+--------+
no       |     15 |      2 |     17
---------+--------+--------+
yes      |     10 |     40 |     50
---------+--------+--------+
Total          25       42       67

Statistics for Table of A_PREF by B_PREF
McNemar's Test
----------------------------
Statistic (S)         5.3333
DF                         1
Asymptotic Pr >  S    0.0209
Exact      Pr >= S    0.0386
```

2.13.3 *The Mainland–Gart test*

The main problem with McNemar's test is the assumption that there is no period effect. Strictly, when this assumption does not hold, the test is invalid. In practice, the consequences are only serious when $n_{12}+n_{13}$ and $n_{22}+n_{23}$ differ substantially, for only then will the period effect favor one of the two treatments (Nam, 1971; Prescott, 1979, 1981). However, since the reason for using the two treatment sequences in the 2×2 cross-over is to allow for a possible period effect, an analysis that assumes this effect is negligible seems particularly inappropriate. We suggest that the following test is to be preferred to McNemar's; in particular, we do not draw conclusions about the examples from the tests above. To derive this alternative test, we can apply the following argument.

We associate with each entry in the 2×4 table a probability ρ_{ij} and obtain Table 2.37.

The odds in favor of a (1,0) response in Group 1 as opposed to a (0,1) response is the ratio of probabilities $\frac{\rho_{13}}{\rho_{12}}$. If there were no carry-over difference or direct treatment effect, we ought to get the same odds in Group 2, i.e., $\frac{\rho_{23}}{\rho_{22}}$. If these two odds were not equal, this would indicate that there was a direct treatment effect. A natural way to express this effect is as the ratio of the

Table 2.37: 2 × 2 Binary cross-over trial.

Group	(0,0)	(0,1)	(1,0)	(1,1)	Total
1 (AB)	ρ_{11}	ρ_{12}	ρ_{13}	ρ_{14}	1
2 (BA)	ρ_{21}	ρ_{22}	ρ_{23}	ρ_{24}	1
Total	$\rho_{.1}$	$\rho_{.2}$	$\rho_{.3}$	$\rho_{.4}$	2

Table 2.38: 2 × 2 Contingency table.

	(0,1)	(1,0)
Group 1	ρ_{12}	ρ_{13}
Group 2	ρ_{22}	ρ_{23}

Table 2.39: Mainland–Gart contingency table.

	(0,1)	(1,0)	Total
Group 1	n_{12}	n_{13}	m_1
Group 2	n_{22}	n_{23}	m_2
Total	$n_{.2}$	$n_{.3}$	$m_.$

odds

$$\phi_\tau = \frac{\rho_{23}}{\rho_{22}} \Big/ \frac{\rho_{13}}{\rho_{12}} = \frac{\rho_{12}\rho_{23}}{\rho_{13}\rho_{22}}.$$

This is just the odds-ratio in the 2 × 2 contingency table with probabilities proportional to those in Table 2.38.

In the absence of a direct treatment effect, there should be no evidence of association in this table. This points to a test for the direct treatment effect in terms of the 2 × 2 contingency table given as Table 2.39.
where $m_1 = n_{12} + n_{13}$ and $m_2 = n_{22} + n_{23}$. To test for this association, we can apply the standard tests for a 2 × 2 contingency table to this table, where evidence of association indicates a direct treatment effect. Mainland (1963), pp. 236–238, derived this test using a heuristic argument based on the randomization of subjects to groups, while Gart (1969) gave a rigorous derivation in which he conditioned on subject effects in a linear logistic model for each individual observation in each period. We return to this view of the analysis in Chapter 6.

2.13.4 Fisher's exact version of the Mainland–Gart test

Cross-over trials are often small, and even with trials of moderate size we have seen in the example that the number of subjects that contribute to the Mainland-Gart table may be small. Hence we need to consider methods of testing association in this table that do not depend on asymptotic results. In tables

Table 2.40: Mainland–Gart table for Example 2.5.

	(0,1)	(1,0)	Total
Group 1	0	6	6
Group 2	4	2	6
Total	4	8	12

with small entries, Fisher's exact test can be used. It is constructed as follows (Stokes et al. (2012), Chapter 2). Conditional on the observed margins we can write down the probability (P) of obtaining any particular arrangement of the table entries. The one-sided significance probability is obtained by adding the probabilities of those tables which show as much or more association than the observed table, where the association in a table is measured by the odds-ratio. The necessary arithmetic can be done relatively simply on a computer. In order to obtain a two-sided test, the usual method is to double the value of P. It can happen that P is greater than one-half and then doubling the value will not produce a meaningful probability. In this situation we have an observed table that lies in the center of the distribution of possible tables and arguably the most sensible two-sided probability for this case is one; certainly there is no evidence of association in the table.

For Example 2.5, the required data are given in Table 2.40.

The SAS `proc freq` commands to apply the Mainland–Gart test are given in the following box.

`proc freq` *code for Mainland–Gart test:*

```
data center2;
input group $ outcome $ count;
datalines;
AB 01 0
AB 10 6
BA 01 4
BA 10 2;
proc freq;
weight count;
tables group*outcome / chisq nocol nopct;
exact chisq;
run;
```

The standard χ^2 test for this table gives the test statistic $X^2 = 6$ on 1 d.f., which has an asymptotic P-value of 0.014. Fisher's exact test gives a P-value of 0.06. So there is some evidence of a direct treatment difference.

`proc freq` *output for Mainland–Gart test:*

```
The FREQ Procedure
Table of GROUP by OUTCOME
GROUP       OUTCOME
Frequency|01       |10       |  Total
---------+--------+--------+
AB       |       0 |       6 |       6
---------+--------+--------+
BA       |       4 |       2 |       6
---------+--------+--------+
Total           4         8        12

WARNING: 100% of the cells have expected counts less than 5
(Asymptotic) Chi-Square may not be a valid test.

Pearson Chi-Square Test
-----------------------------------
Chi-Square                   6.0000
DF                                1
Asymptotic Pr >  ChiSq       0.0143
Exact      Pr >= ChiSq       0.0606
```

2.13.5 Prescott's test

The Mainland–Gart test has the advantage that it does not depend on the randomization of subjects to groups, at least under Gart's logistic model. This advantage is obtained at a price, however; the test does not make use of any additional information that randomization provides and this is reflected in the exclusion from the analysis of the data from subjects who show no preference. Prescott (1981) introduced a test for a direct treatment difference which *does* depend on the randomization for its validity but which can, at the same time, exploit the extra information from the randomization. Under randomization one would then expect Prescott's test to be more sensitive than the Mainland–Gart test and this is confirmed by the limited studies that have been done.

The test makes use of all the data from the trial, although the responses from the subjects who show no preference are combined. The relevant contingency table is then as given in Table 2.41.

Table 2.41: Contingency table for Prescott's test.

Group	(0,1)	(0,0) and (1,1)	(1,0)	Total
1 (AB)	n_{12}	$n_{11}+n_{14}$	n_{13}	$n_{1.}$
2 (BA)	n_{22}	$n_{21}+n_{24}$	n_{23}	$n_{2.}$
Total	$n_{.2}$	$n_{.1}+n_{.4}$	$n_{.3}$	$n_{..}$

Formally, Prescott's test is the test for linear trend in this table (Armitage, 1955), which we met earlier in Section 2.12.6. The test for association in this table, which is on two degrees of freedom, would provide a legitimate test for direct treatments in the absence of direct-by-period interaction and in fact can be used in this way, as, for example, Farewell (1985) suggests. However, this test can be decomposed into two components, each on one degree of freedom: one of which corresponds to Prescott's test. Prescott's test extracts the single degree of freedom that might be expected to show a direct treatment difference if one exists, and in this lies its advantage over the simple test for association on two degrees of freedom.

The SAS `proc freq` commands to apply Prescott's test and the results produced are given in the following boxes. The asymptotic two-sided P-value is 0.021 and the exact two-sided P-value is 0.038, giving evidence of a significant difference in the direct treatments.

`proc freq` *code for Prescott's test:*

```
data center2;
input group $ outcome $ count;
datalines;
AB -1  0
AB  0  28
AB  1  6
BA -1  4
BA  0  27
BA  1  2;
run;
proc freq;
weight count;
tables group*outcome/ cmh
chisq norow nocol nopct trend;
exact chisq;
run;
```

`proc freq` *output for Prescott's test:*

```
The FREQ Procedure
Table of GROUP by OUTCOME
GROUP     OUTCOME
Frequency|-1      |0       |1       |  Total
---------+--------+--------+--------+
AB       |      0 |     28 |      6 |     34
---------+--------+--------+--------+
BA       |      4 |     27 |      2 |     33
---------+--------+--------+--------+
Total           4       55        8      67

Cochran-Armitage Trend Test
--------------------------
Statistic (Z)         2.3156
One-sided Pr >  Z     0.0103
Two-sided Pr > |Z|    0.0206

Statistics for Table of GROUP by OUTCOME

 Mantel-Haenszel Chi-Square Test
 ----------------------------------
 Chi-Square                  5.2819
 DF                               1
 Asymptotic Pr >  ChiSq      0.0215
 Exact      Pr >= ChiSq      0.0380
```

Chapter 3

Higher-order designs for two treatments

3.1 Introduction

In this chapter we consider the properties of higher-order designs for two treatments. By "higher-order" we mean that the design includes either more than two sequence groups or more than two treatment periods or both. In the next chapter we will consider higher-order designs for more than two treatments. In Chapter 5 we illustrate analyses for some of the two-treatment designs introduced below.

The main disadvantages of the standard AB/BA design without baselines are that (a) the test for a carry-over effect or direct-by-period interaction lacks power because it is based on between-subject comparisons and (b) the carry-over effect, the direct-by-period interaction and the group difference are all completely aliased with one another. If higher-order designs are used, however, we are able to obtain within-subject estimators of the carry-over effects or the direct-by-period interaction, and in some designs these estimators are not aliased with each other. We do emphasize, however, that these gains do rest on making very specific assumptions about the nature of the carry-over effects.

Another feature of the higher-order designs is that it is not necessary to assume that the subject effects are random variables in order to test for a difference between the carry-over effects. Although in principle we could recover direct treatment information from the between-subject variability, it is very unlikely to prove worthwhile, due to the large differences between the subjects that are typical in a cross-over trial. Also, the benefits of recovering between-subject information are only realized in large cross-over trials. These issues are explored in detail later in Chapter 5. Consequently, for the purposes of comparing designs, we usually assume that the subject effects are fixed and that the within-subject errors are independent, with mean zero and variance σ^2. In fact, as is shown in Appendix A, as long as we use within-subject contrasts, we get the same estimators of the parameters of interest when we use fixed subject effects and independent within-subject errors as when we use the compound symmetry within-subject covariance structure.

An important feature of this chapter and those following is the way we determine which effects can be estimated from the within-subject contrasts. In order to do this, we first determine how many degrees of freedom are available within-subjects and then determine the contrasts which are associated with these degrees of freedom.

If a design has s sequence groups and p periods, then there are sp group-by-period means, $\bar{y}_{ij.}$. There are $(sp - 1)$ degrees of freedom between these sp means which can be partitioned into $(s - 1)$ between groups, $(p - 1)$ between periods and $(s - 1)(p - 1)$ for the group-by-period interaction effects. This last set contains the degrees of freedom associated with the effects of most interest, i.e., the direct treatments, direct-by-period interaction, the carry-over effects, and so on. Although this set of degrees of freedom can be partitioned in a number of ways, we will always attempt a partition into three basic sets: (a) the direct treatment effects, (b) the direct-by-period interaction and carry-over effects and (c) other effects not of direct interest associated with the group-by-period interaction.

For some designs the effects associated with the degrees of freedom in set (b) will be aliased with other effects, and so there will be a choice of which terms to include in our model. For example, it will not always be possible to obtain unaliased estimates of both the direct-by-period interaction and the carry-over effects. Depending on the design, some, none or all the degrees of freedom in set (b) will have aliases. Occasionally some of these degrees of freedom will be confounded with subjects.

In summary then, our approach will be to identify degrees of freedom which are associated with effects of interest and then to formulate a model which isolates these degrees of freedom. We regard the terms in our model as identifying contrasts of interest between the group-by-period means. Also, our approach takes account of any marginality requirements induced by our model. So, for example, we would not include an interaction effect in the absence of the corresponding main effects. Further, we would not attempt to interpret a main effect in the presence of its corresponding interaction effect. In connection with this last point, we note that it is not unusual in cross-over designs for the carry-over effects to be aliased with the direct-by-period interaction. If the carry-over effects are included in the model and are significant, we must satisfy ourselves that it is unlikely that a direct-by-period interaction could have occurred. Only then would it be sensible to estimate the direct treatment difference in the presence of a carry-over difference.

3.2 "Optimal" designs

In order to choose an optimal design, we must first define the criterion of optimality. The various criteria used to compare cross-over designs with more than two treatments are briefly described in Chapter 4. For two treatments the criterion usually adopted in the literature is that a cross-over design is optimal if it provides minimum variance unbiased estimators of τ and λ, where $\tau = -\tau_1 = \tau_2$ and $\lambda = -\lambda_1 = \lambda_2$.

Table 3.1: Design 3.1.

Sequence	Period	
	1	2
1	A	A
2	B	B
3	A	B
4	B	A

Table 3.2: Design 3.2.

Sequence	Period		
	1	2	3
1	A	B	B
2	B	A	A

Cheng and Wu (1980), Laska et al. (1983), Laska and Meisner (1985) and Matthews (1987) have proved that if a compound symmetry covariance structure, or a fixed subject effect structure, is adopted, then the designs given in Tables 3.1 to 3.5 are optimal. The properties of a number of different two-treatment designs have also been described by Kershner and Federer (1981).

3.3 Balaam's design for two treatments

Design 3.1 as given in Table 3.1 is a special case of one given by Balaam (1968) for comparing t treatments using t^2 experimental subjects. In our version we use only two treatments and assign more than one subject to each sequence group.

Table 3.3: Design 3.3.

Sequence	Period			
	1	2	3	4
1	A	A	B	B
2	B	B	A	A
3	A	B	B	A
4	B	A	A	B

Table 3.4: Design 3.4.

Sequence	Period				
	1	2	3	4	
1	A	B	B	A	A
2	B	A	A	B	B

Table 3.5: Design 3.5.

Sequence	Period					
	1	2	3	4	5	6
1	A	B	B	A	A	B
2	B	A	A	B	B	A
3	A	A	B	B	B	A
4	B	B	A	A	A	B

Let us denote the mean response for the subjects in period j in group i by $\bar{y}_{ij.}$. There are two means in each group and so there are 4 degrees of freedom for within-group comparisons. One of these is associated with the period difference and another with the direct effect. How we use the remaining 2 degrees of freedom depends on the other effects that we think are important in the trial. Balaam was concerned with obtaining a within-subject estimator of the direct-by-period interaction and so associated one of the remaining degrees of freedom with this effect. He did not make use of the other degree of freedom and the contrast associated with this was absorbed into the residual SS. If we include a parameter λ for the carry-over effect, then we can interpret the remaining degree of freedom in a meaningful way. However, we should not forget that λ is completely aliased with the direct-by-period interaction.

In our new parameterization we define $(\tau\lambda)$ to be the direct-by-carry-over interaction. This interaction would be significant if the carry-over effect of a treatment depended on the treatment applied in the immediately following period. Fleiss (1986) has drawn attention to this possibility, suggesting that the carry-over of A when followed by B may not be the same as the carry-over when A is followed by A. See also Senn (1993), Chapter 10, for further discussion on this point.

As usual, we will put the following constraints on our parameters:

$$\tau_1 = -\tau_2 = -\tau$$
$$\pi_1 = -\pi_2 = -\pi$$
$$\lambda_1 = -\lambda_2 = -\lambda.$$

We define the interaction between direct treatment r and carry-over effect m by $(\tau\lambda)_{rm}$ and apply the constraint that

$$(\tau\lambda)_{11} = (\tau\lambda)_{22} = (\tau\lambda)$$
$$(\tau\lambda)_{12} = (\tau\lambda)_{21} = -(\tau\lambda).$$

The expectations of the eight group-by-period means are then as given in Table 3.6, where γ_1, γ_2, γ_3 and γ_4 are unconstrained parameters for Groups 1, 2, 3 and 4, respectively.

Table 3.6: Expectations of $\bar{y}_{ij.}$ for direct-by-carry-over interaction model.

Group	Period 1	Period 2
1 AA	$\gamma_1 - \pi - \tau$	$\gamma_1 + \pi - \tau - \lambda + (\tau\lambda)$
2 BB	$\gamma_2 - \pi + \tau$	$\gamma_2 + \pi + \tau + \lambda + (\tau\lambda)$
3 AB	$\gamma_3 - \pi - \tau$	$\gamma_3 + \pi + \tau - \lambda - (\tau\lambda)$
4 BA	$\gamma_4 - \pi + \tau$	$\gamma_4 + \pi - \tau + \lambda - (\tau\lambda)$

Note that here, and in the rest of this chapter, we will derive the formulae for the least squares estimators of the treatment and interaction parameters by fitting a model to the group-by-period means. It is shown in the appendix that this gives the same estimators of the direct treatment and carry-over effects as fitting the corresponding model to the individual observations, where the group parameters (γ_i) have been replaced by subject parameters (s_{ik}).

When considering the properties of this design, and those described in the following sections, we will assume that n subjects have been randomly assigned to each group. In a real trial the achieved design will usually have unequal group sizes and this will, of course, affect the design's properties. However, assuming equal group sizes will emphasize the good and bad features of the designs and will make comparisons between them much easier.

The OLS estimator of $(\tau\lambda)$ is

$$(\hat{\tau\lambda}) = \frac{1}{4}(-\bar{y}_{11.} + \bar{y}_{12.} - \bar{y}_{21.} + \bar{y}_{22.} + \bar{y}_{31.} - \bar{y}_{32.} + \bar{y}_{41.} - \bar{y}_{42.})$$

and has variance

$$\text{Var}[(\hat{\tau\lambda})] = \frac{\sigma^2}{2n}.$$

If the direct-by-carry-over interaction is removed from the model, the estimators of $\lambda|\tau$ and $\tau|\lambda$ are

$$\hat{\lambda}|\tau = \frac{1}{2}(\bar{y}_{11.} - \bar{y}_{12.} - \bar{y}_{21.} + \bar{y}_{22.}) \qquad \text{and}$$

$$\hat{\tau}|\lambda = \frac{1}{4}(\bar{y}_{11.} - \bar{y}_{12.} - \bar{y}_{21.} + \bar{y}_{22.} - \bar{y}_{31.} + \bar{y}_{32.} + \bar{y}_{41.} - \bar{y}_{42.}).$$

The variances of these are

$$\text{Var}[\hat{\lambda}|\tau] = \frac{\sigma^2}{n} \text{ and } \text{Var}[\hat{\tau}|\lambda] = \frac{\sigma^2}{2n}.$$

Of course, the above estimator of τ is only sensible if we are certain that there is no direct-by-period interaction and we wish to estimate τ adjusted for λ. This is the advantage that this design has over the 2×2 cross-over: we can obtain a within-subjects estimate of τ in the presence of a carry-over effect. We also note that only Groups 1 and 2 are used to estimate $\lambda|\tau$.

If the carry-over effect is dropped from the model, then the estimator of τ is

$$\hat{\tau} = \frac{1}{4}(-\bar{y}_{31.} + \bar{y}_{32.} + \bar{y}_{41.} - \bar{y}_{42.})$$

and has variance

$$\text{Var}[\hat{\tau}] = \frac{\sigma^2}{4n}.$$

If there is no carry-over effect, we note that, as in the AB/BA design, only two groups are used to estimate τ.

As the analysis of a cross-over trial will almost certainly be done using a computer, it is not necessary to know the formulae for the OLS estimators for the general case of unequal group sizes. However, should these be required, they can easily be obtained (see the appendix).

We will illustrate the analysis of data from a trial that used Balaam's design in Section 5.5.1.

3.4 Effect of preliminary testing in Balaam's design

In Section 2.7 of Chapter 2, we considered the effects of preliminary testing in the AB/BA design. In this section we repeat what was done there for Balaam's design. Using the results given in Section 3.3, the corresponding estimators for Balaam's design are as follows, where we assume that there are n subjects in each of the four sequence groups.

$$S = 2\hat{\lambda}|\tau \sim N(\lambda_d, \frac{4\sigma^2}{n})$$

$$F = 2\hat{\tau}|\lambda \sim N(\tau_d, \frac{2\sigma^2}{n})$$

and

$$D = 2\hat{\tau} \sim N(\tau_d - \frac{\lambda_d}{2}, \frac{\sigma^2}{n}),$$

where $\lambda_d = \lambda_1 - \lambda_2$ and $\tau_d = \tau_1 - \tau_2$.

We see that these are the same as in Section 2.7, except that the ρ that occurs in the formulae in Section 2.7 is missing. The ρ disappears because all of the estimators for Balaam's design are calculated using only within-subjects information. If we now use TS to refer to the procedure of using $\hat{\lambda}_d|\tau$ in the preliminary test and then using either $\hat{\tau}_d|\lambda$ if the test is significant and $\hat{\tau}_d$ otherwise, we can use the same notation as in Section 2.7.

Using the same values for the parameters as in Section 2.7 ($\sigma = \sqrt{(n)}$, $n = 20$, $\frac{\lambda_d\sqrt{n}}{\sigma} = -11$ to 11, $\alpha_1 = 0.10$ and $\alpha_2 = 0.05$), the corresponding plots of the MSE and coverage probability are given in Figures 3.1 and 3.2, respectively. Compared to Figure 2.9, we see a similar pattern in Figure 3.1; however, the size of the bias of both PAR (constant = 2) and TS have been reduced.

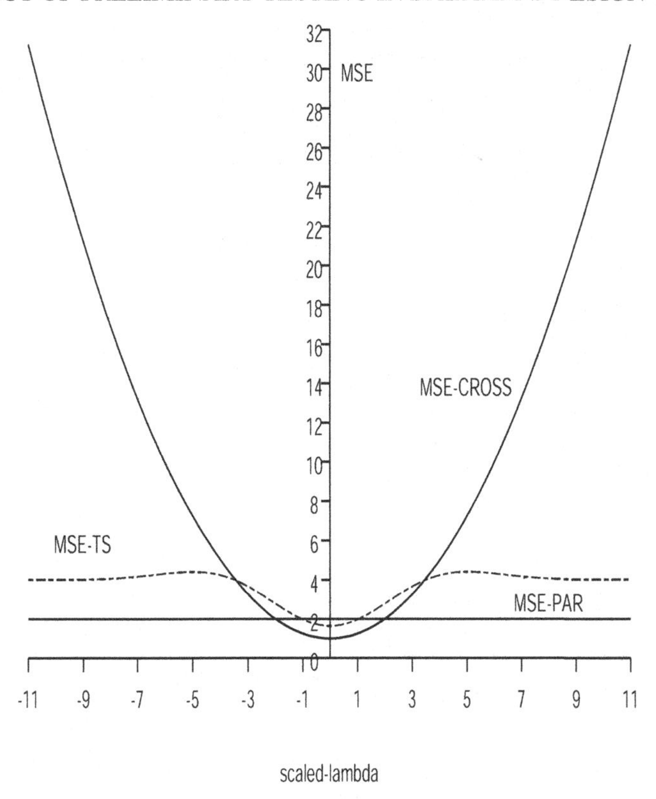

Figure 3.1: Mean squared errors of PAR, CROSS and TS.

Looking now at Figure 3.2, and comparing it to Figure 2.10, we see that as for the MSE, the effects of preliminary testing are less severe in Balaam's design. When $\lambda_d = 0$, the coverage probability is 0.93 (rather than 0.95), i.e., the probability of the Type I error is 0.07 (rather than 0.05). The coverage probability reaches a minimum of 0.78 at $\lambda_d = 3.6$. Therefore, as for the AB/BA design, the preliminary test for a carry-over difference has a detrimental effect on the test for a direct treatment difference.

The power curves for Balaam's design are plotted in Figure 3.3 for $\lambda_d =$ 0, 1 and 5. Unlike the curve for TS in Figure 2.11, the corresponding curve in Figure 3.3 is much more like that for PAR. When $\tau_d = 0$, the power (i.e., significance level) is 0.167, i.e., higher than 0.05. This, of course, is an extreme situation where there is a very large carry-over difference in the absence of a direct treatment difference. When calculated for $\lambda_d = 1$, the significance level is 0.093. It is more likely that a carry-over difference will occur in the presence of a direct treatment difference. If we look at the right panel of Figure 3.3 for values of $\tau_d\sqrt{(n)}/\sigma \geq 2$ (i.e., the carry-over is equal to or smaller than half the

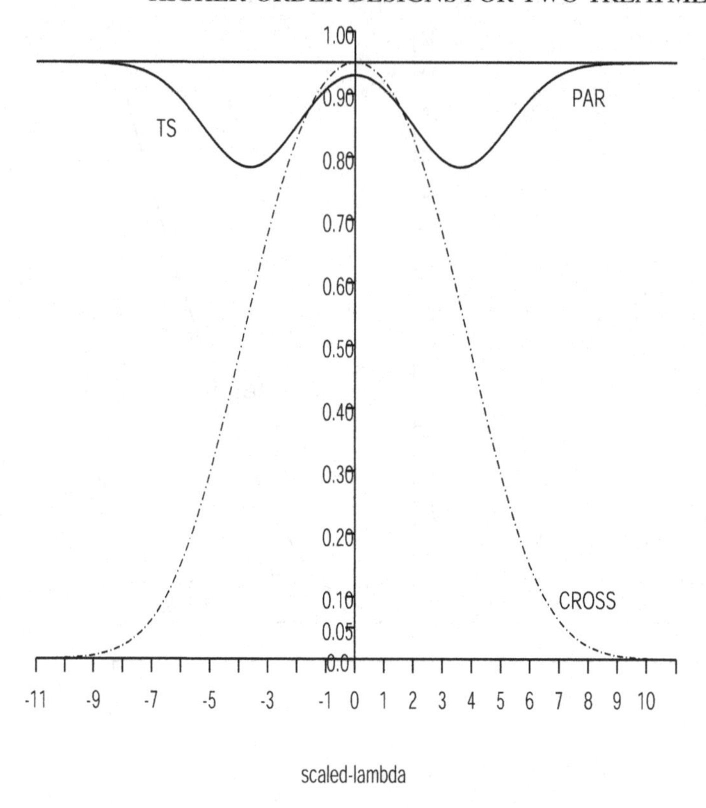

Figure 3.2: Coverage probability.

direct treatment difference), we see that the power curves for TS and CROSS are virtually indistinguishable. The contours of the power values in the (τ_d,λ_d) space are given in Figure 3.4.

In summary, provided the simple carry-over assumption is appropriate, in particular that there is no treatment-by-carry-over interaction, then Balaam's design has the advantage over the AB/BA design of allowing a within-subjects test of a direct treatment difference in the presence of a significant carry-over difference and is therefore useful when differential carry-over effects are anticipated. Although preliminary testing has a detrimental effect on the MSE, coverage probability and power, the consequences are not as severe as for the AB/BA design. Unless a carry-over difference can occur in the absence of a direct treatment difference, the power of the TS method is close to that of the CROSS procedure when the carry-over difference is less than half that of the direct treatment difference. If differential carry-over effects can be ruled out at the planning stage or by the use of suitable wash-out periods, then the AB/BA design is the appropriate two-period design to use.

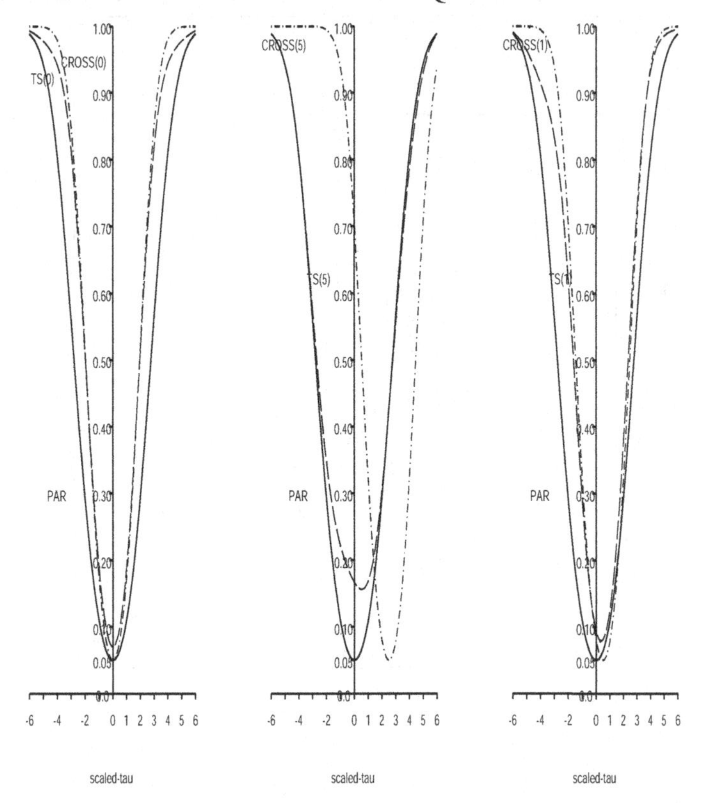

Figure 3.3: Power curves for PAR, CROSS and TS (left panel $\lambda_d = 0$, middle panel $\lambda_d = 5\sigma/\sqrt(n)$, right panel $\lambda_d = \sigma/\sqrt(n)$).

3.5 Three-period designs with two sequences

As noted in Section 3.2, the three-period design that is optimal for estimating $\tau|\lambda$ and $\lambda|\tau$ is the one reproduced in Table 3.7 and now labeled as Design 3.2.1. We introduce the new labeling to aid the comparison of different designs. We label a design using the code $p.s.i$, where p is the number of periods, s is the number of sequence groups and i is an index number to distinguish different designs with the same p and s.

Table 3.7: Design 3.2.1.

Sequence	Period		
	1	2	3
1	A	B	B
2	B	A	A

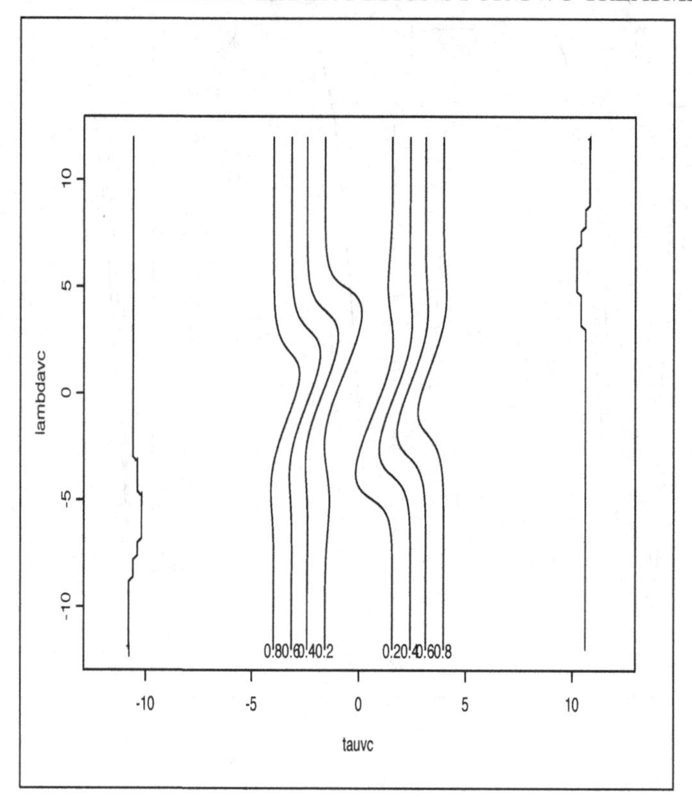

Figure 3.4: Contours of power for TS.

It will be noted that all the optimal designs listed earlier in Section 3.2 are made up of one or more pairs of **dual** sequences. A dual of a sequence is obtained by interchanging the A and B treatment labels. So, for example, the dual of ABB is BAA. From a practical point of view, the only designs worth considering are those which are made up of one or more equally replicated pairs of dual sequences. Designs which have equal replication on each member of a dual pair are called **dual balanced**. Although optimal designs are not necessarily dual balanced, there will always be a dual-balanced optimal design (Matthews (1990)). Also, as will be seen Chapter 5, if a design is made up of a dual pair, then a simple and robust analysis is possible. This simple analysis can also be extended to designs which contain more than one dual pair, as will also be seen in Chapter 5. Therefore, here and in the following, we will only consider designs made up of dual sequences. It will be noted that all the optimal designs listed in Section 3.2 are dual balanced.

Examples of the analysis of higher-order two-treatment designs are given in Chapter 5.

Table 3.8: Design 3.2.2.

Sequence	Period		
	1	2	3
1	A	B	A
2	B	A	B

Table 3.9: Design 3.2.3.

Sequence	Period		
	1	2	3
1	A	A	B
2	B	B	A

The only other three-period designs with two sequences which contain a dual pair are Designs 3.2.2 and 3.2.3, which are given in Tables 3.8 and 3.9, respectively.

Let us now consider the properties of Design 3.2.1 and let $\bar{y}_{ij.}$ denote the mean for period j of group i, where $j = 1,2$ or 3 and $i = 1$ or 2. Within each group there are 2 degrees of freedom associated with the differences between the period means, giving a total of 4 for both groups. Of these, 2 are associated with the period differences, 1 is associated with the direct treatment difference and 1 is associated with the direct-by-period interaction. The carry-over difference is aliased with one component of the direct-by-period interaction and so we can, in our model for the within-subject responses, either include a carry-over parameter or an interaction parameter. For convenience, we will include the carry-over parameter.

The expectations of the six group-by-period means are given in Table 3.10, where the period effects are denoted by π_1, π_2 and π_3 and the constraint $\pi_1 + \pi_2 + \pi_3 = 0$ has been applied. The other parameters are as defined previously. For Design 3.2.1 the OLS estimators of $\hat{\lambda}|\tau$ and $\hat{\tau}|\lambda$ are

$$\hat{\lambda}|\tau = \frac{1}{4}(-\bar{y}_{12.} + \bar{y}_{13.} + \bar{y}_{22.} - \bar{y}_{23.})$$

$$\hat{\tau}|\lambda = \frac{1}{8}(-2\bar{y}_{11.} + \bar{y}_{12.} + \bar{y}_{13.} + 2\bar{y}_{21.} - \bar{y}_{22.} - \bar{y}_{23.})$$

and

$$\hat{\tau} = \hat{\tau}|\lambda$$

where we assume that each group contains n subjects. The variances of these estimators are $\text{Var}[\hat{\lambda}|\tau] = \sigma^2/(4n)$, $V[\hat{\tau}|\lambda] = (3\sigma^2)/(16n)$ and $\text{Cov}[\hat{\tau}|\lambda, \hat{\lambda}|\tau] = 0$.

Table 3.10: The expectations of $\bar{y}_{ij.}$ for Design 3.2.1.

Group	Period		
	1	2	3
1 ABB	$\gamma_1+\pi_1-\tau$	$\gamma_1+\pi_2+\tau-\lambda$	$\gamma_1-\pi_1-\pi_2+\tau+\lambda$
2 BAA	$\gamma_2+\pi_1+\tau$	$\gamma_2+\pi_2-\tau+\lambda$	$\gamma_2-\pi_1-\pi_2-\tau-\lambda$

Table 3.11: The variances and covariances for the three-period designs (in multiples of $\frac{\sigma^2}{n}$).

Design	$\text{Var}[\hat{\lambda}\|\tau]$	$\text{Var}[\hat{\tau}\|\lambda]$	$\text{Cov}[\hat{\tau}\|\lambda,\hat{\lambda}\|\tau]$
3.2.1	0.2500	0.1875	0.0000
3.2.2	1.0000	0.7500	0.7500
3.2.3	1.0000	0.2500	0.2500

For the case of unequal group sizes $n_1 \neq n_2$, the estimators of $\hat{\lambda}|\tau$ and $\hat{\tau}|\lambda$ are the same as given above. The formulae for their variances, however, need to be modified in the obvious way. That is,

$$\text{Var}[\hat{\lambda}|\tau] = \frac{\sigma^2}{8}\left(\frac{1}{n_1}+\frac{1}{n_2}\right) \text{ and } \text{Var}[\hat{\tau}|\lambda] = \frac{3\sigma^2}{32}\left(\frac{1}{n_1}+\frac{1}{n_2}\right).$$

The advantages of using Design 3.2.1 can be appreciated if we compare the variances of the estimators obtained from this design with those obtained from Designs 3.2.2 and 3.2.3. These variances and covariances are given in Table 3.11, in multiples of σ^2/n. It can be seen that the variances are up to four times larger in Design 3.2.2 and 3.2.3. Also, the estimators are not uncorrelated in these designs. It should be noted that Matthews (1990) proved that $\text{Cov}[\hat{\tau}|\lambda,\hat{\lambda}|\tau] = 0$ for any optimal two-treatment design with more than two periods.

In most cross-over trials there will be a run-in baseline measurement on each subject prior to the start of the first treatment period. As with Balaam's design we could either include this baseline in our model or use it as a covariate. If we include the baseline in our model, we find we get the same estimator of $\lambda|\tau$ but a different estimator of $\tau|\lambda$. Although the new estimator of $\tau|\lambda$ makes use of baselines, its variance is only slightly reduced: without baselines the variance is $0.1875\sigma^2/n$ as compared to $0.1818\sigma^2/n$ with baselines. In fact, if there had also been a wash-out period between each of the three treatment periods (and we include pre-period baselines in our model), the conclusions would have been the same. The estimator of $\lambda|\tau$ does not change and the variance of $\hat{\tau}|\lambda$ is only reduced to $0.1765\sigma^2/n$. These variance calculations illustrate a general result proved by Laska et al. (1983) which states that when three or more periods are used, baselines taken before each period are of little or no use for increasing the precision of the estimators. However, the run-in baseline can sometimes be usefully included as a covariate (see Chapter 5).

Unlike Balaam's design, Design 3.2.1 does not provide sufficient degrees of freedom for a direct-by-carry-over interaction to be included in the model. If, however, additional information on the nature of the carry-over effect is available, then our model can be altered to take account of it. For example, if we know that a treatment cannot carry over into itself, and there is no other form of direct-by-period interaction, then our model can be modified so that λ appears only in Period 2. The OLS estimators of the parameters are then

$$\hat{\lambda}|\tau = \frac{1}{2}(-\bar{y}_{12.} + \bar{y}_{13.} + \bar{y}_{22.} - \bar{y}_{23.}) \text{ with } \mathrm{Var}[\hat{\lambda}|\tau] = \frac{\sigma^2}{n}$$

and

$$\hat{\tau}|\lambda = \frac{1}{4}(-\bar{y}_{11.} + \bar{y}_{13.} + \bar{y}_{21.} - \bar{y}_{23.}) \text{ with } \mathrm{Var}[\hat{\tau}|\lambda] = \frac{\sigma^2}{4n}.$$

3.6 Three-period designs with four sequences

Although Design 3.2.1 is optimal in the sense that it minimizes the variances of the OLS estimators of $\lambda|\tau$ and $\tau|\lambda$, it does have certain disadvantages. For example, the estimators of the carry-over effect and the direct-by-period interaction are aliased with one another, and it is not possible to test for a direct-by-carry-over interaction. The use of additional sequences can overcome these disadvantages and so it is useful to consider the properties of designs with more than two groups.

There are three different four-group designs which can be constructed by using different pairings of the dual designs given in Section 3.5. These new designs are labeled as 3.4.1, 3.4.2 and 3.4.3 and are given in Tables 3.12, 3.13 and 3.14, respectively.

There are 11 degrees of freedom between the 12 group-by-period means and following our usual practice we associate 3 of these with the group effects, 2 with the period effects and 6 with the group-by-period interaction. These last 6 are the ones of most interest to us and we would like to associate them with the direct treatment effect, the direct-by-period interaction and the carry-over

Table 3.12: Design 3.4.1.

Sequence	Period		
	1	2	3
1	A	B	B
2	B	A	A
3	A	B	A
4	B	A	B

Table 3.13: Design 3.4.2.

Sequence	Period		
	1	2	3
1	A	B	B
2	B	A	A
3	A	A	B
4	B	B	A

Table 3.14: Design 3.4.3.

Sequence	Period		
	1	2	3
1	A	B	A
2	B	A	B
3	A	A	B
4	B	B	A

effects. However, the 2 degrees of freedom for the direct-by-period interaction are aliased with the degrees of freedom for the first-order carry-over effect and the second-order carry-over effect. The second-order carry-over is the differential treatment effect that lasts for two periods after the treatments are administered. If we choose to include two interaction parameters in our model, then there are 3 degrees of freedom left which are associated with uninteresting group-by-period interaction contrasts. If we include parameters for the two different sorts of carry-over effect, however, then we can associate 1 of the remaining 3 degrees of freedom with the interaction between direct treatments and the first-order carry-over effects. The remaining 2 degrees of freedom are then associated with uninteresting group-by-period interaction contrasts. Whichever parameterization is chosen, the uninteresting degrees of freedom are added to those of the residual SS. Although we choose to include the carry-over parameters, it should be remembered that these parameters are aliased with the direct-by-period interaction parameters and so apparently significant carry-over effects may be caused by the presence of more general interaction effects.

As always we will compare the designs for the special case of $n_1 = n_2 = n_3 = n_4 = n$. General formulae for the case of unequal group sizes can easily be obtained from the results in Appendix A.

In each of Designs 3.4.1, 3.4.2 and 3.4.3 we wish to allocate effects of interest to the 11 degrees of freedom between the group-by-period means. As said earlier, 3 of these are associated with the group effects, 2 are associated with the period effects, 4 are associated with various treatment effects and 2 are associated with the interaction of groups and periods. Let us label the effects associated with these last 6 degrees of freedom as $\tau, \lambda, \theta, (\tau\lambda), (\gamma\pi)_1$ and $(\gamma\pi)_2$, where these refer, respectively, to the direct treatment effect, the first-order carry-over effect, the second-order carry-over effect, the interaction between the direct treatments and the first-order carry-over effects and two particular group-by-period interaction contrasts. These last two contrasts are, of course, not of great interest in themselves and we have included them only in order that the full partition of the 11 degrees of freedom can be seen. It turns out that these two contrasts are orthogonal to each other and to the other effects in the full model.

Let us consider Design 3.4.1 in detail. The OLS estimators of $(\gamma\pi)_1$ and $(\gamma\pi)_2$ are

$$(\hat{\gamma\pi})_1 = \frac{1}{4}(-\bar{y}_{11.} + \bar{y}_{12.} + \bar{y}_{31.} - \bar{y}_{32.})$$

and

$$(\hat{\gamma\pi})_2 = \frac{1}{4}(-\bar{y}_{21.} + \bar{y}_{22.} + \bar{y}_{41.} - \bar{y}_{42.}).$$

It will be convenient to represent estimators using the notation $\mathbf{c}^\top\bar{\mathbf{y}}$ where $\mathbf{c}$ is a vector of contrast coefficients and $\bar{\mathbf{y}} = (\bar{y}_{11.}, \bar{y}_{12.}, \ldots, \bar{y}_{43.})^\top$. So, for example,

$$(\hat{\gamma\pi})_1 = \frac{1}{4}[-1,1,0,0,0,0,1,-1,0,0,0,0]^\top\bar{\mathbf{y}}$$

and

$$(\hat{\gamma\pi})_2 = \frac{1}{4}[0,0,0,-1,1,0,0,0,0,1,-1,0]^\top\bar{\mathbf{y}}.$$

We now consider the remaining effects τ, λ, θ and $(\tau\lambda)$. Whether or not all of these effects need to be included will depend on the particular trial and on the amount of prior knowledge that exists about the nature of the treatment effects. However, for the sake of completeness, we will consider models containing all of the effects τ, λ, θ and $(\tau\lambda)$.

When testing for these effects, we begin with $(\tau\lambda)$. If this effect is significant, it means that there is evidence of an interaction between the direct treatment and first-order carry-over effects. In the presence of such an interaction it would not be sensible to continue and test for a second-order carry-over effect.

When testing for significant effects, we consider them in the order $(\tau\lambda), \theta, \lambda$ and τ. We assume that the model under consideration always contains parameters for the groups and periods.

In the presence of θ, λ and τ the OLS estimator of $(\tau\lambda)$ is

$$(\hat{\tau\lambda})|\theta, \lambda, \tau = \frac{1}{8}[-1,-1,2,-1,-1,2,1,1,-2,1,1,-2]^\top\bar{\mathbf{y}}$$

with

$$\text{Var}[(\hat{\tau\lambda})|\theta, \lambda, \tau] = \frac{3\sigma^2}{8n}.$$

If $(\tau\lambda)$ cannot be dropped from the model, then we would not test any of the remaining effects. To test τ and λ would break marginality rules and to test θ would not be sensible in the presence of rather unusual first-order carry-over effects.

If $(\tau\lambda)$ can be dropped from the model, then

$$\hat{\theta}|\lambda,\tau = \frac{1}{8}[1,-5,4,-1,5,-4,7,1,-8,-7,-1,8]^{\mathsf{T}}\bar{\mathbf{y}}$$

with

$$\text{Var}[\hat{\theta}|\lambda,\tau] = \frac{39\sigma^2}{8n}.$$

If θ cannot be dropped from the model, then we would presumably be interested in estimating $\tau|\theta,\lambda$. The estimator is

$$\hat{\tau}|\theta,\lambda = \frac{1}{8}[-1,-1,2,1,1,-2,1,1,-2,-1,-1,2]^{\mathsf{T}}\bar{\mathbf{y}}$$

with

$$\text{Var}[\hat{\tau}|\theta,\lambda] = \frac{3\sigma^2}{8n}.$$

If θ can be dropped from the model, then

$$\hat{\lambda}|\tau = \frac{1}{26}[-2,-3,5,2,3,-5,-1,-2,3,1,2,-3]^{\mathsf{T}}\bar{\mathbf{y}}$$

with

$$\text{Var}[\hat{\lambda}|\tau] = \frac{2\sigma^2}{13n}$$

and

$$\hat{\tau}|\lambda = \frac{1}{52}[-8,1,7,8,-1,-7,-4,5,-1,4,-5,1]^{\mathsf{T}}\bar{\mathbf{y}}$$

with

$$\text{Var}[\hat{\tau}|\lambda] = \frac{3\sigma^2}{26n}.$$

Also

$$\text{Cov}[\hat{\tau}|\lambda,\hat{\lambda}|\tau] = \frac{3\sigma^2}{52n}.$$

If λ can be dropped from the model, then

$$\hat{\tau} = \frac{1}{16}[-2,1,1,2,-1,-1,-1,2,-1,1,-2,1]^{\mathsf{T}}\bar{\mathbf{y}}$$

with

$$\text{Var}[\hat{\tau}] = \frac{3\sigma^2}{32n}.$$

Table 3.15: Variances of the estimators (in multiples of $\frac{\sigma^2}{n}$).

Effect	Design 3.4.1	Design 3.4.2	Design 3.4.3
$(\tau\lambda)\|\theta,\lambda,\tau$	0.3750	0.1250	0.3750
$\theta\|\lambda,\tau$	4.8750	1.9375	1.0000
$\tau\|\theta,\lambda$	0.3750	0.4375	0.4375
$\lambda\|\tau$	0.1538	0.1935	0.3750
$\tau\|\lambda$	0.1154	0.0968	0.1875
τ	0.0938	0.0938	0.0938

A similar derivation can be given for Designs 3.4.2 and 3.4.3.

Of most interest to potential users of these three designs is how they differ in terms of the precision with which they estimate the various effects. Therefore, in Table 3.15 we give the variances of the estimators obtained from each design.

Clearly, no single design is optimal for all effects. As all three designs are equally good at estimating τ in the absence of the other parameters, we might choose to use Design 3.4.2, as it has the smallest variance of $\hat{\tau}|\lambda$. However, as Design 3.4.1 is better at estimating $\lambda|\tau$, the choice is not clear cut. Our opinion is that in most situations it is not possible from statistical considerations alone to choose the optimal design. Depending on the circumstances, the choice of the design to use will depend on the effects of most interest, the amount of prior knowledge and the practicalities of conducting the trial. We will say more on the choice of an optimal three-period design in Section 3.8.

Chapter 5 has an example of the analysis of a three-period design with four sequences.

3.7 A three-period six-sequence design

If we join together Designs 3.2.1, 3.2.2 and 3.2.3, we obtain the design in Table 3.16, which we label as Design 3.6.1.

Table 3.16: Design 3.6.1.

Sequence	Period		
	1	2	3
1	A	B	B
2	B	A	A
3	A	B	A
4	B	A	B
5	A	A	B
6	B	B	A

The advantage of this design is that it provides unaliased estimators of the carry-over and the direct-by-period interaction effects. However, the design is less attractive from a practical point of view because it requires the management of six different groups of subjects.

We will not give the details of the contrasts which can be estimated using Design 3.6.1; the variances of the effects of interest will be given in the next section.

3.8 Which three-period design to use?

Here we compare the three-period designs described in the previous sections with a view to deciding which one to use. Let us suppose that N subjects are available and that they can be equally divided among two, four or six sequence groups. That is, the size of each group is $N/2$ if one of Designs 3.2.1, 3.2.2 or 3.2.3 is used, the size is $N/4$ if one of Designs 3.4.1, 3.4.2 or 3.4.3 is used and the size is $N/6$ if Design 3.6.1 is used. The variances of the various effects which can be estimated in each design are given in Tables 3.17 and 3.18.

If one is interested in estimating all the effects, then clearly Design 3.6.1 is the one to choose. If $(\tau\lambda)$ is of particular interest, then Design 3.4.2 is the one to choose. The best design for estimating θ is 3.4.3. However, in most trials θ and $(\tau\lambda)$ are unlikely to be significantly large and so we would choose our design on its ability to estimate $\lambda|\tau$ and $\tau|\lambda$. The design which estimates these effects most efficiently is Design 3.2.1.

However, as Ebbutt (1984) pointed out, Design 3.4.1 might be preferred because it is harder for the subjects and the clinician to break the randomization code. Subjects in Design 3.2.1 always receive the same treatments in the last two periods and this feature might bias the clinician's assessment of the subject's response. Also, Design 3.4.1 does permit additional effects to be tested should they become of interest when the trial is completed. If the trial has to be stopped at the end of the second period, then both designs revert to

Table 3.17: Variances of the estimators (in multiples of σ^2/N).

Effect	τ	$\tau\|\lambda$	$\lambda\|\tau$	$(\tau\lambda)\|\tau,\lambda,\theta$
Design 3.2.1	0.375	0.375	0.500	-
Design 3.2.2	0.375	1.500	2.000	-
Design 3.2.3	0.375	0.500	2.000	-
Design 3.4.1	0.375	0.462	0.616	1.500
Design 3.4.2	0.375	0.387	0.774	0.600
Design 3.4.3	0.375	0.750	1.500	1.500
Design 3.6.1	0.375	0.463	0.794	0.675

Table 3.18: Variances of the estimators (in multiples of σ^2/N).

Effect	$\theta\|\tau,\lambda$	$\tau\|\lambda,\theta$	$(\tau\pi)_1$	$(\tau\pi)_2$
Design 3.2.1	-	-	-	-
Design 3.2.2	-	-	-	-
Design 3.2.3	-	-	-	-
Design 3.4.1	19.500	1.500	-	-
Design 3.4.2	7.750	1.750	-	-
Design 3.4.3	4.000	1.750	-	-
Design 3.6.1	5.017	1.088	1.750	1.813

being the standard 2×2 trial. Finally, a point in favor of Design 3.4.2 is that if the trial is stopped after the second period, we are left with Balaam's design, which permits a within-subjects estimate of λ to be obtained.

Of course, any remarks we make concerning the choice of design to use must depend on the assumptions we make about the parameters in the model. If we change the assumptions, then it is quite likely that the "optimal" design will change too. Fleiss (1986), it will be recalled, questioned whether it was sensible to always assume that the carry-over of treatment A into treatment B, for example, is the same as the carry-over of treatment A into itself. As a special case of this we consider the model in which we set to zero the carry-over of a treatment into itself. The variances of the estimators $\hat{\tau}|\lambda$ and $\hat{\lambda}|\tau$ are then as given in Table 3.19. (The full model used contains terms for the subjects, periods, direct treatments and carry-overs.) We see that, although Design 3.2.1 is still optimal, the best four-sequence design is now Design 3.4.1 as opposed

Table 3.19: Variances of the estimators (in multiples of σ^2/N) assuming that a treatment cannot carry over into itself.

Effect	$\tau\|\lambda$	$\lambda\|\tau$
Design 3.2.1	0.500	2.000
Design 3.2.2	1.500	2.000
Design 3.2.3	0.375	-
Design 3.4.1	0.750	1.500
Design 3.4.2	0.857	3.428
Design 3.4.3	1.714	3.428
Design 3.6.1	0.938	2.250

to the earlier choices of Design 3.4.2 (for direct effects) and Design 3.4.1 (for carry-over effects). Also, in Design 3.2.3, $\lambda|\tau$ is no longer estimable.

More generally, we note that under the extra assumption, the variances of the effects are larger than they were previously (with the exception of Design 3.2.2). This would have implications when deciding on the ideal size of the trial.

3.9 Four-period designs with two sequences

Trials which include four treatment periods are, by their very nature, likely to be more expensive to conduct than their two- and three-period alternatives. Also, the longer a trial lasts the greater will be the chance of subjects dropping out for reasons unconnected with the treatments. Therefore, if a four-period trial is to be used, it must offer substantial improvements over trials with fewer periods.

It will be recalled that the main reason for using three periods is to obtain a within-subjects estimator of the carry-over effect, λ. However, in order to obtain an estimator which is not aliased with the direct-by-period interaction, a design with six sequences is needed. If it is thought that the monitoring and organization of six different groups of subjects will be difficult, then a four-period design might be attractive if it uses fewer than six sequences. If, on the other hand, a direct-by-period interaction is thought unlikely to occur, then a four-period design will be attractive if it provides estimators of τ and λ (and perhaps $(\tau\lambda)$ and θ), which have substantially smaller variances than could be achieved by using three periods.

As in the previous sections, we only consider designs made up of dual sequences. We will consider, in turn, the properties of the designs with two, four and six sequences and then return to consider the remarks made above.

Although the optimal design for estimating $\lambda|\tau$ and $\tau|\lambda$ is the four-group Design 3.3 given in Section 3.2, we first consider the properties of the various two-group dual designs. This is because these designs have the attractive and important property of permitting a simple and robust analysis, as illustrated in Section 5.8.2.1 for a three-period design. We will also consider using more than four groups in order to see what practical advantages this might have over the optimal four-group design.

If we discard the sequences AAAA and BBBB, then there are seven different two-sequence designs and they are given in Tables 3.20 to 3.26.

In each of these designs there are 6 degrees of freedom within-subjects and 3 of these are associated with the period effects and 3 are associated with τ, λ and θ. In Designs 4.2.1 and 4.2.4, θ is not estimable and in the remaining designs λ and θ are aliased with the direct-by-period interaction. The variances associated with each of the seven designs are given in Table 3.27, where we assume that there are n subjects in each group. Of these designs the one

Table 3.20: Design 4.2.1.

Sequence	Period			
	1	2	3	4
1	A	A	B	B
2	B	B	A	A

Table 3.21: Design 4.2.2.

Sequence	Period			
	1	2	3	4
1	A	B	A	B
2	B	A	B	A

which provides minimum variance estimators of τ and $\tau|\lambda$ is Design 4.2.3. The design which is best for estimating $\theta|\tau,\lambda$ is Design 4.2.6.

If for some reason θ was of prime interest, Design 4.2.6 would be the one to use. It should also be noted that although Design 4.2.1 provides estimators of τ and λ which have variances equal to those of Design 4.2.3, θ is not estimable in Design 4.2.1.

3.10 Four-period designs with four sequences

By taking the seven two-sequence designs in pairs we obtain 21 different four-group designs. Each of these provides 12 degrees of freedom within-subjects and we can associate 3 of these with the period effects, 4 with τ, λ, θ and $(\tau\lambda)$, respectively, and 3 with the direct-by-period interaction effects, which we label as $(\tau\pi)_1$, $(\tau\pi)_2$ and $(\tau\pi)_3$, respectively. The remaining 2 degrees of freedom are associated with uninteresting group-by-period contrasts.

Table 3.22: Design 4.2.3.

Sequence	Period			
	1	2	3	4
1	A	B	B	A
2	B	A	A	B

Table 3.23: Design 4.2.4.

Sequence	Period			
	1	2	3	4
1	A	B	A	A
2	B	A	B	B

Table 3.24: Design 4.2.5.

Sequence	Period			
	1	2	3	4
1	A	A	B	A
2	B	B	A	B

Table 3.25: Design 4.2.6.

Sequence	Period			
	1	2	3	4
1	A	B	B	B
2	B	A	A	A

Table 3.26: Design 4.2.7.

Sequence	Period			
	1	2	3	4
1	A	A	A	B
2	B	B	B	A

We label the four-group design obtained by joining together Designs 4.2.a and 4.2.b as Design 4.4.ab for given a and b. Only 7 of the 21 designs provide unaliased estimators of τ, λ, θ, $(\tau\lambda)$, $(\tau\pi)_1$, $(\tau\pi)_2$ and $(\tau\pi)_3$, and these are Designs 4.4.14, 4.4.16, 4.4.25, 4.4.27, 4.4.35, 4.4.37 and 4.4.67. Assuming that n subjects are in each group, the design which provides minimum variance estimators of τ, $\tau|\lambda$ and $\lambda|\tau$ is Design 4.4.13, given in Table 3.28, and is seen to be Design 3.3 as given in Section 3.2. That is, it is the optimal design for four periods. (Consequently, $\text{Cov}[\hat{\tau}|\lambda, \hat{\lambda}|\tau] = 0$.)

However, as is often the case, if other effects are of prime importance, then Design 4.4.13 is not necessarily the one to choose. The design which minimizes the sum of the variances of the estimators of $(\tau\pi)_1$, $(\tau\pi)_2$ and $(\tau\pi)_3$ is Design 4.4.67. However, if $(\tau\lambda)|\tau,\lambda,\theta$ is of prime interest, then Design 4.4.13 is again optimal. If $\theta|\tau,\lambda$ is of prime interest, then we would choose Design 4.4.36. The variances of the estimators obtained from Designs 4.4.13, 4.4.36 and 4.4.67 are given in Tables 3.29 and 3.30.

In practice, of course, trials are planned to minimize the chances of treatment carry-over and direct-by-period interaction. Under these conditions Design 4.4.13 is clearly the one to use. Not only does it provide the most precise estimators of τ and λ but it also provides unaliased estimators of nearly all the other effects. If for some reason the fourth period had to be abandoned, then Design 4.4.13 reduces to the three-period Design 3.4.2, which provides

Table 3.27: Variances (in multiples of σ^2/N) of effects obtained from Designs 4.2.1–4.2.7.

Effect	τ	$\tau\|\lambda$	$\lambda\|\tau$	$\theta\|\tau,\lambda$	$\tau\|\lambda,\theta$
Design 4.2.1	0.1250	0.1375	0.2000	-	0.1375
Design 4.2.2	0.1250	0.6875	1.0000	1.0000	0.7500
Design 4.2.3	0.1250	0.1375	0.2000	0.5556	0.3056
Design 4.2.4	0.1667	0.2292	0.2500	-	0.2292
Design 4.2.5	0.1667	0.2292	0.2500	3.0000	1.2500
Design 4.2.6	0.1667	0.1719	0.1875	0.2500	0.1719
Design 4.2.7	0.1667	0.1875	0.7500	1.0000	0.2500

Table 3.28: Design 4.4.13.

Sequence	Period			
	1	2	3	4
1	A	A	B	B
2	B	B	A	A
3	A	B	B	A
4	B	A	A	B

the minimum variance estimator of $\tau|\lambda$. If the third and fourth periods are lost, then Design 4.4.13 reduces to Balaam's design.

3.11 Four-period designs with six sequences

By choosing all possible triples of the seven two-group designs listed in Section 3.9, we can obtain 35 different six-group designs. We will not list them all here but will refer to a particular design by using the label 4.6.abc, which

Table 3.29: Variances of the estimators (in multiples of σ^2/n).

Effect	τ	$\tau\|\lambda$	$\lambda\|\tau$	$\theta\|\tau,\lambda$	$\tau\|\lambda,\theta$
Design 4.4.13	0.0625	0.0625	0.0909	0.5238	0.1935
Design 4.4.36	0.0714	0.0719	0.0915	0.1460	0.0840
Design 4.4.67	0.0833	0.0833	0.1429	0.1810	0.0884

Table 3.30: Variances of the estimators (in multiples of σ^2/n).

Effect	$(\tau\lambda)\|\tau,\lambda,\theta$	$(\tau\pi)_1$	$(\tau\pi)_2$	$(\tau\pi)_3$
Design 4.4.13	0.0909	0.2500	0.5250	-
Design 4.4.36	0.3333	0.1804	-	-
Design 4.4.67	0.1250	0.4219	0.2969	0.2969

Table 3.31: Design 4.6.136.

Sequence	Period			
	1	2	3	4
1	A	A	B	B
2	B	B	A	A
3	A	B	B	A
4	B	A	A	B
5	A	B	B	B
6	B	A	A	A

Table 3.32: Design 4.6.146.

Sequence	Period			
	1	2	3	4
1	A	A	B	B
2	B	B	A	A
3	A	B	A	A
4	B	A	B	B
5	A	B	B	B
6	B	A	A	A

indicates that the design has been formed by joining together Designs 4.2.a, 4.2.b and 4.2.c. As usual we assume that there are n subjects in each group.

If our model includes only terms for the groups, periods, treatments and carry-over, then the design which provides the minimum variance estimator of $\tau|\lambda$ is Design 4.6.136. The designs which provide minimum variance estimators of $\lambda|\tau$ are 4.6.146 and 4.6.156. Designs 4.6.136 and 4.6.146 are listed in Tables 3.31 and 3.32.

A number of other designs provide values of $\text{Var}[\hat{\tau}|\lambda]$ which are not much larger than that of Design 4.6.136. The index numbers of these designs are 123, 137, 134, 135, 146 and 156.

The variances of the estimated effects obtained from Designs 4.6.136 and 4.6.146 are given in Tables 3.33 and 3.34. Overall, the two designs are very

Table 3.33: Variances (in multiples of σ^2/n) of effects obtained from Designs 4.6.136 and 4.6.146.

Effect	τ	$\tau\|\lambda$	$\lambda\|\tau$	$\tau\|\lambda,\theta$	$\theta\|\tau,\lambda$
Design 4.4.136	0.0455	0.0456	0.0608	0.0641	0.1415
Design 4.4.146	0.0500	0.0500	0.0606	0.0552	0.1301

Table 3.34: Variances (in multiples of σ^2/n) of effects obtained from Designs 4.6.136 and 4.6.146.

Effect	$(\tau\lambda)\|\tau,\lambda,\theta$	$(\tau\pi)_1$	$(\tau\pi)_2$	$(\tau\pi)_3$
Design 4.4.136	0.0682	0.4255	0.2420	0.4368
Design 4.4.146	0.1071	0.2269	0.3237	0.1786

Table 3.35: The variances of the estimators (in multiples of σ^2/N).

Effect	τ	$\tau\|\lambda$	$\lambda\|\tau$	$\theta\|\tau,\lambda$	$\tau\|\lambda,\theta$
Design 4.2.3	0.2500	0.2750	0.4000	-	0.6112
Design 4.2.6	0.3334	0.3438	0.3750	-	0.3438
Design 4.4.13	0.2500	0.2500	0.3636	0.3636	0.7740
Design 4.4.36	0.2856	0.2876	0.3600	1.3333	0.3360
Design 4.4.67	0.3332	0.3332	0.5716	0.5000	0.3536
Design 4.6.136	0.2730	0.2736	0.3648	0.4092	0.3846
Design 4.6.146	0.3000	0.3000	0.3636	0.6426	0.3312

similar in terms of these variances, with no design having the minimum variance for all effects. Overall, Design 4.6.136 is the one we recommend, unless the direct-by-period interactions are of prime interest. Design 4.6.146 provides estimators of the interactions which have a smaller total variance, although even in this design the precision of estimation is quite low.

We compare the two-, four- and six-group designs in the next section.

3.12 Which four-period design to use?

Here we compare the four-period designs described in the previous sections with a view to deciding which one to use. As done in Section 3.8, we suppose that N subjects are available and that they can be equally divided among two, four or six sequence groups. That is, the size of each group is $N/2$ if one of Designs 4.2.3, 4.2.6 is used, the size is $N/4$ if one of Designs 4.4.13, 4.4.36 or 4.4.67 is used and the size is $N/6$ if Design 4.6.136 or Design 4.6.146 is used. The variances of the various effects which can be estimated in each design are given in Tables 3.35 and 3.36.

If the only effects of interest are τ and λ, then clearly Design 4.4.13 is the one to choose. This design is, of course, optimal in the sense considered in Section 3.2. However, this design is not as good at estimating $(\tau\lambda)$ or θ, for example, as Design 4.4.67. If all effects are of interest, including the direct-by-period interactions, then Design 4.4.67 is a good overall design to use. Also, it is clear from Tables 3.35 and 3.36 that there is no real advantage to be gained

Table 3.36: The variances of the estimators (in multiples of σ^2/N).

Effect	$\theta\|\lambda,\tau$	$(\tau\lambda)\|\tau,\lambda,\theta$	$(\tau\pi)_1$	$(\tau\pi)_2$	$(\tau\pi)_3$
Design 4.2.3	1.1112	-	-	-	-
Design 4.2.6	0.5000	-	-	-	-
Design 4.4.13	2.0952	0.3636	1.0000	2.1000	-
Design 4.4.36	0.5840	1.3333	0.7216	-	-
Design 4.4.67	0.7240	0.5000	1.6876	1.1876	1.1876
Design 4.6.136	0.8490	0.4092	2.5530	1.4520	2.6208
Design 4.6.146	0.7806	0.6426	1.3614	1.9422	1.0716

from using six sequence groups. If only two groups can be used, then Design 4.2.3 should be used, unless θ is of particular interest, when Design 4.2.6 should be used. Design 4.2.3, it will be noted, provides similar variances to the "optimal" Design 4.4.13. Also, it will be recalled that two-group designs consisting of a dual pair permit a simple and robust analysis. This makes Designs 4.2.3 and 4.2.6 quite attractive if we suspect a nonparametric analysis might be needed.

As already noted in Section 3.8, we must not forget that the final choice of design will depend on the assumptions we make about the parameters in the model. So, for example, if we only retain terms in the model for subjects, periods, direct and carry-over effects and set to zero the carry-over of a treatment into itself, as done in Section 3.8, we find that:

1. Design 4.4.13 is no longer optimal; Design 4.4.16 is now optimal for direct effects and Design 4.4.36 is optimal for carry-over effects.
2. Of the two-group designs, Designs 4.2.1 and 4.2.6 are optimal for direct effects and Design 4.2.3 is optimal for carry-over effects.

3.13 Which two-treatment design to use?

When comparing the designs we will assume that N subjects can be made available for the trial. How large N needs to be will depend on (1) how efficient our chosen design is at estimating the effects of interest and (2) the anticipated size of the within-subject variance σ^2. One design, D1 say, is more efficient at estimating an effect than another design, D2 say, if the variance of the estimated effect is smaller in design D1. Often a reasonable estimate of σ^2 can be made by using results from earlier trials on the treatments or from trials involving similar treatments.

The choice between the designs described in this chapter is complicated slightly because we are comparing designs of different sizes: Balaam's design requires $2N$ measurements to be taken (two for each subject), whereas the designs which use three or four periods require $3N$ and $4N$ measurements, respectively. Therefore, in practice we need to weigh the possible increase in precision obtained from using an extra period against the expense of taking additional measurements on each subject.

Let us assume that the maximum value of N has been decided upon from practical considerations. The next things to be decided are the maximum number of periods and sequences that can be used. The maximum number of periods will depend on the nature of the trial. If the treatments to be compared require a long time before their effect can assessed, then the total time for the trial may be too long if more than two or three periods are used. In other trials the treatment effects can be assessed quite quickly and so there is more freedom to use up to four periods. Generally, we can increase the precision with which we estimate the direct treatment and carry-over effects by using more periods. However, this "replication in time" may not be as cost effective as using additional subjects. The choice, if we have any, between using more periods or subjects, will depend, among other things, on the relative costs of recruiting subjects and the costs of taking repeated measurements on the subjects. If repeat measurements are costly, then we would be inclined to use more subjects and fewer periods. However, if the major cost is one of recruitment, then we would want to keep each subject for as many periods as is practical and ethical. However, we should always bear in mind that the longer a trial lasts the greater the chance that subjects will drop out. We have not mentioned wash-out periods, as they do not help increase the precision of estimation when three or more periods are used. If they are thought to be necessary, to "rest" the subjects between treatments, for example, then this needs to be taken into account when calculating the total time of the trial.

The choice of the number of sequences will depend on the effects we wish to estimate or test for. If we are sure that there is no possibility of direct-by-period or second-order carry-over, then fewer sequences will be needed than would otherwise be the case. More sequences may also be thought desirable as a means of disguising as much as possible the randomization code used to allocate subjects to sequences. Clearly, the choice of design involves many different and sometimes conflicting decisions. In the following we will base our comparison of the designs on the precision with which they estimate the effects of interest.

We remind the reader at this point that most of the optimal design results that have been calculated in this setting rest on the assumption that there is no treatment-by-carry-over interaction. If this is not an appropriate assumption, for example, if it were not expected that a carry-over would occur from a treatment into itself, then the relative worth of a design needs to be re-considered. We emphasize again that the efficiency of a design can depend critically on the model assumed for the analysis. If alternative carry-over models were thought to be more relevant in any particular setting, then the efficiencies of designs can be re-calculated in a straightforward way using the tools introduced earlier in this chapter, and the conclusions summarized below can then be modified accordingly.

If only two periods can be used, then we have no choice but to use Balaam's design, described in Section 3.3. Compared to the designs with three periods, however, the precision of this design is quite low: using an extra period, for example, reduces the variance of $\hat{\lambda}|\tau$ from $4\sigma^2/N$ to $0.5\sigma^2/N$ if Design 3.2.1 is used.

Let us now consider the choice between the three- and four-period designs. If we wish to estimate all the effects, including the direct-by-period interactions, then only Designs 3.6.1 and 4.4.67 need to be considered. The extra precision obtained by using Design 4.4.67 makes it the natural choice if four periods can be used. The increased precision is not great, however, except for θ. If subjects are cheap to recruit, it might be better to increase the number of subjects and use Design 3.6.1. Of course, comparisons involving the six-sequence designs are rather academic, as we would not seriously plan to conduct a cross-over trial if large carry-over or interaction effects were anticipated.

If treatment-by-period interactions are not anticipated but we still need to retain a check on θ and $\tau\lambda$, then the choice of design is between 3.4.2 and 4.4.67. The logical choice here is Design 4.4.67 unless using four periods poses a problem. However, as will be seen below, Design 4.4.67 is not a good overall choice.

If τ and λ are the only anticipated effects (as is usually the case), then our choice is between 3.2.1 and 4.4.13. Excluding cost considerations, the natural choice here is 4.4.13, as using the extra period produces a large increase in precision and permits additional effects to be estimated.

One other consideration that might be important is the consequences of the trial having to be stopped before all the periods have been completed.

Let us consider the four-period designs. If only the first three periods of Design 4.4.67 are used, then the third and fourth sequences become AAA and BBB, respectively. As such sequences provide no within-subject comparisons of the treatments, we have lost the advantages of using the cross-over principle. If only the first two periods of Design 4.4.67 are used, then the design becomes Balaam's design.

If Design 4.4.13 is used, however, then its first three periods make up Design 3.4.2, which provides good estimators of $\tau|\lambda$ and $\lambda|\tau$. The first two periods of Design 4.4.13 also make up Balaam's design. Therefore, we would prefer Design 4.4.13 over Design 4.4.67 if the possibility of the trial ending prematurely was a serious consideration.

Of the three-period designs, Design 3.2.1 is the natural choice.

If we had to pick a single design to recommend, then we would choose Design 4.4.13. However, if it was important to use only two groups, in order to use the robust analysis, for example, then Design 3.2.1 would be a good choice. Its four-period competitor is Design 4.2.3, which provides a more precise estimate of $\tau|\lambda$. However, compared to an increase of 33% in the number of measurements entailed in adding the fourth period, the increase in precision is probably not cost effective. If Design 4.2.3 is used, however, it is worth noting that its first three periods make up Design 3.2.1. In other words, if we did change our mind about using four periods, then stopping early would not be a problem.

As stated at the beginning of this chapter, examples of analyses of some of the designs described in this chapter are given in Chapter 5.

Chapter 4

Designing cross-over trials for three or more treatments

4.1 Introduction

The aims of this chapter are

1. to review the large number of designs which have been proposed in the literature,
2. to compare them with a view to recommending which ones should be used and
3. to illustrate the use of a computer algorithm to construct designs.

The majority of the literature on cross-over designs assumes a very simple model for the direct and carry-over effects and that is the model we used in the previous chapters. In this model there is a unique carry-over effect for each treatment and that carry-over effect does not depend on the following treatment, if there is one, or on the magnitude or nature of the treatment which produces it. Let us label the t treatments as A, B, C, ..., and the corresponding direct effects as $\tau_1, \tau_2, \tau_3, \ldots, \tau_t$. In this simple model the corresponding carry-over effects are denoted by $\lambda_1, \lambda_2, \lambda_3, \ldots, \lambda_t$. So, for example, if a subject received the treatment sequence BAC, the simple model for the direct and carry-over effects in these three periods would be τ_2, $\tau_1 + \lambda_2$ and $\tau_3 + \lambda_1$, respectively.

In recent times this simple model for the carry-over effects has been questioned (see, for example, Senn (1993, 2002), Chapter 10) and methods of constructing designs for alternative models have been suggested (see, for example, Jones and Donev (1996)). The more useful methods involve some form of computer search for the best design. Some alternative models that have been suggested by Jones and Donev (1996) include the situations where (1) there is no carry-over effect from a placebo treatment, (2) there is no carry-over effect if the treatment is followed by itself and (3) the carry-over effect produced by a treatment depends on the treatment applied in the following period. These are all specific forms of a direct treatment-by-carry-over interaction.

In Sections 4.2 to 4.7 we review and illustrate the main methods of constructing designs for the simple carry-over effects model. In Section 4.8 we look at extensions of the simple model for carry-over effects and in Section

4.9 we review some methods for the construction of designs using computer search algorithms and illustrate the use of one algorithm that has been written to accompany this book.

Compared with trials for two treatments, the most fundamental difference that arises when trials for three or more treatments are planned is that we must decide which contrasts are to be estimated with the highest precision.

Quite often we will want to plan the trial so that all simple differences between the treatments are estimated with the same precision. A design which provides this feature is said to possess **variance balance**, that is $\text{Var}[\hat{\tau}_i - \hat{\tau}_j] = v\sigma^2$, where v is constant for all $i \neq j$. As we shall see, variance-balanced designs cannot be constructed for all values of n and p, where n is the number of subjects and p is the number of periods. As a compromise we may consider using a design which has **partial balance**.

In a partially balanced design the value of $\text{Var}[\hat{\tau}_i - \hat{\tau}_j]$ depends on which treatments are being compared. If the design has two associate classes, then there are only two different variances depending on the choice of i and j. If the two variances are not much different, then the design has similar properties to one that is variance balanced.

A further possibility when no variance-balanced design exists is to use a **cyclic** design. Although these designs can have up to $[t/2]$ different contrast variances, where $[t/2]$ is the greatest integer less than or equal to $t/2$, some have the attractive property that these variances are not very different.

If one of the treatments, A say, is a control or standard treatment, the aim of the trial might be to compare each of B, C, D, etc., with A, the comparisons between B, C, D, etc., being of less interest. In this situation we would want to ensure that the contrasts which involve A are estimated with the highest achievable precision, possibly at the expense of estimating the other contrasts with low precision.

If the treatments are increasing doses of the same drug and we wish to discover the dose that gives the highest response, then we would want to estimate the linear, quadratic, cubic, etc., components of the response function. These components can be expressed as contrasts and we would want the components of most interest to be estimated most precisely. For example, the linear and quadratic components would be of most interest if we were estimating the maximum response, with the higher-order components being of interest only to check on the adequacy of the fitted model.

In another situation we might have four treatments, for example, made up of the four combinations of two different drugs (A and B), each present at a low and a high level (labeled as 1 and 2). The four treatments could then be more appropriately labeled as AB_{11}, AB_{12}, AB_{21} and AB_{22}, where AB_{11} indicates that the treatment is made up of the low level of A and the low level of B and AB_{21} indicates that the treatment is made up of the high level of A and the low level of B, etc. In this 2×2 factorial structure the contrasts of interest are the interaction and main effects. That is, we would want to discover if the effect of changing A (or B) from its low to its high level depends on the level of B (or A). If it does not, then we would want to estimate the average effect of changing A (or B). If the effects of the two drugs are well known when used separately, then the purpose of the trial might be to obtain a precise estimate of the interaction, the main effects being of little interest. Cyclic designs, among others, can also be useful for this situation.

The points made above, concerning the choice of contrasts, should have made it clear that we cannot choose among the large number of available designs until the purposes of the trial have been carefully decided. In order to choose the most appropriate design, we need at least to know the following:

1. the contrasts of interest and their relative importance,
2. the maximum number of periods that can be used and
3. the maximum number of subjects that could be made available for the trial.

Having found a design which meets these requirements, we can then check that, based on a prior estimate of the within-subject variance, the design is likely to be large enough to detect differences between the treatments of the size we think is important.

The chapter is organized as follows. In Section 4.2 we consider designs that are variance balanced. This section includes consideration of designs with $p = t$, $p < t$ and $p > t$ and the definitions of balanced and strongly balanced designs. In addition, we look at designs with many periods and designs which are nearly balanced and nearly strongly balanced. These latter designs fill in gaps where balanced and strongly balanced designs do not exist. In Section 4.3 we review some of the literature on the optimality of cross-over designs and in Section 4.4 we give tables of recommended designs. In Section 4.5 we review designs which are partially balanced. Like the nearly balanced designs, these designs fill in gaps where the values of (t, p, n) are such that a balanced design does not exist. In Section 4.6 we consider the case where one treatment is a control to be compared with all the others and in Section 4.7 we consider designs for factorial sets of treatments. In Section 4.8 we consider extensions of the simple model for carry-over effects and in Section 4.9 we illustrate the construction of designs using an R package especially written to accompany this book. This package includes a facility to easily access most, if not all, of the designs mentioned in this chapter and to search for new designs. As time passes, the catalog of designs that can be accessed by the package will be enlarged.

4.2 Variance-balanced designs

Variance balance, it will be recalled, means that $\text{Var}[\hat{\tau}_i - \hat{\tau}_j]$ is the same for all $i \neq j$. An alternative definition is that all normalized treatment contrasts are estimated with the same variance. Such a design is appropriate when we wish to compare each treatment equally precisely with every other treatment.

Table 4.1: Latin square design for four treatments (18.18, 12.50).

Sequence	Period			
	1	2	3	4
1	A	B	C	D
2	B	C	D	A
3	C	D	A	B
4	D	A	B	C

In order to simplify the following description of the different types of variance-balanced designs that have been suggested in the literature, we have divided the designs into groups according to whether (i) $p = t$, (ii) $p < t$ or (iii) $p > t$.

Plans of all the most useful cross-over designs known up to 1962 were given by Patterson and Lucas (1962).

When we give the plan of a design, we will give it in its most convenient form. The design given in the plan must be randomized before being used. The efficiencies of a design, which we will define shortly, will be given in the title of the table containing the design.

4.2.1 Designs with $p = t$

Orthogonal Latin squares

If carry-over effects are not present, then variance balance can easily be achieved by using t subjects in an arbitrarily chosen Latin square design. An example of such a design for four treatments is given in Table 4.1. A Latin square is a $t \times t$ arrangement of t letters such that each letter occurs once in each row and once in each column. In our context this means that each subject should receive each treatment and that over the whole design each treatment should occur once in each period. As this design provides only $(t-1)(t-2)$ d.f. for the residual SS, a number of randomly chosen Latin squares are needed if t is small. To obtain 10 d.f. for the residual SS for $t = 3$, for example, we would need 15 subjects arranged in 5 randomly chosen squares. Further information on the construction, enumeration, randomization and other properties of Latin squares is given in Kempthorne (1983) and Federer (1955), for example.

In the absence of carry-over effects the Latin square is optimal in the sense that it not only accounts for the effects of subjects and periods, but it also provides the minimum value of $\text{Var}[\hat{\tau}_i - \hat{\tau}_j]$. This minimum value is $2\sigma^2/r$, where r is the replication of each treatment. The replication of a treatment is the number of times it occurs in the complete design. This minimum value can be used as a yardstick by which other designs can be compared. The **efficiency** (expressed as a percentage) with which a design estimates the contrast $\tau_i - \tau_j$

is defined to be

$$E_t = \frac{2\sigma^2/r}{\text{Var}[\hat{\tau}_i - \hat{\tau}_j]} \times 100.$$

The subscript t is used to indicate that the treatments have not been adjusted for carry-over effects. By definition, $E_t = 100$ for the Latin square design. If all pairwise contrasts $\tau_i - \tau_j$ have the same efficiency, then E_t defines the efficiency of the design. Designs of the same or of different size can be compared in terms of their efficiencies. Naturally, we should use the most efficient design if at all possible, as this makes the best use of the available subjects.

In the presence of carry-over effects we define efficiency exactly as above but with $\text{Var}[\hat{\tau}_i - \hat{\tau}_j]$ now denoting the difference between two treatments adjusted for carry-over effects. We label this efficiency as E_d to distinguish it from E_t, which is calculated using the unadjusted effects.

Similarly, we define

$$E_c = \frac{2\sigma^2/r}{\text{Var}[\hat{\lambda}_i - \hat{\lambda}_j]} \times 100$$

as the efficiency of $\text{Var}[\hat{\lambda}_i - \hat{\lambda}_j]$. It should be noted that in this definition r is the treatment replication. As the carry-over effects appear only in the last $p-1$ periods, they have a smaller replication than r. We will keep to the above definition, however, to maintain consistency with Patterson and Lucas (1962).

The R package *Crossover* (Rohmeyer (2014)) can be used to calculate the efficiencies of a cross-over design.

For information we will always include the values of the efficiencies of a design, in the order E_d, E_c, in the title of the table giving the plan of the design. So, for example, we can see from Table 4.1 that the efficiencies of the design are $E_d = 18.18$ and $E_c = 12.50$.

Let us now return to the design given in Table 4.1. Although this design has maximum efficiency in the absence of carry-over effects, it is not as efficient at estimating the direct treatment effects as it could be. To achieve the highest possible efficiency, the design must be **balanced**. The term balance refers to the combinatorial properties that the design must possess. In a balanced design, not only does each treatment occur once with each subject, but, over the whole design, each treatment occurs the same number of times in each period and the number of subjects who receive treatment i in some period followed by treatment j in the next period is the same for all $i \neq j$. The design in Table 4.1 is not balanced because treatment A is followed three times by treatment B and treatment B is never followed by treatment A.

For the remainder of this section it can be taken (with some exceptions which we will point out) that when we refer to a design as balanced it is also variance balanced.

Balance can be achieved by using a complete set of **orthogonal** Latin squares. Orthogonal Latin squares are defined in John (1971), Chapter 6, for

Table 4.2: Orthogonal Latin square design for three treatments (80.00, 44.44).

Sequence	Period		
	1	2	3
1	A	B	C
2	B	C	A
3	C	A	B
4	A	C	B
5	B	A	C
6	C	B	A

example. This use of orthogonal squares was first pointed out by Cochran et al. (1941), and the designs given by them for three and four treatments are reproduced in Tables 4.2 and 4.3, respectively. Here, and in the following, different squares are separated in the tables by lines. In Table 4.3, for example, we can see that each treatment follows every other treatment twice. A complete set of $t \times t$ orthogonal Latin squares contains $t-1$ squares and complete sets exist for values of t that are prime or are powers of a prime. A notable exception is therefore $t = 6$. To use a complete set, at least $t(t-1)$ subjects are needed for the trial, and this can be a disadvantage for large t if subjects are difficult or expensive to recruit.

When constructing sets of orthogonal squares for values of t other than those illustrated here, it will be noted that the squares need to be arranged so that their first columns are in the same alphabetical order. That is, in our notation, the sequence corresponding to the first period in each square is the same.

Table 4.3: Orthogonal Latin square design for four treatments (90.91, 62.50).

Sequence	Period			
	1	2	3	4
1	A	B	C	D
2	B	A	D	C
3	C	D	A	B
4	D	C	B	A
5	A	D	B	C
6	B	C	A	D
7	C	B	D	A
8	D	A	C	B
9	A	C	D	B
10	B	D	C	A
11	C	A	B	D
12	D	B	A	C

Randomization

As with all the designs in this book, we must, having chosen the treatment sequences, randomly assign them to the subjects. The simplest way to randomize a cross-over trial is to

1. randomly assign the treatments to the letters A, B, C, ...,
2. randomly assign the treatment sequences to the subjects.

If the trial is large, it may include subjects from a number of different treatment centers. If this is the case, then after step 1 above, step 2 would be undertaken for each center separately. If the sequences are to be taken from a Latin square design and there is a choice of square, then the square is first chosen at random from the available set and then steps 1 and 2 are applied.

Sometimes only a single replicate of the design is used, but it is made up of a number of smaller, self-contained, sub-designs, e.g., the orthogonal squares design is made up of $t-1$ Latin squares. If the single replicate is to be assigned to subjects from different centers, then after step 1 above each sub-design (or sets of sub-designs, if more sub-designs than centers) should be randomly assigned to a different center and then step 2 undertaken at each center.

Obviously, the precise form of the randomization will depend on the design and the circumstances in which it will be used. The basic rule is that, if at all possible, we randomly allocate subjects to sequences in a way which takes account of any known sources of systematic variation.

Williams designs

Although using orthogonal Latin squares has additional advantages, as we will note below, they require more subjects than is necessary to achieve balance. Williams (1949) showed that balance could by achieved by using only one particular Latin square if t is even and by using only two particular squares if t is odd. For more than three treatments, therefore, the designs suggested by Williams require fewer subjects than the those based on complete sets of orthogonal squares. Although Williams (1949) described the steps needed to construct one of his designs, a more easily remembered algorithm has been given by Sheehe and Bross (1961). Bradley (1958) also gave a simple algorithm, but only for even values of t and Hedayat and Afsarinejad (1978) gave a formula for deciding on $d(i,j)$ where $d(i,j)$ is the treatment to be applied to subject i in period j.

The steps in Sheehe and Bross's algorithm are as follows:

1. Number the treatments from 1 to t.
2. Start with a cyclic $t \times t$ Latin square. In this square the treatments in the ith row are $i, i+1, , \ldots, t, 1, 2, \ldots, i-1$.
3. Interlace each row of the cyclic Latin square with its own mirror image (i.e., its reverse order). For example, if $t = 4$, the first row of the cyclic square is

Table 4.4: Balanced Latin square design for four treatments (90.91,62.50).

Subject	Period			
	1	2	3	4
1	A	D	B	C
2	B	A	C	D
3	C	B	D	A
4	D	C	A	B

$1,2,3,4$. Its mirror image is $4,3,2,1$. When the two sequences are interlaced we get $1,4,2,3,3,2,4,1$.

4. Slice the resulting $t \times 2t$ array down the middle, to yield two $t \times t$ arrays. The columns of each $t \times t$ array correspond to the periods, the rows are the treatment sequences, and the numbers within the square are the treatments.
5. If t is even, we choose any one of the two $t \times t$ arrays. If t is odd, we use both arrays.

The design for $t = 4$ obtained by using this algorithm and choosing the left-hand square is given in Table 4.4. The efficiencies of this design are, of course, the same as those given for the orthogonal squares design given in Table 4.3. However, the Williams design requires fewer subjects, and this may be an advantage in certain circumstances. For example, if sufficient power can be obtained using only 16 subjects, then the Williams square, replicated four times, could be used: designs based solely on complete sets of orthogonal squares, however, require multiples of 12 subjects.

To see the gain in efficiency obtained by using a Williams design, rather than an arbitrarily chosen Latin square, compare the efficiencies of the designs in Tables 4.1 and 4.4.

Sometimes we may need to decide between using a number of replicates of a Williams square and using a complete set of orthogonal squares. One advantage of using the complete set is that, as Williams (1950) proved, they are balanced for all preceding treatments. That is, they are balanced for first-, second-, ..., $(p-1)$th-order carry-over effects. Using the complete set therefore enables other effects to be conveniently tested should they be of interest. The disadvantage of using a complete set is that it consists of $t(t-1)$ different sequences and so the chance of a sequence being incorrectly administered through mishap is increased. Also, the loss of subjects from the complete set is likely to be more damaging, as its combinatorial structure is more complex.

Minimal designs

Hedayat and Afsarinejad (1975) considered the construction of **minimal balanced** (MB) designs. These are balanced designs which use the minimum possible number of subjects. They referred to a cross-over design for t treatments, n subjects and p periods as an RM(t,n,p) design. They noted that for even t, MB RM(t,t,t) designs exist and can be constructed using the method of Sheehe and Bross (1961), for example. For odd values of t they noted that no MB RM(t,t,t) is possible for $t = 3$, 5 and 7, but such a design does exist for $t = 21$. Hedayat and Afsarinejad (1978) later added that MB RM(t,t,t) designs for $t = 9$, 15 and 27 had been found and gave plans of them.

For all odd values of t and $n = 2t$, MB RM$(t,2t,t)$ designs exist and are Williams designs, which can again be easily constructed using the Sheehe and Bross algorithm. In addition, Hedayat and Afsarinejad (1975) showed how to construct MB RM$(t,2t,p)$ designs when t is a prime power. Methods of constructing MB designs for $p < t$ were described by Afsarinejad (1983). However, these designs are not variance balanced except in a few special cases.

Further results on Williams designs

Williams designs are special cases of what have been called **sequentially counter balanced** Latin squares (Isaac et al. (1999)) or **row complete** Latin squares (Bailey (1984)). Isaac et al. (1999) describe a range of methods of constructing such designs for even t, including the algorithm of Sheehe and Bross (1961), which we have already described. They note that for a given t the designs constructed by the various methods may or may not be unique. If a design for t subjects is written so that the treatments in the first period are in alphabetical order and the treatments for the first subject are in alphabetical order, the design is said to be in **standard order**. If two apparently different designs for the same t when written in standard order (if necessary by relabeling the treatments and reordering rows) are identical, then they are essentially the same design. For $t = 4$ there is only one design which is in standard order. For $t = 6$ there are two standard squares and these are given in Table 4.5. These designs have been constructed using methods described by Isaac et al. (1999), who also note that there are at most eight standard designs for $t = 8$.

When randomizing a design for the cases where there is more than one standard square, a square is first chosen at random from those available. Then the steps in the randomization described earlier are followed.

As already noted earlier, for odd t no single sequentially counterbalanced square exists for $t = 3, 5$ and 7, although single squares have been found by computer search for $t = 9, 15, 21$ and 27 (Hedayat and Afsarinejad, 1975, 1978). Archdeacon et al. (1980) gave methods of constructing such designs for odd t and their design for $t = 9$ is given in Table 4.6.

To provide an alternative when single sequentially balanced squares for odd t do not exist, Russell (1991) gave a method of construction for what might be termed nearly sequentially counterbalanced squares. In these squares each treatment is preceded by all but two treatments once, by one of the remaining two twice and not at all by the remaining treatment. Examples of such squares for $t = 5$ and 7 are given in Tables 4.7 and 4.8, respectively. The efficiencies of the pairwise comparisons of the direct treatments adjusted for carry-over effects are either 83.86 or 78.62 for the design in Table 4.7 and 92.62, 92.55 or 90.18 for the design in Table 4.8.

Table 4.5: Two balanced Latin squares for six treatments (96.55, 77.78).

Standard square 1						
Subject	Period					
	1	2	3	4	5	6
1	A	B	C	D	E	F
2	B	D	A	F	C	E
3	C	A	E	B	F	D
4	D	F	B	E	A	C
5	E	C	F	A	D	B
6	F	E	D	C	B	A

Standard square 2						
Subject	Period					
	1	2	3	4	5	6
1	A	B	C	D	E	F
2	B	D	F	A	C	E
3	C	F	B	E	A	D
4	D	A	E	B	F	C
5	E	C	A	F	D	B
6	F	E	D	C	B	A

Table 4.6: Balanced Latin square design for nine treatments (98.59, 86.42).

Subject	Period								
	1	2	3	4	5	6	7	8	9
1	A	B	C	D	E	F	G	H	I
2	B	D	A	F	C	I	H	G	E
3	C	F	E	G	D	B	I	A	H
4	D	G	F	I	B	H	E	C	A
5	E	A	I	C	H	D	F	B	G
6	F	H	B	E	I	G	A	D	C
7	G	I	D	H	F	A	C	E	B
8	H	C	G	B	A	E	D	I	F
9	I	E	H	A	G	C	B	F	D

Using multiple Latin squares

When, as is usually the case, more than t subjects are to be used in the trial, a choice has to be made how this will be achieved. Let us assume that the total number of subjects to be used is N, an integer multiple of t.

If the design contains t (or $2t$) sequences, it is common practice in pharmaceutical trials to randomly allocate $n = N/t$ (or $n = N/(2t)$ for N even) subjects to each of the sequences. This simplifies the design and lessens the risk of subjects receiving the treatments in an incorrect order. Also, the combinatorial and

Table 4.7: Russell nearly balanced Latin square design for five treatments (83.86 or 78.62, 63.73 or 59.75).

Subject	Period				
	1	2	3	4	5
1	A	B	C	D	E
2	B	D	E	C	A
3	C	E	B	A	D
4	D	C	A	E	B
5	E	A	D	B	C

Table 4.8: Russell nearly balanced Latin square design for seven treatments (92.62, 92.55 or 90.18, 77.50, 77.44 or 75.46).

Subject	Period						
	1	2	3	4	5	6	7
1	A	B	C	D	E	F	G
2	B	F	G	A	D	C	E
3	C	G	D	F	B	E	A
4	D	A	F	E	G	B	C
5	E	D	B	G	C	A	F
6	F	C	E	B	A	G	D
7	G	E	A	C	F	D	B

variance properties of the design are more robust to subjects dropping out or failing to complete all t periods.

For odd t where no single sequentially counterbalanced square exists (e.g., for $t = 3, 5$ and 7), this means that the number of subjects must be a multiple of $2t$, which may be inconvenient.

To alleviate this problem, we can use the designs suggested by Newcombe (1996). He gave sets, each containing three $t \times t$ Latin squares, such that the $3t$ sequences in the set formed a balanced design. In these designs each treatment precedes every other treatment, except itself, equally often. Prescott (1999) later give a systematic method of construction of these triples. Examples of designs for $t = 5$ and $t = 7$ obtained using Prescott's method of construction are given in Tables 4.9 and 4.10, respectively.

Locally balanced designs

Anderson and Preece (2002) gave methods for constructing **locally balanced** designs for odd t. These are designs for $t(t-1)$ patients that are not only balanced in the conventional sense, but also have additional local balance properties. An example of such a design for $t = 7$ is given in Table 4.11. These additional properties of balance are:

1. The patients can be grouped into $(t-1)/2$ groups of size $2n$ so that, for each $i \neq j$, exactly two patients per group receive treatment i immedi-

Table 4.9: Prescott triple Latin square design for five treatments (94.94, 72.00).

Subject	Period				
	1	2	3	4	5
1	A	B	D	E	C
2	B	C	E	A	D
3	C	D	A	B	E
4	D	E	B	C	A
5	E	A	C	D	B
6	A	C	E	D	B
7	B	D	A	E	C
8	C	E	B	A	D
9	D	A	C	B	E
10	E	B	D	C	A
11	A	E	D	B	C
12	B	A	E	C	D
13	C	B	A	D	E
14	D	C	B	E	A
15	E	D	C	A	B

ately after treatment j. This means that each group forms a single copy of a Williams design for $2n$ patients. The efficiencies of this sub-design are (97.56, 81.63).

2. The design for Periods 1 to $(t+1)/2$ has each carry-over from treatment i to treatment j exactly once in each of the groups. This ensures that if patients drop out of the trial after period $(t+1)/2$, the remaining design is still reasonably efficient. For example, in the extreme situation where the trial that used the design in Table 4.11 only completed the first four periods, the remaining design would have efficiencies of (79.84, 57.03).

3. Each of the $t(t-1)$ sequences of two different treatments must, at each stage of the trial, be allocated to exactly one of the $t(t-1)$ patients. In Table 4.11, for example, the sequence pair BC occurs in Periods (1,2) for Patient 1, in Periods (2,3) for Patient 36, in Periods (3,4) for Patient 24, in Periods (4,5) for Patient 23, in Periods (5,6) for Patient 39 and in Periods (6,7) for Patient 4. Therefore, should the trial be stopped in any period after Period 2, each carry-over effect will have occurred with the same number of patients.

4. If the trial is stopped after $(t+1)/2$ periods, the remaining design forms a balanced incomplete block design, with the patients as blocks. In such a design each pair of treatments is administered the same number of times to the patients, although not necessarily in successive periods. For example, in Table 4.11, each pair of treatments is administered to 12 patients.

Table 4.10: Prescott triple Latin square design for seven treatments (97.56, 81.63).

Subject	Period						
	1	2	3	4	5	6	7
1	A	B	F	D	E	G	C
2	B	C	G	E	F	A	D
3	C	D	A	F	G	B	E
4	D	E	B	G	A	C	F
5	E	F	C	A	B	D	G
6	F	G	D	B	C	E	A
7	G	A	E	C	D	F	B
8	A	C	G	E	D	F	B
9	B	D	A	F	E	G	C
10	C	E	B	G	F	A	D
11	D	F	C	A	G	B	E
12	E	G	D	B	A	C	F
13	F	A	E	C	B	D	G
14	G	B	F	D	C	E	A
15	A	G	F	C	D	B	E
16	B	A	G	D	E	C	F
17	C	B	A	E	F	D	G
18	D	C	B	F	G	E	A
19	E	D	C	G	A	F	B
20	F	E	D	A	B	G	C
21	G	F	E	B	C	A	D

4.2.2 *Designs with $p < t$*

Designs obtained from orthogonal squares

All the designs described in the previous section are such that each subject receives every treatment. In practice this may not be possible for ethical or practical reasons. Even if all treatments could be administered, it is sometimes desirable to use a smaller number to decrease the chances of subjects dropping out of the trial. A number of balanced designs for $p < t$ have been suggested in the literature and we will describe and compare them in the following subsections. As in the previous section, we will include the efficiencies of the design in the title of the table containing the design.

The simplest method of obtaining a balanced design with $p < t$ is to delete one or more periods from the full design obtained from a complete set of orthogonal Latin squares. This method was first suggested by Patterson (1950) and described in more detail by Patterson (1951, 1952). If we remove the last period from the design given in Table 4.3, for example, we will get a design for three periods with $E_d = 71.96$ and $E_c = 41.98$.

Table 4.11: Anderson and Preece locally balanced design for seven treatments (97.56, 81.63).

Subject	Period						
	1	2	3	4	5	6	7
1	B	C	E	A	D	F	G
2	C	D	F	B	E	G	A
3	D	E	G	C	F	A	B
4	E	F	A	D	G	B	C
5	F	G	B	E	A	C	D
6	G	A	C	F	B	D	E
7	A	B	D	G	C	E	F
8	G	F	D	A	E	C	B
9	A	G	E	B	F	D	C
10	B	A	F	C	G	E	D
11	C	B	G	D	A	F	E
12	D	C	A	E	B	G	F
13	E	D	B	F	C	A	G
14	F	E	C	G	D	B	A
15	C	E	B	A	G	D	F
16	D	F	C	B	A	E	G
17	E	G	D	C	B	F	A
18	F	A	E	D	C	G	B
19	G	B	F	E	D	A	C
20	A	C	G	F	E	B	D
21	B	D	A	G	F	C	E
22	F	D	G	A	B	E	C
23	G	E	A	B	C	F	D
24	A	F	B	C	D	G	E
25	B	G	C	D	E	A	F
26	C	A	D	E	F	B	G
27	D	B	E	F	G	C	A
28	E	C	F	G	A	D	B
29	D	G	F	A	C	B	E
30	E	A	G	B	D	C	F
31	F	B	A	C	E	D	G
32	G	C	B	D	F	E	A
33	A	D	C	E	G	F	B
34	B	E	D	F	A	G	C
35	C	F	E	G	B	A	D
36	E	B	C	A	F	G	D
37	F	C	D	B	G	A	E
38	G	D	E	C	A	B	F
39	A	E	F	D	B	C	G
40	B	F	G	E	C	D	A
41	C	G	A	F	D	E	B
42	D	A	B	G	E	F	C

Table 4.12: One of Patterson's incomplete designs for seven treatments (79.84, 57.03).

Subject	Period			
	1	2	3	4
1	A	B	D	G
2	B	C	E	A
3	C	D	F	B
4	D	E	G	C
5	E	F	A	D
6	F	G	B	E
7	G	A	C	F
8	A	G	E	B
9	B	A	F	C
10	C	B	G	D
11	D	C	A	E
12	E	D	B	F
13	F	E	C	G
14	G	F	D	A

Although more than one period can be removed, we should always ensure that the design we use has at least three periods. This is because designs with two periods have low efficiencies and should be avoided if possible. Two-period designs can, however, form a useful basic design to which extra periods are added. Extra-period designs are described below. Designs obtained from complete sets of orthogonal squares are also balanced for second-order carry-over effects and this property is retained when periods are removed.

Designs obtained from Youden squares and other methods

Patterson (1951) noted that a design which uses $4t$ subjects can always be constructed when a $4 \times t$ Youden square exists. (John (1971), for example, gives a definition of a Youden square.) Patterson also gave a design for $t = 7$ which uses 14 subjects. This design, which is given in Table 4.12, can be divided into two blocks of seven subjects, as indicated. This design is also of the cyclic type: the sequences for Subjects 2 to 7 are obtained by cycling the treatments for Subject 1, and the sequences for Subjects 9 to 14 are obtained by cycling the treatments for Subject 8. In this cycling the treatments are successively changed in the order ABCDEFGA, etc. A number of the incomplete designs given by Patterson and Lucas (1962) for other values of t can be constructed using this cyclic method of construction.

Patterson (1952) extended his earlier results and gave designs which use fewer than $t(t-1)$ units for the special case of prime $t = 4n+3$, where n is a positive integer. In addition to the design given here in Table 4.12, he also gave a design for $t = 7$ which uses 21 subjects.

Designs obtained from balanced incomplete block designs

A number of different types of cross-over design can be constructed by starting with a non-cross-over incomplete block design. An incomplete design is such that each subject receives only one treatment and the subjects are grouped into b homogeneous blocks of size $p < t$. (We added the qualification non-cross-over to emphasize that the incomplete block designs we are referring to are the traditional ones which have been used in agriculture, for example, for many years. In these designs each experimental unit in a block receives a single treatment.) Patterson (1952) noted that balanced cross-over designs can be constructed by starting with a **balanced incomplete block design** (BIB design). In a BIB design each treatment is replicated the same number of times and each pair of treatments occurs together in the same block α times, where α is a constant integer. An example of a BIB for $t = 4$, $b = 4$ and $p = 3$ is (123), (124), (134) and (234). Each block of the design is enclosed by brackets and it can be seen that each pair of treatments occurs together in two blocks. To build a balanced cross-over design we take each block of the BIB in turn and construct a balanced cross-over design for the p treatments in that block. These blocks are then joined together to give a balanced cross-over design for t treatments, p periods and bp subjects. If we take the BIB used as our example above, then the corresponding balanced cross-over design we need for each block is the one given earlier in Table 4.2. We replace each block of the BIB with this three-treatment design and relabel the treatments where necessary. For example, the treatments in the third block are (134) and so in the cross-over design for three treatments which corresponds to this block, we relabel 1 as A, 2 as C and 3 as D, to get the six sequences to be included in the final cross-over design for four treatments and three periods. The complete design for 24 subjects is given in Table 4.13.

It should be noted that a design which uses 12 subjects and which has the same efficiencies as the design in Table 4.13 can be obtained by removing the last period from the orthogonal squares design for four treatments.

Other designs with $p < t$

For completeness we mention some designs that have been suggested in the literature. These designs are generally not as efficient as the ones mentioned previously and so we do not devote much space to them here.

The two-period Balaam design described in Chapter 3 is a special case of the design suggested by Balaam (1968) for two or more treatments. The sequences in this more general design consist of all possible pairings of one treatment with another, including the pairing of a treatment with itself. These designs consist, as Balaam pointed out, of the first two periods of the designs suggested by Berenblut (1964). Balaam introduced his designs for use in animal experiments where a wash-out period is used to eliminate any carry-over effects. The designs are such that they permit a within-subject test of the direct-by-period interaction. In our situation, where carry-over effects are included in the model, the Balaam designs, like all designs which use only two periods,

Table 4.13: Incomplete design for four treatments obtained using a BIB (71.96, 41.98).

Subject	Period		
	1	2	3
1	A	B	C
2	B	C	A
3	C	A	B
4	A	C	B
5	B	A	C
6	C	B	A
7	A	B	D
8	B	D	A
9	D	A	B
10	A	D	B
11	B	A	D
12	D	B	A
13	A	D	C
14	C	A	D
15	D	A	C
16	A	D	C
17	C	A	D
18	D	C	A
19	B	C	D
20	C	D	B
21	D	B	C
22	B	D	C
23	C	B	D
24	D	C	B

do not have high efficiencies. We have included them mainly for completeness and to draw attention to them again when we consider designs for $p > t$.

A different type of design, known as the switch-back, was introduced by Lucas (1957) for use in cattle feeding trials. He assumed that there were no carry-over effects or direct-by-period interactions. These designs are an extension of those described by Brandt (1938) for two treatments. These designs use the two different sequences ABAB ... and BABA .... That is, in the third period the animal switches back to the treatment it received in the first period, then switches back to the treatment it received in the second period, and so on. In Lucas' extension the design lasts for three periods and the treatment applied in the third period is the same as the treatment applied in the first period. In general, these designs consist of all possible $t(t-1)$ pairings of the treatments, which make up the sequences in the first two periods. He also gave, for odd t, designs which use only $t(t-1)/2$ animals. However, these are not balanced for the adjusted treatment effects in our model. A feature of the Lucas designs is that they can be divided into blocks of t subjects.

Extra-period designs with $p < t$

Extra-period designs are obtained by adding an additional period to an existing cross-over design. In this extra period each subject receives the treatment he or she received in the last period of the original design. Adding the extra period has the effect of increasing the efficiency of estimation $\lambda_i - \lambda_j$ and of causing the carry-over effects to become orthogonal to both subjects and direct effects. The origins of the idea of adding extra periods are described below, where extra-period designs for $p > t$ are considered. If $p < t - 1$, then adding an extra period still gives a design with $p < t$.

If we add an extra period to one of Balaam's two-period designs, we find that $E_d = E_c$. If it were not for their low efficiencies, the extra-period Balaam designs would therefore be ideal for the situation where exactly the same precision is required for both carry-over and direct effects. Also, the orthogonality of the carry-over and direct effects makes the design quite easy to analyze. These extra-period designs are therefore a possible alternative to the tied-double-change-over designs to be described below.

4.2.3 Designs with $p > t$

Extra-period designs

In general, the balanced designs described so far are such that the efficiency, E_c of the carry-over effects is much lower than the efficiency E_d of the direct effects. This, as Lucas (1957) pointed out, is mainly because the carry-over effects are nonorthogonal to the direct effects and subjects. This nonorthogonality can be removed, and the efficiency of the carry-over effects increased, if we use a design in which each carry-over effect occurs the same number of times with each subject and the same number of times with each direct effect. The simplest way to achieve this is to (a) take a balanced design for p periods and (b) repeat in period $p+1$ the treatment a subject received in period p. This way of increasing precision was first noted by F. Yates in a seminar in 1947 and by Patterson (1951) at the end of a paper concerned mainly with the analysis and design of trials with $p < t$. Lucas (1957), however, gave the first formal description of adding an extra period.

Extra-period designs for $t = 3$ and 4 are given in Tables 4.14 and 4.15, respectively. The design for $t = 3$ is obtained by adding an extra period to the complete set of orthogonal squares and the design for $t = 4$ is obtained by adding on an extra period to the Williams square, where now the square is written in standard order (i.e., the first row and column are in alphabetical order).

The change in the relative sizes of E_d and E_c which results from adding the extra period can be illustrated by comparing the efficiencies of the extra-period designs in Tables 4.14 and 4.15 with the efficiencies of their parent designs

Table 4.14: Balanced extra-period design for three treatments (93.75, 75.00).

Subject	Period			
	1	2	3	4
1	A	B	C	C
2	B	C	A	A
3	C	A	B	B
4	A	C	B	B
5	B	A	C	C
6	C	B	A	A

Table 4.15: Balanced extra-period design for four treatments (96.00, 80.00).

Subject	Period				
	1	2	3	4	5
1	A	B	C	D	D
2	B	D	A	C	C
3	C	A	D	B	B
4	D	C	B	A	A

in Tables 4.2 and 4.4, respectively. The increase in efficiency arises because the extra-period designs are **completely balanced**, i.e., each treatment follows every treatment, *including itself*, the same number of times. Therefore, each carry-over effect occurs the same number of times with each direct effect. In the cross-over literature complete balance is synonymous with **strong balance**, and we will use this latter term. As with the term balance, we will take it as understood that complete balance implies variance balance.

Apart from the increase in efficiency, extra-period designs also have the advantage of permitting a more convenient analysis because the direct effects are orthogonal to the carry-over effects. In other words, the estimates of the direct effects are the same whether or not the carry-over effects are present in the fitted model.

Trials which use extra-period designs are, however, by their very definition, going to take longer to complete than trials which use the minimum number of periods. They are going to be more expensive and time consuming and so are likely to prove useful only when carry-over effects are strongly suspected and need to be estimated with relatively high efficiency. If carry-over effects are not present, then the extra-period designs are not as efficient at estimating the direct effects as their parent designs. This is because the direct effects are not orthogonal to subjects in the extra-period designs. Also, some bias may creep into the process of measuring the response if those undertaking the measurements realize that the last two treatments administered to each subject are the same.

As we noted earlier, balanced designs for $p < t$ can also be constructed by adding an extra period. Also, repeating twice the treatment used in the last period of a balanced design will increase the precision with which the second-order effects are estimated. This was noted by Linnerud et al. (1962), for example.

4.2.4 *Designs with many periods*

If we can use a design with considerably more than t periods, then strongly or **nearly strongly balanced** designs can be constructed. This latter term was introduced by Kunert (1983) and will be defined shortly. Here we give a selection of methods of constructing such designs.

4.2.4.1 *Quenouille, Berenblut and Patterson designs*

Quenouille (1953) gave a method of constructing strongly balanced designs and an example of one of these for $t = 3$ is given in Table 4.16. It can be seen that the sequences for Subjects 2 to 6 are obtained by cyclically shifting the sequence for Subject 1. The sequences for Subjects 8 to 12 are similarly obtained from sequence 7 and the sequences for Subjects 14 to 18 are similarly obtained from the sequence for Subject 13. The design is therefore completely

Table 4.16: Quenouille design for $t = 3$ (100.00, 80.56).

Subject	Period					
	1	2	3	4	5	6
1	A	A	B	B	C	C
2	C	A	A	B	B	C
3	C	C	A	A	B	B
4	B	C	C	A	A	B
5	B	B	C	C	A	A
6	A	B	B	C	C	A
7	A	A	C	C	B	B
8	B	A	A	C	C	B
9	B	B	A	A	C	C
10	C	B	B	A	A	C
11	C	C	B	B	A	A
12	A	C	C	B	B	A
13	A	B	C	B	A	C
14	C	A	B	C	B	A
15	A	C	A	B	C	B
16	B	A	C	A	B	C
17	C	B	A	C	A	B
18	B	C	B	A	C	A

Table 4.17: Berenblut's design for $t = 3$ (100.00, 85.94).

Subject	Period							
	1	2	3	4	5	6	7	8
1	A	D	C	B	B	C	D	A
2	B	A	D	C	C	D	A	B
3	C	B	A	D	D	A	B	C
4	D	C	B	A	A	B	C	D
5	D	D	B	B	A	C	C	A
6	A	A	C	C	B	D	D	B
7	B	B	D	D	C	A	A	C
8	C	C	A	A	D	B	B	D
9	C	D	A	B	D	C	B	A
10	D	A	B	C	A	D	C	B
11	A	B	C	D	B	A	D	C
12	B	C	D	A	C	B	A	D
13	B	D	D	B	C	C	A	A
14	C	A	A	C	D	D	B	B
15	D	B	B	D	A	A	C	C
16	A	C	C	A	B	B	D	D

and concisely defined by the three sequences (AABBCC), (AACCBB) and (ABCBAC). Quenouille also gave an alternative set of three sequences for $t =$ 3 and three alternative pairs of sequences for $t = 4$. One pair of sequences for $t = 4$, for example, is (AABBCCDD) and (ACBADBDC). By cyclically shifting each of these sequences in turn, a design for four treatments using sixteen subjects and eight periods is obtained.

Berenblut (1964) showed that designs like those of Quenouille, which have direct effects orthogonal to carry-over effects and subjects, can be obtained by using t treatments, $2t$ periods and t^2 different sequences. Therefore, for $t = 4$, for example, they require fewer subjects than the designs suggested by Quenouille. A set of instructions for constructing a Berenblut design was given by Namboordiri (1972) and is somewhat easier to understand than the original set of instructions given by Berenblut (1964). The design for $t = 4$ obtained using these instructions is given in Table 4.17.

Berenblut (1967b) described how to analyze his designs and Berenblut (1967a) described a design appropriate for comparing equally spaced doses of the same drug which uses only eight subjects and four periods. This design is not balanced but does have the property that the linear, quadratic and cubic contrasts of the direct effects are orthogonal to the linear and cubic contrasts of the carry-over effects. This design would be useful for comparing equally spaced doses of the same drug when carry-over effects are thought most unlikely but if present can be detected by a comparison of the low and high dose levels.

Berenblut (1968) noted that his 1964 designs are such that in addition to the properties already described, the direct-by-carry-over interaction is orthogonal to the direct and carry-over effects. He then described a method of constructing designs for $t = 4$ and 5 which have the same properties as his 1964 designs but only require $2t$ subjects. Each of these designs is constructed by combining two suitably chosen Latin squares. These designs are appropriate when the treatments correspond to equally spaced doses, the direct effects have a predominantly linear component and the carry-over effects are small in comparison to the direct effects and proportional to them. The designs are such that (a) the linear component of the carry-over effect is orthogonal to the linear, quadratic, etc., components of the direct effect and (b) the linear direct-by-linear carry-over interaction is orthogonal to each component of the direct effect.

Patterson (1970) pointed out that although the Berenblut (1964) design, when used for four equally spaced treatments, is suitable for the estimation of the direct and carry-over effects, other designs may be preferred for the estimation of the linear direct-by-linear carry-over interaction. He gave a method of constructing a family of designs which contained within it the designs of Berenblut (1964), and also showed how the subjects in his designs could be divided into blocks of eight or four, with a minimum loss of information due to confounding. He also noted that the Berenblut (1967a) design which uses eight subjects has low efficiency for estimating the linear-by-linear interaction and suggested that if economy of subjects and periods is important, then it is better to reduce the number of treatment levels to three and to use one of his or Berenblut's designs for three treatments. Patterson (1973) described a way of extending the Quenouille (1953) method so that a larger collection of designs can be obtained.

4.2.4.2 *Federer and Atkinson's designs*

Federer and Atkinson (1964) described a series of designs for r periods and c subjects, where $r = tq + 1$, $c = ts$, $sq = k(t-1)$ and q, s and k are positive integers. These designs, which they called **tied-double-change-over designs**, are such that the variances of the direct and carry-over effects approach equality as the number of periods increases. If the number of periods is kept to a minimum, then these designs require $t(t-1)$ subjects and $(t+1)$ periods.

Atkinson (1966) proposed a series of designs for the situation where the effect of consecutive applications of a treatment is the quantity of interest. The designs are obtained by taking a Williams design and repeating each column (i.e., period) k times, where $k \geq 2$. The effect of repeating periods is to increase the efficiency of the estimation of the carry-over effects at the expense of the direct effects. It should be noted that, unlike Atkinson, we are assuming that the design consists of all $2t$ periods. The analysis given by Atkinson assumed that the data from the first $k-1$ periods would not be used.

Table 4.18: Anderson training-schedule design for seven treatments (97.41, 89. 95).

Subject	Period													
	1	2	3	4	5	6	7	8	9	10	11	12	13	14
1	A	B	E	C	G	F	D	C	B	F	A	D	E	G
2	B	C	F	D	A	G	E	D	C	G	B	E	F	A
3	C	D	G	E	B	A	F	E	D	A	C	F	G	B
4	D	E	A	F	C	B	G	F	E	B	D	G	A	C
5	E	F	B	G	D	C	A	G	F	C	E	A	B	D
6	F	G	C	A	E	D	B	A	G	D	F	B	C	E
7	G	A	D	B	F	E	C	B	A	E	G	C	D	F
8	A	G	D	F	B	C	E	F	G	C	A	E	D	B
9	B	A	E	G	C	D	F	G	A	D	B	F	E	C
10	C	B	F	A	D	E	G	A	B	E	C	G	F	D
11	D	C	G	B	E	F	A	B	C	F	D	A	G	E
12	E	D	A	C	F	G	B	C	D	G	E	B	A	F
13	F	E	B	D	G	A	C	D	E	A	F	C	B	G
14	G	F	C	E	A	B	D	E	F	B	G	D	C	A
15	A	D	F	G	E	B	C	G	D	B	A	C	F	E
16	B	E	G	A	F	C	D	A	E	C	B	D	G	F
17	C	F	A	B	G	D	E	B	F	D	C	E	A	G
18	D	G	B	C	A	E	F	C	G	E	D	F	B	A
19	E	A	C	D	B	F	G	D	A	F	E	G	C	B
20	F	B	D	E	C	G	A	E	B	G	F	A	D	C
21	G	C	E	F	D	A	B	F	C	A	G	B	E	D
22	A	E	C	B	D	G	F	B	E	G	A	F	C	D
23	B	F	D	C	E	A	G	C	F	A	B	G	D	E
24	C	G	E	D	F	B	A	D	G	B	C	A	E	F
25	D	A	F	E	G	C	B	E	A	C	D	B	F	G
26	E	B	G	F	A	D	C	F	B	D	E	C	G	A
27	F	C	A	G	B	E	D	G	C	E	F	D	A	B
28	G	D	B	A	C	F	E	A	D	F	G	E	B	C
29	A	C	B	E	F	D	G	E	C	D	A	G	B	F
30	B	D	C	F	G	E	A	F	D	E	B	A	C	G
31	C	E	D	G	A	F	B	G	E	F	C	B	D	A
32	D	F	E	A	B	G	C	A	F	G	D	C	E	B
33	E	G	F	B	C	A	D	B	G	A	E	D	F	C
34	F	A	G	C	D	B	E	C	A	B	F	E	G	D
35	G	B	A	D	E	C	F	D	B	C	G	F	A	E
36	A	F	G	D	C	E	B	D	F	E	A	B	G	C
37	B	G	A	E	D	F	C	E	G	F	B	C	A	D
38	C	A	B	F	E	G	D	F	A	G	C	D	B	E
39	D	B	C	G	F	A	E	G	B	A	D	E	C	F
40	E	C	D	A	G	B	F	A	C	B	E	F	D	G
41	F	D	E	B	A	C	G	B	D	C	F	G	E	A
42	G	E	F	C	B	D	A	C	E	D	G	A	F	B

Anderson design

An example of a balanced design for $t = 7$, 14 periods and 42 subjects is given in Table 4.18. This design was constructed by Ian Anderson of the University of Glasgow to provide a training schedule for 42 rugby football players. Each player has to accomplish each of seven tasks once, and then once again. No player is to have a repeated carry-over. In addition, in each consecutive pair of periods, each carry-over effect is to occur once.

Nearly strongly balanced designs

Although strongly balanced designs have attractive properties, they do not exist for all combinations of values of t, n and p. If the numbers of subjects

Table 4.19: Nearly strongly balanced design for $t = 8$ (99.90 or 99.79, 93.26 or 93.16).

Subject	Period															
	1	2	3	4	5	6	7	8	9	10	11	12	13	14	15	16
1	A	B	H	C	G	D	F	E	E	F	D	G	C	H	B	A
2	B	C	A	D	H	E	G	F	F	G	E	H	D	A	C	B
3	C	D	B	E	A	F	H	G	G	H	F	A	E	B	D	C
4	D	E	C	F	B	G	A	H	H	A	G	B	F	C	E	D
5	E	F	D	G	C	H	B	A	A	B	H	C	G	D	F	E
6	F	G	E	H	D	A	C	B	B	C	A	D	H	E	G	F
7	G	H	F	A	E	B	D	C	C	D	B	E	A	F	H	G
8	H	A	G	B	F	C	E	D	D	E	C	F	B	G	A	H
9	B	H	C	G	D	F	E	E	F	D	G	C	H	B	A	A
10	C	A	D	H	E	G	F	F	G	E	H	D	A	C	B	B
11	D	B	E	A	F	H	G	G	H	F	A	E	B	D	C	C
12	E	C	F	B	G	A	H	H	A	G	B	F	C	E	D	D
13	F	D	G	C	H	B	A	A	B	H	C	G	D	F	E	E
14	G	E	H	D	A	C	B	B	C	A	D	H	E	G	F	F
15	H	F	A	E	B	D	C	C	D	B	E	A	F	H	G	G
16	A	G	B	F	C	E	D	D	E	C	F	B	G	A	H	H

and periods are both multiples of t, then nearly strongly balanced designs, constructed using the methods of Bate and Jones (2006), can be used. These designs also include the balanced and strongly balanced designs as special cases. We do not give details of the methods of construction here, but give some examples. The motivation for these designs was the question of whether a design used by McNulty (1986) was optimal in terms of its efficiency of estimation. The design used by McNulty is given in Chapter 5 and was for 8 treatments, 16 periods and 16 subjects. This design is made up of four repeats of a Williams design for 8 treatments, 8 periods and 8 subjects. The sequences in Periods 9 to 16 for Subjects 1 to 8 are a copy of those used in Periods 1 to 8, respectively. The sequences in Periods 1 to 16 for Subjects 9 to 16 are a copy of those for Subjects 1 to 8. The background to the trial that used this design and an analysis of some of the data collected in it are given in Chapter 5. Bate and Jones showed that this design is suboptimal and constructed the universally optimal (as defined below) design given in Table 4.19. In this design the efficiencies of the pairwise direct comparisons are either 99.90 or 99.79 and the efficiencies of the pairwise carry-over comparisons are either 93.26 or 93.16. In McNulty's design these are 97.88 or 96.23 for the direct comparisons and 91.38 or 89.84 for the carry-over comparisons. An example of a nearly strongly balanced design for $t = 5$, 10 periods and 15 subjects is given in Table 4.20.

4.3 Optimality results for cross-over designs

Here we briefly review some results concerning the optimality of cross-over designs with three or more treatments. In the general (i.e., not necessarily cross-over) design case, optimality criteria are usually defined in terms of functions of the information matrix of the design or the variance-covariance matrix

Table 4.20: Nearly strongly balanced design for $t = 5$ (99.87 or 99.75, 88.89 or 88.78).

Subject	Period									
	1	2	3	4	5	6	7	8	9	10
1	A	C	B	E	D	D	E	B	C	A
2	B	D	C	A	E	E	A	C	D	B
3	C	E	D	B	A	A	B	D	E	C
4	D	A	E	C	B	B	C	E	A	D
5	E	B	A	D	C	C	D	A	B	E
6	C	B	E	D	D	E	B	C	A	A
7	D	C	A	E	E	A	C	D	B	B
8	E	D	B	A	A	B	D	E	C	C
9	A	E	C	B	B	C	E	A	D	D
10	B	A	D	C	C	D	A	B	E	E
11	B	E	D	D	E	B	C	A	A	C
12	C	A	E	E	A	C	D	B	B	D
13	D	B	A	A	B	D	E	C	C	E
14	E	C	B	B	C	E	A	D	D	A
15	A	D	C	C	D	A	B	E	E	B

V of $(t-1)$ orthogonal and normalized contrasts between the t treatments. A good design is one which makes **V** "small" in some sense. Different ways of defining "small" have led to different optimality criteria:

1. the D-optimal design minimizes the determinant of **V**;
2. the A-optimal design minimizes the average variance of the $(t-1)$ orthonormal contrasts; and
3. the E-optimal design minimizes the maximum variance of the $(t-1)$ orthonormal contrasts.

Kiefer (1975) subsumed these criteria and others into his criterion of universal optimality: the universal (U)-optimal design is also D-, A- and E- optimal. Later, Hedayat and Afsarinejad (1978) considered the optimality of *uniform* cross-over designs. In a uniform design each treatment occurs equally often in each period and for each subject; each treatment appears in the same number of periods. They proved that uniform balanced designs are U-optimal for the estimation of the direct effects and for the first-order carry-over effects. (These designs, it will be realized, are the ones we described earlier in the section on minimal balanced designs.) Consequently, the Williams designs, and the MB $RM(t,t,t)$ designs which exist, are U-optimal. The rest of this short review is based mainly on Matthews (1988), Section 3.2.

Cheng and Wu (1980) extended Hedayat and Afsarinejad's results and in particular were able to prove, for i a positive integer, that (a) balanced uniform designs are U-optimal for the estimation of first-order carry-over effects over all $RM(t,it,t)$ designs where no treatment precedes itself and (b) if a design is obtained from a balanced uniform design by repeating the last period, then it is U-optimal for the estimation of direct and carry-over effects over all $RM(t,it,t+1)$ designs.

Result (b) of Cheng and Wu is particularly useful because it provides a more rigorous justification for the extra-period designs suggested by Lucas (1957). Kunert (1984) proved that if a balanced uniform $RM(t,t,t)$ design exists, then it is U-optimal for the estimation of the direct treatment effects.

Cheng and Wu were also able to prove that a *strongly* balanced uniform $RM(t,n,p)$ design is U-optimal for the estimation of direct and carry-over effects. Finally, we note that Sen and Mukerjee (1987) extended some of the results of Cheng and Wu to the case where the direct-by-carry-over interaction parameters are also included in the model. They proved that strongly balanced uniform designs were also U-optimal for the estimation of the direct effects in the presence of these interaction parameters. This follows from the orthogonality of the direct effects, the carry-over effects and the interaction parameters.

For a more recent review of methods that can be used to construct uniform designs, see Bate and Jones (2008).

Rather than continuing to give more theoretical results on the construction of optimal cross-over designs, we refer the reader to the excellent book by Bose and Dey (2009), which contains many of the most useful theoretical results. Also, for an updated review of developments in the design of cross-over trials, see Bose and Dey (2013).

For completeness, we note that some earlier reviews of the optimality results for cross-over designs have been given by Stufken (1996). See also Afsarinejad (1990), Hedayat and Zhao (1990), Stufken (1991), Kunert (1991), Jones et al. (1992), Collombier and Merchermek (1993), Matthews (1990, 1994a,b), Kushner (1997a,b, 1998, 1999) and Martin and Eccleston (1998).

Before we leave this section we should emphasize that when planning a trial there will be a number of different criteria that we will want the design to satisfy. Optimal design theory concentrates our attention on a particular aspect of the designs, e.g., average variance, and ignores the rest. Therefore the investigator who is planning a trial should try to achieve what we term *practical optimality*. This requires taking into account such things as:

1. the likelihood of drop-outs if the number of periods is large;
2. whether or not the staff who will run the trial will be able to successfully administer the treatments correctly if the design plan is at all complicated;
3. whether those who have to make use of the results of the trial will find it difficult to interpret the results obtained from a rather complicated design.

Although this list could be extended, it is long enough to make the point that in the planning of a trial every aspect must be carefully reconciled. Also, if we change the model we assume for the data to be collected in the trial, then we should not be surprised if the optimal design changes, too.

4.4 Which variance-balanced design to use?

It should be clear from Section 4.2 that there are a great many balanced designs to choose from. In Tables 4.21 to 4.23 we give the efficiencies of a selection of designs for $t \leq 9$. The purpose of Tables 4.21 to 4.23 is to illustrate the

Table 4.21: Balanced designs for $t = 3$ and 4.

t	Design	p	n	E_d	E_c
3	PL1	2	6	18.75	6.25
3	BAL	2	9	25.00	12.50
3	WD	3	6	80.00	44.44
3	LSB	3	6	21.67	18.06
3	PL30(EP)	3	9	66.67	55.56
3	BAL(EP)	3	9	44.44	44.44
3	WD(EP)	4	6	93.75	75.00
3	FA(1,2)	4	6	75.00	60.00
3	ATK	6	6	86.21	69.44
3	BER	6	9	100.00	80.55
3	QUE	6	18	100.00	80.55
3	FA(2,1)	7	3	76.53	66.96
3	ATK	7	6	92.60	81.03
4	PL3	2	12	22.22	8.33
4	BAL	2	16	25.00	12.50
4	PL4	3	12	71.96	41.98
4	PL32(EP)	3	12	59.26	51.85
4	LSB	3	12	21.16	18.52
4	BAL(EP)	3	16	44.44	44.44
4	BIB	3	24	71.96	41.98
4	WD	4	6	90.91	62.50
4	PL33(EP)	4	6	83.33	68.75
4	OLS	4	12	90.91	62.50
4	WD(EP)	5	4	96.00	80.00
4	OLS(EP)	5	12	96.00	80.00
4	FA(1,3)	5	12	87.11	72.59
4	ATK	8	4	83.64	71.88
4	BER	8	16	100.00	85.94
4	FA(2,3)	9	12	88.89	80.00

Table 4.22: Balanced designs for $t = 5$ and 6.

t	Design	p	n	E_d	E_c
5	PL7	2	20	23.44	9.38
5	BAL	2	25	25.00	12.50
5	PL36(EP)	3	20	55.66	50.00
5	PL8	3	20	67.90	40.74
5	LSB	3	20	20.83	18.75
5	BAL(EP)	3	25	44.44	44.44
5	PL9	4	20	85.38	59.76
5	PL37(EP)	4	20	78.13	65.63
5	WD	5	10	94.74	72.00
5	PT	5	15	94.74	72.00
5	PL38(EP)	5	20	90.00	76.00
5	OLS	5	20	94.74	72.00
5	FA(1,1)	6	5	13.89	11.90
5	WD(EP)	6	10	97.22	83.33
5	OLS(EP)	6	20	97.22	83.33
5	FA(1,4)	6	20	97.06	76.27
6	PL12	2	30	24.00	10.00
6	BAL	2	36	25.00	12.50
6	PL41(EP)	3	30	53.33	48.89
6	LSB	3	30	20.61	18.89
6	BAL(EP)	3	36	44.44	44.44
6	PL13	5	30	91.00	69.76
6	WD	6	6	96.55	77.78
6	PL24(EP)	6	30	93.33	80.56
6	WD(EP)	7	6	97.96	85.71

features of the designs which were noted in Section 4.2 and to provide information that can be used to choose a design for particular values of t, p and n. In Tables 4.21 to 4.23 the designs have been identified using the following abbreviations: PLNN — design NN from Patterson and Lucas (1962); BAL — Balaam (1968); WD — Williams (1949); OLS — Orthogonal Latin squares; FA(q,s) — Federer and Atkinson (1964) with parameters q and s; LSB — Lucas (1957); ATK — Atkinson (1966); BER — Berenblut (1964); QUE — Quenouille (1953); BIB — constructed using a balanced incomplete block design; ADST - Archdeacon et al. (1980); PT — triple Latin square design from Prescott (1999); (EP) — design is of the extra-period type.

Tables 4.21 to 4.23 illustrate quite clearly some of the points already made in Sections 4.2 and 4.3:

1. The two-period designs, the switch-back designs and Balaam's designs have low efficiencies and should be avoided if at all possible.

Table 4.23: Balanced designs for $t = 7$, 8 and 9.

t	Design	p	n	E_d	E_c
7	PL16	2	42	24.30	10.44
7	BAL	2	49	25.00	12.50
7	PL17	3	21	63.82	39.51
7	LSB	3	42	20.44	18.98
7	PL43(EP)	3	42	51.85	48.15
7	BAL(EP)	3	49	44.44	44.44
7	PL19	4	14	79.84	57.03
7	PL44(EP)	4	21	72.92	62.50
7	PL46(EP)	5	14	84.00	72.00
7	PL21	5	21	88.49	68.27
7	PL48(EP)	6	21	90.74	78.70
7	PL23	6	42	93.89	76.00
7	WD	7	14	97.56	81.63
7	PT	7	21	97.56	81.63
7	PL23(EP)	7	42	95.24	83.67
7	OLS	7	42	97.56	81.63
7	WD(EP)	8	14	98.44	87.50
8	WD	8	8	98.18	84.38
8	WD(EP)	9	8	98.76	88.89
9	ADST	9	9	98.59	86.42
9	ADST(EP)	10	9	99.00	90.00

2. For $p = t$, the minimal balanced designs are optimal and (b) for $p = t + 1$, the corresponding extra-period designs are optimal. (This, of course, illustrates the optimality results of Cheng and Wu (1980).)
3. For $p \neq t$ or $p \neq t + 1$, the choice of design depends on p and n. So, for example, if $3 \leq p < t \leq 7$ and we ignore any restrictions on n, good choices of design, in the notation $(t, p, n,$ design), are (4,3,12,PL4); (5,4,20,PL9); (5,3,20,PL8); (6,5,30,PL13); (6,3,30,PL41(EP)); (7,6,42,PL23); (7,5,21,PL21); (7,4,14,PL19); (7,3,21,PL17).

If no balanced design can be chosen to fit in with our particular choice of t, p and n, and there is no possibility of changing this choice, then the partially balanced designs which we describe in the next section may provide useful alternatives.

4.5 Partially balanced designs

It sometimes happens that, although a balanced design is required, it is not possible to construct one for the available number of subjects and the chosen values of t and p. In these circumstances a useful compromise is to use a partially balanced (PB) design. Even if a balanced design can be constructed, PB designs may be preferred, as they are such that $p < t$ and they usually require far fewer subjects. The characteristic feature of a PB design is that $\text{Var}[\hat{\tau}_i - \hat{\tau}_j]$ (and $\text{Var}[\hat{\lambda}_i - \hat{\lambda}_j]$) depends on the pair of treatments, i and j, being compared. In balanced designs these variances are constant. In this section we will describe a number of methods of constructing partially balanced designs and at the end give a table of useful designs. This table can be used to help pick a suitable design for a given trial.

Before we can sensibly explain how to construct PB cross-over designs, we must first define what is meant by a **PB incomplete block design** (PBIB, for short) as used in non-cross-over experiments. By a non-cross-over experiment we mean one in which each subject receives only one of the t treatments. In an incomplete block design the experimental units are grouped into b homogeneous blocks of size p, where $p < t$. One way of characterizing a PBIB is in terms of how many associate classes it has. If a PBIB has m associate classes, then there will be m different values for $\text{Var}[\hat{\tau}_i - \hat{\tau}_j]$ (where $\hat{\tau}_i$ and $\hat{\tau}_j$ here refer to treatment estimators in the non-cross-over design). For convenience we will refer to these designs as PBIB (m) designs. The simplest and potentially most useful designs are the PBIB(2) designs and these have been extensively cataloged by Clatworthy (1973). In these designs the treatments are assigned to the blocks in such a way that each treatment occurs 0 or 1 times in each block and each pair of treatments occurs together in the same block either α_1 times or α_2 times where $\alpha_1 \neq \alpha_2$. If we assume that $\alpha_1 > \alpha_2$, then the pairs of treatments that occur together in α_1 blocks are first associates and the other pairs are second associates. The efficiency of comparisons between first associates is higher than that of comparisons between second associates. Clatworthy's catalog not only gives the plans of a great many PBIB(2) designs but also the corresponding efficiencies, E_1 and E_2, of treatment differences between first- and second-associates, respectively, and $\bar{E}$, the average efficiency of the design.

The average efficiency is defined as

$$\bar{E} = \sum_{i=1}^{t-1} \sum_{j=i+1}^{t} \frac{2E_{ij}}{t(t-1)},$$

where E_{ij} is the efficiency of the estimated difference between treatments i and j.

The average efficiency is a useful measure for comparing designs which have two or more associate classes. Unless a design with a particular pattern of pair-wise efficiencies is required, the design of choice will be the one with the highest average efficiency.

Also given by Clatworthy is the association scheme of each design, which specifies which pairs of treatments are first associates and which pairs are second associates.

Table 4.24: Biswas and Raghavarao design for $t = 4$, $p = 3$.

Subject	Period		
	1	2	3
1	A	B	C
2	B	A	C
3	A	B	D
4	B	A	D
5	C	D	A
6	D	C	A
7	C	D	B
8	D	C	B

To illustrate the above points let us look at the design labeled as S1 in Clatworthy's catalog. This design is for $t = 6$, $b = 3$ and $p = 4$ and is of the group-divisible type. The blocks of the design are (ADBE), (BECF) and (CFAD) and its association scheme can be written as

A D
B E
C F

The treatments in the same row of this scheme are first associates and those in the same column are second associates.

The above definition of a PBIB(2) is extended in an obvious way to PBIB(m) designs. A more formal definition of a PBIB(m) and numerous related references can be found in Raghavarao (1971), Chapter 8.

In the following we describe some PB cross-over designs that have been suggested by various authors. At the end of this section we give a table of useful designs.

Biswas and Raghavarao (1998) also gave methods of constructing group divisible designs and their design for $t = 4$, $k = 3$ is given in Table 4.24.

The PB designs of Patterson and Lucas

In this method, which was first described by Patterson and Lucas (1962), we take a PBIB(2) from Clatworthy's catalog and replace each block of the design by a balanced cross-over design for p treatments. This is the same method that was used in Section 4.2 to construct balanced cross-over designs using BIB designs.

To illustrate the method let us take the PBIB(2) design S1 which was described in the previous subsection. Each block of this design contains four treatments and so we need to find a balanced cross-over design for four treatments. Such a design was given earlier in Table 4.4. We replace each block of the PBIB(2) design with the design given in Table 4.4, and relabel the treatments so that they correspond to those in the block under consideration. The

Table 4.25: PB design constructed from PBIB(2) design S1.

Subject	Period			
	1	2	3	4
1	A	D	B	E
2	D	E	A	B
3	B	A	E	D
4	E	B	D	A
5	B	E	C	F
6	E	F	B	C
7	C	B	F	E
8	F	C	E	B
9	C	F	A	D
10	F	D	C	A
11	A	C	D	F
12	D	A	F	C

complete cross-over design is then as given in Table 4.25. If we always use a Williams design as our balanced design, then the final cross-over designs for p periods will require bp subjects if p is even and $2bp$ subjects if p is odd. The efficiencies of the design in Table 4.25 are $E_{d1} = 90.91$, $E_{d2} = 78.29$, $E_{c1} = 62.50$ and $E_{c2} = 56.51$, where $E_{d1}(E_{c1})$ is the efficiency of the estimated difference between two first-associate direct (carry-over) effects and $E_{d2}(E_{c2})$ is the efficiency of the estimated difference between second-associate direct (carry-over) effects. Naturally, the association scheme of the parent PBIB(2) design will also apply to the cross-over design constructed from it and the efficiencies of the final design will reflect those of the parent design used to construct it.

In a similar way to that done previously we define $\bar{E}_d$ as the average efficiency of the direct treatment comparisons and $\bar{E}_c$ as the average efficiency of the carry-over comparisons.

As with the balanced designs, if necessary, the treatments in the last period of a partially balanced design can be repeated in an extra period to increase the relative efficiency of the estimated carry-over effects.

It will be recalled that if periods are removed from a balanced design which is made up of a complete set of orthogonal Latin squares, the depleted design is still balanced. We can therefore repeat the above construction procedure using a depleted design obtained from a complete set of Latin squares. Unfortunately, as the complete set of squares for p periods requires $p(p-1)$ subjects, the final cross-over design will be very large if p is bigger than 3 or 4. When $p = 3$ in the original set of squares, however, we can, as done by Patterson and Lucas, apply the procedure to construct a number of PB cross-over designs which require only two periods. Of course, as already noted in Section 4.2, two-period designs have low efficiencies and should, if possible, be avoided. However, these two-period designs provide yet another set of designs to which an extra period can be added.

The cyclic PB designs of Davis and Hall

Davis and Hall (1969) proposed a series of PB cross-over designs which were obtained from cyclic incomplete block designs (CIBDs). A CIBD is constructed by cyclically developing one or more generating sequences of treatments. For example, if for $t = 6$ a generating sequence is (0132), where 0 represents treatment A, 1 represents treatment B, and so on, then the blocks generated are (0132), (1243), (2354), (3405), (4510) and (5021). We see in this example that the entries in a block are obtained by adding 1 to the entries of the previous block, subject to the restriction that numbers above 5 are reduced modulo 5. In our notation the blocks of the design are then (ABDC), (BCED), (CDFE), (DEAF), (EFBA) and (FACB). Davis and Hall's method is to consider the blocks of the CIBD as the treatment sequences to be applied to the subjects. From the large number of CIBDs available in the literature they selected those which required fewer units than the PB designs of Patterson and Lucas and which had comparable efficiencies. A feature of the selected designs is that, although there may be up to $[t/2]$ associate classes, the efficiencies of the estimated differences between pairs of treatments do not differ very much from each other.

As an example, we give in Table 4.26 the design obtained when the generating sequences are (0132) and (0314). The first sequence which was used as our illustration in the previous paragraph does not generate a useful cross-over design when used alone: when used in conjunction with the second sequence, however, a useful design results. This design has three associate classes.

Table 4.26: PB cyclic design generated by (0132) and (0314).

Subject	Period			
	1	2	3	4
1	A	B	D	C
2	B	C	E	D
3	C	D	F	E
4	D	E	A	F
5	E	F	B	A
6	F	A	C	B
7	A	D	B	E
8	B	E	C	F
9	C	F	D	A
10	D	A	E	B
11	E	B	F	C
12	F	C	A	D

Table 4.27: Numbers of treatments, periods and subjects.

Series	Number of treatments	Number of periods	Number of subjects
R1	$v = 2q$ ($q >= 4$ and even)	$q+1$	$2q$
R2	$v = 3q$ ($q >= 3$ and odd)	$q+1$	$6q$
T1	$v = q(q-1)/2$ ($q >= 5$ and odd)	$q-1$	$q(q-1)$
T2	$v = q(q-1)/2$ ($q >= 4$ and even)	$q-1$	$2q(q-1)$

The PB designs of Blaisdell and Raghavarao

Blaisdell (1978) and Blaisdell and Raghavarao (1980) described the construction of four different series of PB cross-over designs. Two of the series, which they labeled as R1 and R2, have three associate classes and the other two, which they labeled as T1 and T2, have two associate classes. The association scheme of the R1 and R2 designs is the rectangular scheme defined by Vartak (1955) and the association scheme of the T1 and T2 designs is the triangular scheme defined by Bose and Shimamoto (1952). The number of treatments, periods and subjects required by each of the four series is given in Table 4.27.

It can be seen that the R1 designs are for $8, 12, 16, \ldots,$ treatments, the R2 designs are for $9, 15, 21, \ldots$ treatments, the T1 designs are for $10, 21, 36, \ldots$ treatments and the T2 designs are for $6, 15, 28, \ldots$ treatments. As it is unusual for clinical trials to compare large numbers of treatments, it is clear that the four series of designs are of limited usefulness in the clinical trials context. The average efficiencies ($\bar{E}_d$,$\bar{E}_c$) of their designs for $t = 6$, 8 and 9 are, respectively, (63.57, 39.73), (80.38, 51.26) and (70.94, 41.28).

The cyclic designs of Iqbal and Jones

Iqbal and Jones (1994) gave tables of efficient cyclic designs for $t \leq 10$. These, like the designs of Davis and Hall described earlier, are such that they require t or a multiple of t subjects and the sequences are obtained by developing one or more sets of generating sequences. As an example, we give in Table 4.28 their design for $t = 9$ and $p = 8$. As with the designs of Davis and Hall, the designs of Iqbal and Jones are such that the set of values for the variances of the pairwise differences between the treatments may contain two or more values.

Tables of design

In Tables 4.29 and 4.30 we give a useful list of partially balanced designs. Alongside each set of values of t, p and n (the number of subjects), we give the source of the design, its average efficiencies and, for the cyclic designs, the generating sequences. The source of the design is given as (1) PB2(N) — a Patterson and Lucas, two-associate class, design constructed using design N, (2) DH — a Davis and Hall design, (3) IJ — an Iqbal and Jones design, (4) R

Table 4.28: Iqbal and Jones cyclic design generated by (06725381).

Subject	Period							
	1	2	3	4	5	6	7	8
1	A	G	H	C	F	D	I	B
2	B	H	I	D	G	E	A	C
3	C	I	A	E	H	F	B	D
4	D	A	B	F	I	G	C	E
5	E	B	C	G	A	H	D	F
6	F	C	D	H	B	I	E	G
7	G	D	E	I	C	A	F	H
8	H	E	F	A	D	B	G	I
9	I	F	G	B	E	C	H	A

— a nearly balanced design due to Russell (1991) and (5) BR — a Biswas and Raghavarao design.

4.6 Comparing test treatments to a control

Pigeon (1984) and Pigeon and Raghavarao (1987) proposed some designs for the situation where one treatment is a *control* or standard and is to be compared to t test treatments (i.e., there are $t+1$ treatments in the trial). The characteristic feature of these **control balanced** designs is that pairwise comparisons between the control and the test treatments are made more precisely than pairwise comparisons between the test treatments. The precision of comparisons between the test treatments has been sacrificed in order to achieve high precision on comparisons with the control.

An example of a control balanced design for $t = 3$ is given in Table 4.31, where X denotes the control treatment and A, B and C denote the test treatments. If τ_x is the direct effect of the control treatment and λ_x is the corresponding carry-over effect, then the variance properties of the control balanced designs are (for $i \neq j \neq x$):

$$\text{Var}[\hat{\tau}_x - \hat{\tau}_i] = c_1\sigma^2\,, \quad \text{Var}[\hat{\tau}_i - \hat{\tau}_j] = c_2\sigma^2,$$
$$\text{Var}[\hat{\lambda}_x - \hat{\lambda}_i] = c_3\sigma^2, \quad \text{Var}[\hat{\lambda}_i - \hat{\lambda}_j] = c_4\sigma^2$$

where c_1, c_2, c_3 and c_4 are such that $c_1 < c_2 < c_3 < c_4$. The values of c_1, c_2, c_3 and c_4 for the design in Table 4.31 are 0.372, 0.491, 0.648 and 0.818, respectively.

A number of methods of constructing control balanced designs were described by Pigeon and Raghavarao, and their paper should be consulted for details.

We can change each of the control balanced designs into an extra-period design with similar variance properties by repeating the treatment given in the last period. This has the effect of making the direct and carry-over effects

Table 4.29: Some PB cross-over designs for $t \leq 9$ and $p \leq t$.

t	p	n	Source	$\bar{E}_d$	$\bar{E}_c$	Generating sequence
4	3	8	BR	70.30	35.05	
5	3	10	IJ	61.44	38.09	(013)(032)
5	3	30	PB2(C12)	66.85	40.59	
5	4	5	IJ	77.31	54.12	(0143)
5	4	10	IJ	84.00	58.55	(0143)(0412)
5	5	5	R	81.24	61.74	
6	3	12	DH	58.42	34.22	(034)(051)
6	3	18	IJ	62.74	38.46	(014)(021)(031)
6	3	24	PB2(SR18)	63.57	39.73	
6	3	36	PB2(R42)	64.55	39.88	
6	3	48	PB2(SR19)	93.57	39.73	
6	4	6	IJ	76.25	53.30	(0154)
6	4	12	DH	81.32	57.44	(0132)(0314)
6	4	18	IJ	81.05	56.91	(0132)(02253)(0142)
6	4	24	PB2(R94)	81.56	57.96	
6	4	36	PB2(SR35)	81.87	58.06	
6	4	48	PB2(R96)	81.98	58.10	
6	5	6	DH	85.86	65.64	(01325)
6	5	12	IJ	87.60	67.18	(01542)(022541)
7	3	14	DH	62.42	35.57	(031)(045)
7	4	21	IJ	77.33	54.65	(0124)(0251)(0631)
7	5	7	DH	80.29	61.11	(02315)
7	5	14	IJ	85.79	66.16	(01632)(02564)
7	6	7	IJ	90.50	73.19	(014652)
7	6	21	IJ	93.23	75.44	(014652)(016325)
7	7	7	R	91.78	76.80	

orthogonal and reducing the variances of the carry-over effects. The values of $c_i, i = 1,2,3$ and 4, for some of the control balanced designs for up to five test treatments are given in Table 4.32.

Optimality results for designs that compare test treatments with controls have been given by Hedayat et al. (1988).

4.7 Factorial treatment combinations

It is not unusual in drug-trial work to administer treatments that are made up of combinations of more than one drug. Among the reasons for doing this are to determine if a combination of drugs is more efficacious than using a single drug; to investigate the joint actions of drugs that are usually prescribed for

Table 4.30: Some PB cross-over designs for $t \leq 9$ and $p \leq t$, continued.

t	p	n	Source	$\bar{E}_d$	$\bar{E}_c$	Generating sequence
8	3	16	DH	54.59	31.99	(041)(065)
8	3	48	PB2(R54)	61.68	39.02	
8	4	8	IJ	63.19	40.21	(0467)
8	4	16	DH	77.28	54.87	(0214)(0153)
8	4	24	IJ	77.49	54.99	(0612)(0254)(0273)
8	4	32	PB2(SR36)	76.93	55.80	
8	4	40	PB2(R97)	78.04	56.18	
8	4	48	PB2(SR38)	77.99	56.16	
8	5	8	DH	78.67	59.06	(01325)
8	5	16	IJ	77.49	54.99	(01532)(03746)
8	6	24	PB2(S18)	91.71	74.59	
8	7	8	IJ	93.15	78.13	(0342157)
8	7	24	IJ	95.12	79.81	(0546731)(0132647) (0342715)
9	3	18	DH	54.74	31.18	(038)(067)
9	3	54	PB2(SR23)	60.28	38.67	
9	4	9	IJ	63.43	45.36	(0352)
9	4	18	DH	74.36	53.61	(0142)(0526)
9	4	27	IJ	76.22	54.69	(0137)(0317)(0851)
9	4	36	PB2(LS26)	76.23	55.40	
9	5	9	DH	63.43	45.36	(0352)
9	5	18	IJ	85.14	65.96	(01724)(08475)
9	6	9	IJ	85.86	69.12	(013286)
9	6	18	PB2(S21)	89.36	73.15	
9	6	36	PB2(LS72)	90.20	73.59	
9	6	54	PB2(SR65)	90.44	73.72	
9	7	9	IJ	90.57	76.02	(0152764)
9	7	18	IJ	92.82	78.05	(0236187)(0184632)
9	8	9	IJ	94.83	81.63	(06725381)

different conditions; and that one drug is being used to combat an unpleasant side-effect of another. In this section we will consider treatments that are made up of all possible combinations of the chosen drug dose levels. In the terminology of factorial experiments, each drug is a **factor** and can be administered at a number of different **levels**. A treatment made up by combining one dose level from each of the drugs is called a **factorial treatment combination**.

To take our brief introduction to factorial experiments a little further, consider, as an example, a trial in which the four treatments are (1) no treatment (2) drug A at a fixed dose, (3) drug B at a fixed dose and (4) drugs A and B together at the same fixed doses as in treatments (2) and (3). Here the two

Table 4.31: A control balanced design for $t = 3$.

Subject	Period 1	2	3
1	X	A	B
2	X	B	C
3	X	C	A
4	A	X	C
5	B	X	A
6	C	X	B
7	A	C	X
8	B	A	X
9	C	B	X

Table 4.32: Variances of contrasts in Pigeon's designs.

t	p	n	c_1	c_2	c_3	c_4
3	3	9	0.3720	0.4909	0.6477	0.8182
3	3	21	0.1666	0.1896	0.2882	0.3214
3	3	30	0.1147	0.1367	0.1989	0.2308
4	3	28	0.1540	0.2037	0.2608	0.3333
4	3	38	0.1159	0.1440	0.1957	0.2368
4	3	36	0.1174	0.1741	0.1992	0.2812
4	4	16	0.1665	0.1995	0.2395	0.2832
4	4	36	0.0775	0.0844	0.1110	0.1203
5	3	20	0.2628	0.3482	0.4368	0.5625
5	3	30	0.1704	0.2698	0.2839	0.4286
5	4	40	0.0784	0.1044	0.1118	0.1461
5	5	25	0.0972	0.1110	0.1272	0.1445

factors are the drugs A and B and each factor takes the levels no dose or the fixed dose for that drug. A standard way of labeling the treatment combinations is to use 0 to indicate that the factor (i.e., drug) is being used at its lower level (i.e., no dose in our example) and to use a 1 to indicate that the factor is being used at its higher level (i.e., at the fixed dose level). The four treatments, in the order listed above, can then be denoted by 00, 10, 01 and 11, respectively. In a different trial, the labels 0 and 1 might actually represent low dose and high dose rather than absence and presence.

Clearly this system of labeling can be extended to more than two factors and/or to more than two levels. For example, if there are three drugs, the first of which can be administered at three equally spaced doses (no dose, low dose, high dose) and the second and third can be administered at two doses (no dose, fixed dose), then the first factor has three levels and the other two factors have two levels. If we label the levels of the first drug as 0, 1 and 2, and label the levels of the other two drugs as 0 and 1, then the twelve factorial treatment combinations are 000, 001, 010, 011, 100, 101, 110, 111, 200, 201, 210 and 211. By convention we would call this trial a $3 \times 2 \times 2$ factorial. The trial used as our example at the beginning of this section is a 2×2 factorial.

In a factorial experiment the contrasts between the treatments that are of most interest are the main effects and interactions of the factors. In order to explain these terms a little more fully let us again refer to our 2×2 example. It will be recalled that the four treatment combinations are 00, 10, 01 and 11. Let us denote the corresponding direct effects of these combinations as τ_1, τ_2, τ_3 and τ_4, respectively. The three direct contrasts of interest are then as follows:

1. the main effect of drug A = $\frac{1}{2}(-\tau_1 + \tau_2 - \tau_3 + \tau_4)$;
2. the main effect of drug B = $\frac{1}{2}(-\tau_1 - \tau_2 + \tau_3 + \tau_4)$;
3. the interaction of drugs A and B = $\frac{1}{2}(\tau_1 - \tau_2 - \tau_3 + \tau_4)$.

By convention we label these contrasts as A_d, B_d and $A_d \times B_d$, respectively, where the d indicates that we are taking contrasts of the direct effects.

We can see that the main effect A_d is a measure of the change brought about by changing the levels of drug A, averaged over the levels of drug B, i.e., $A_d = \frac{1}{2}[(\tau_2 - \tau_1) + (\tau_4 - \tau_3)]$. Similarly, B_d is a measure of the change brought about by changing the levels of drug B averaged over the levels of drug A. The interaction $A_d \times B_d$ is a measure of how changing the levels of A depends on the level chosen for B, i.e., $\frac{1}{2}(\tau_2 - \tau_1) - \frac{1}{2}(\tau_4 - \tau_2)$. (Of course, $A_d \times B_d$ is also a measure of how changing the levels of B depends on A.)

The attraction of the factorial experiment is that it allows us the possibility of detecting interactions and in the absence of interactions, to obtain information on the separate effects of each drug (i.e., the main effects) using a single trial.

So far in this section we have not mentioned the carry-over effects. In our 2×2 example there are four treatments and we would, as usual, include the carry-over effects λ_1, λ_2, λ_3 and λ_4 in our fitted model. If there is evidence of significant carry-over, then we can obtain a better understanding of the form it takes by looking at the carry-over main effects and interactions. These contrasts, which are labeled using the subscript c, are as follows:

1. $A_c = \frac{1}{2}(-\lambda_1 + \lambda_2 - \lambda_3 + \lambda_4)$;
2. $B_c = \frac{1}{2}(-\lambda_1 - \lambda_2 + \lambda_3 + \lambda_4)$;
3. $A_c \times B_c = \frac{1}{2}(\lambda_1 - \lambda_2 - \lambda_3 + \lambda_4)$.

That is, they correspond exactly to the contrasts used for the direct effects.

A crucially important feature of the factorial experiment is that there is a well-defined structure among the treatment combinations. For example, the treatments can be subdivided into sets which have the same level of a particular factor, e.g., (00,01) and (10,11) in our 2×2 example. When there is structure we are usually no longer interested in all pairwise differences between the treatments but in particular differences or particular contrasts. Naturally, we will want a design which estimates the contrasts of interest with as high an efficiency as possible. For example, if the separate effects of the two drugs in our 2×2 experiment are well known and it is their joint effect that is of interest, then the main effects are of much less interest than the interaction. A design which estimates the interaction with as high an efficiency as possible would then be the design of choice. In order to achieve high efficiency of estimation of the contrasts of interest, we will usually be happy to accept a low efficiency on the contrasts of little or no interest. If this is the case, then the balanced and completely balanced designs will not be the most suitable designs. In these designs the main effects and interactions are estimated with equal efficiency.

The type of design we seek for factorial experiments must take account of the structure of the treatments, the need to estimate effects with different efficiencies and the need to retain a sufficient degree of balance to keep the data analysis relatively simple. The designs which come closest to satisfying these requirements are the ones which possess **factorial structure**. A design is said to possess factorial structure if and only if

1. estimates of the direct treatment contrasts belonging to different factorial effects are orthogonal;
2. estimates of the carry-over treatment contrasts belonging to different factorial effects are orthogonal;
3. estimates of direct treatment contrasts and estimates of carry-over contrasts belonging to different factorial effects are orthogonal.

This definition is taken from Fletcher and John (1985) and is a generalization of one given by Cotter et al. (1973) for non-cross-over block designs.

The attractiveness of factorial structure is enhanced by the availability of a large number of cross-over designs that possess this structure. Fletcher and John (1985) showed that the generalized cyclic designs (GC/n designs, for short) of John (1973) provide a flexible class of cross-over designs that possess factorial structure.

Fletcher (1987) considered the construction of cross-over designs using GC/n designs and gave a list of suitable designs for up to six periods for the 2×2, 2×3, 2×4, 3×3, 4×4, $2 \times 2 \times 2$ and $3 \times 3 \times 3$ factorial experiments. Fletcher's designs are such that the main effects are estimated with a higher efficiency than the interactions. An example of one of the Fletcher (1987) designs for the 2×2 factorial is given in Table 4.33.

Lewis et al. (1988) constructed cross-over designs for factorial experiments by joining together one or more **bricks**. A brick is made up of one or more GC/n cross-over designs. By combining different bricks, designs that have different patterns of efficiencies can be obtained. Jones (1985) used a similar technique to construct block designs for non-cross-over experiments. Lewis et al. (1988) gave a selection of designs for the 2×2, 2×3, 2×4, and 3×3

Table 4.33: Generalized cyclic design for the 2×2 factorial.

Subject	Period		
1	00	01	11
2	01	00	10
3	10	11	01
4	11	10	00

factorials that used three or four periods. In some of these designs the interactions are estimated with higher efficiencies than the main effects.

From a historical point of view we should note that Seath (1944) described a three-period 2×2 factorial for comparing two different diets for dairy cows. Also, Patterson (1952) showed that designs for the 2×2 and $2 \times 2 \times 2$ experiments could be obtained by using some or all of the subjects from a balanced design constructed from a set of mutually orthogonal Latin squares. Patterson also showed how confounding can be introduced into the design by arranging the subjects into blocks which correspond to the Latin squares or rectangles.

Russell and Dean (1998) constructed efficient designs for factorial experiments that require a relatively small number of subjects. Lewis and Russell (1998) considered designs with carry-over effects from two factors.

In the case of a two-factor experiment it may be the case that the levels of one factor need to be administered for a longer period than the levels of the other. An illustration of such a situation is given by Altan et al. (1996). An example of such a design for a 2×2 factorial trial with four periods is given in Table 4.34 and was given by Biswas (1997). See also Raghavarao and Xie (2003) and Dean et al. (1999)

4.8 Extending the simple model for carry-over effects

The simple model for carry-over effects which we have used so far in this book states that the first-order carry-over effect of a treatment is additive and a constant for that treatment. It implies, for instance, that the carry-over effect of a treatment is always present and that the carry-over of a treatment given in a previous period does not depend on the treatment in the current period. So, for

Table 4.34: Split-plot design for the 2×2 factorial.

Subject	Period			
1	00	01	10	11
2	00	01	11	10
3	01	10	00	11
4	01	10	00	11

example, in the two-period Balaam design (Section 3.3) for two treatments, which has sequences AB, BA, AA and BB, the simple model assumes that the carry-over of A from the first period in sequence AB is the same as the carry-over from the first period in sequence AA. The validity of such an assumption has long been questioned (see Fleiss (1986), for example). A situation where the simple model may not be true is when A is an effective drug that reaches its maximum effect in every period and has a strong additive carry-over effect, but B is a relatively ineffective treatment. In the second period of the sequence AA, the strong carry-over effect of A has no impact on the observed response to A, because A cannot be increased any more as it has already reached its maximum effect. However, in the sequence AB, the strong carry-over effect of A will increase (or decrease) the observed response to B in the second period. In another situation, when one of the treatments is a placebo, there is no reason to expect a pharmacological carry-over effect into a following period as there should be no active drug ingredients in the placebo. Hence a realistic model for pharmacological carry-over effects in a trial that contains a placebo treatment would not include a carry-over parameter for placebo, but there may be carry-over parameters for the other active treatments. Senn (1993), Chapter 10 has argued forcefully that simple mathematical models of the type so far used in this book are unrealistic and any optimality properties claimed for designs based on these models should be treated with caution. Kunert and Stufken (2002) and Afsarinejad and Hedayat (2002) give optimality results and construction methods for a more general model for carry-over effects. In this model there are two types of carry-over effect: self and mixed. A self carry-over effect is the carry-over effect of a treatment into a following period that contains the same treatment that produced the carry-over effect. A mixed/simple carry-over effect is a carry-over effect of a treatment into a following period that contains a different treatment.

Jones and Donev (1996) described a series of alternative models for the direct treatment and carry-over effects: *Placebo* where there is no carry-over from a placebo treatment, *No carry-over into self* where a treatment does not carry-over into itself and *Treatment decay* where there is no carry-over from a treatment into the following period if the latter period contains a different treatment, but if the following treatment contains the same treatment there is a negative carry-over effect. This last model is meant to represent, in a simple way, the phenomenon of treatments becoming less effective if they are used repeatedly. We more formally define these models and some others shortly.

However, while all models are strictly wrong, some may be useful approximations to reality. At the moment there is no body of strong empirical evidence to suggest that the conclusions obtained from simple models have seriously misled those who interpret the results from cross-over trials. Although this gives some reassurance, we should not be complacent. We should strive to use improved models for treatment and carry-over effects and to construct or search for designs which are optimal for these models. Indeed some progress has been made already and in the next section we will briefly review some of these developments.

4.9 Computer search algorithms

Although mathematical results which prove the optimality of classes of designs under some more general assumptions about the carry-over effects will be useful and of interest, it is likely that computer search algorithms will be of more practical use.

Jones and Donev (1996) described an exchange-interchange algorithm that searched for optimal cross-over designs for an arbitrary model for treatment and carry-over effects. They illustrated the use of the algorithm using a variety of examples and models. (See also Donev and Jones (1995) and Donev (1997).) Previously Eccleston and Street (1994) described a computer algorithm that searched for optimal designs based on the simple additive model for treatment and carry-over effects. Eccleston and Whitaker (1999) described a computer search algorithm based on simulated annealing that optimized a multi-objective function, but again based on the simple model for carry-over effects. Jones and Wang (1999) considered methods of constructing optimal cross-over designs for the situation where each subject in each period has a series of blood samples taken and the concentration of drug in the blood is modeled as a nonlinear function of time using pharmacokinetic compartmental models. Fedorov et al. (2002) described an approach to constructing optimal cross-over designs for nonlinear models for pharmacokinetic data that takes into account various costs related to taking the repeated blood samples.

John and Russell (2003) gave formulae for updating the direct and carry-over efficiency factors of a cross-over design as the result of interchanging two treatments. They assumed the simple additive model for treatments and carry-over effects. They also described a computer search algorithm that used these updating formulae. John and Russell (2002) described a unified theory for the construction of cross-over designs under a variety of models for the direct and carry-over effects. John and Whitaker (2002) developed this work further and described a computer algorithm that searches for cross-over designs that minimize or maximize a criterion based on the average variance of estimated pairwise differences between direct effects.

The R package *Crossover* (Rohmeyer (2014)), developed by Kornelius Rohmeyer to accompany this book, provides a graphical user interface (GUI) to select a design from a catalog and then to give its average efficiency and the efficiencies and variances of all pairwise comparisons of the treatments. The user can choose from a range of models for the carry-over effects, which are described below and are the models suggested by Jones and Donev (1996) and also used by John and Whitaker (2002). The designs in the catalog include some of those listed in the previous tables, but more designs will be added to the catalog over time.

The package also offers the option of searching for an optimal design, i.e., one that maximizes the average efficiency of the treatment comparisons, under the different carry-over models. The optimal design is searched for using a hill climbing interchange algorithm (see Rohmeyer and Jones (2015) for more details). The algorithm also allows the user a choice of models for the correlation structure of the within-subject errors: independence, compound symmetry and autoregressive. The latter two structures are defined by a single parameter ρ.

The different models for the carry-over effects included in the package are those suggested by Jones and Donev (1996), where β_{ij} is the model for treatments and carry-over effects for periods $j-1$ and j, $j>1$, in sequence i (John and Russell (2003)):

1. Additive:
$$\beta_{ij} = \tau_{d(i,j)} + \lambda_{d(i,j-1)}$$
2. Self adjacency:
$$\beta_{ij} = \begin{cases} \tau_{d(i,j)} + \lambda_{d(i,j-1)} & \text{if } d(i,j) \neq d(i,j-1) \\ \tau_{d(i,j)} + \lambda'_{d(i,j-1)} & \text{if } d(i,j) = d(i,j-1) \end{cases}$$
3. Proportionality:
$$\beta_{ij} = \tau_{d(i,j)} + R\tau_{d(i,j-1)}$$
4. Placebo model (first $t_0 < t$ treatments are placebos):
$$\beta_{ij} = \begin{cases} \tau_{d(i,j)} & \text{if } d(i,j-1) \leq t_0 \\ \tau_{d(i,j)} + \lambda_{d(i,j-1)} & \text{otherwise} \end{cases}$$
5. No carry-over into self:
$$\beta_{ij} = \begin{cases} \tau_{d(i,j)} & \text{if } d(i,j) = d(i,j-1) \text{ or } j = 1 \\ \tau_{d(i,j)} + \lambda_{d(i,j-1)} & \text{otherwise} \end{cases}$$
6. Treatment decay:
$$\beta_{ij} = \begin{cases} \tau_{d(i,j)} - \lambda_{d(i,j-1)} & \text{if } d(i,j) = d(i,j-1) \\ \tau_{d(i,j)} & \text{otherwise} \end{cases}$$
7. Interaction:
$$\beta_{ij} = \tau_{d(i,j)} + \lambda_{d(i,j-1)} + \gamma_{d(i,j),d(i,j-1)}$$
8. Second-order carry-over:
$$\beta_{ij} = \tau_{d(i,j)} + \lambda_{d(i,j-1)} + \theta_{d(i,j-2)}, \quad j > 2$$

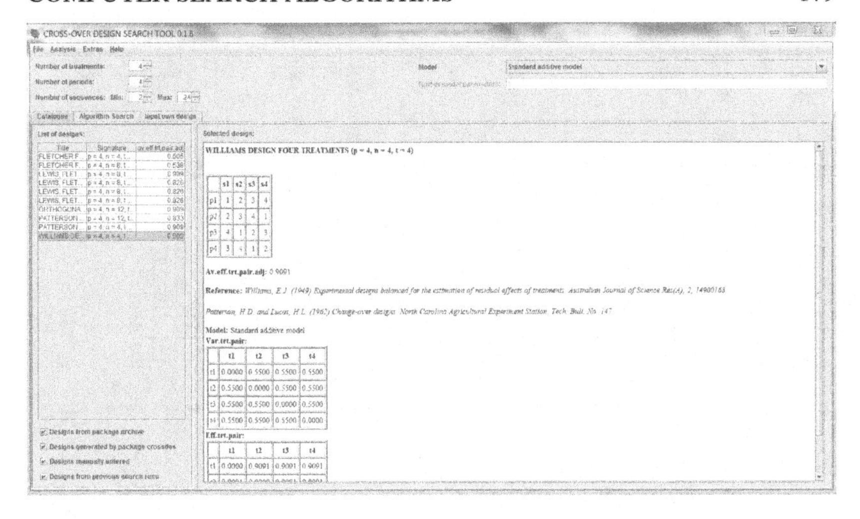

Figure 4.1: Screenshot from *Crossover* R package GUI: searching the catalog for a design with $t = 4$.

Using the catalog in the GUI

As an example of using the GUI we show in Figure 4.1 a screenshot for the case where a design for $t = 4$ treatments is required. Here the user enters the number of periods $p = 4$ and a minimum and maximum number of sequences (e.g., $s = 4$ and $s = 24$, respectively). We should note that, due to limitations of space on the page, this screenshot and the following three do not show the full extent of the image seen in the GUI.

As well as specifying values for t, p and s, the user also has to choose a model for the carry-over effects. Here the Standard Additive Model (model 1 in the list above) is chosen. We see that a choice of 10 designs is offered and the Williams design with 4 sequences has been selected. On the right of the figure we see the design, its average efficiency (0.9091) and the variances of each of the pairwise treatment comparisons. The GUI also displays the pairwise efficiencies (partly shown in Figure 4.1). Because this design is balanced, all the pairwise efficiencies are equal and, of course, equal the average efficiency of 0.9091.

It is also possible to directly input a design into the GUI and calculate its efficiencies and variances, but we do not illustrate that here.

Using the search algorithm in the GUI

As well as making it easy to choose among a set of alternative designs, the GUI also has an option to search for an efficient design. This option is particularly useful when there is not a design in the catalog for the given values of t, p and s, or if the designs in the catalog do not have a high enough efficiency and the user wishes to see if a better one can be found. To illustrate this option we will look for a design for $t = 6$, $p = 4$ and $s = 24$. Using the GUI, we can see

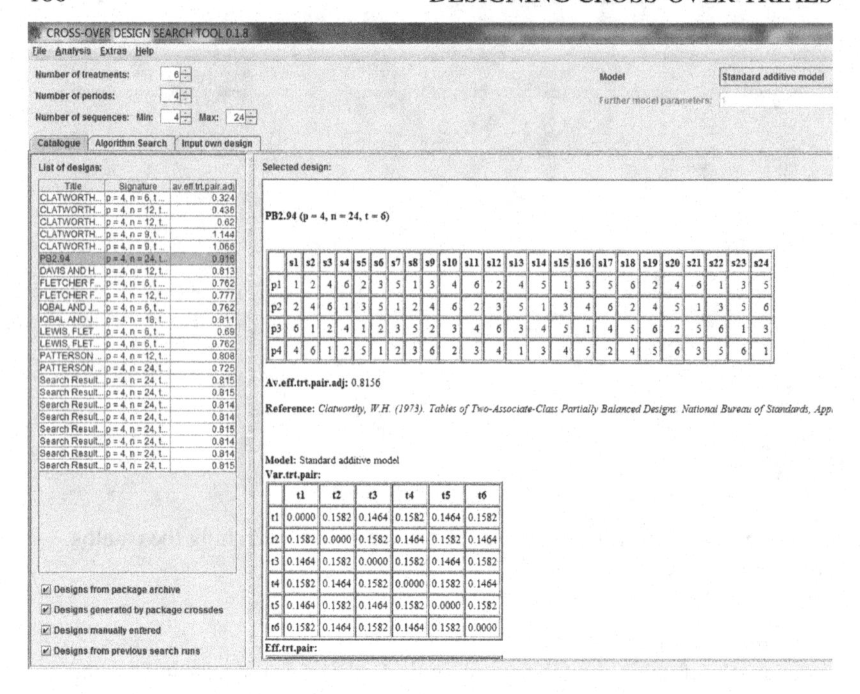

Figure 4.2: Screenshot from *Crossover* R package GUI: possible designs in the catalog for $t = 6$ and $p = 4$.

that there is a design in the catalog, PB2.94, which has an average efficiency of 0.8156 (see Figure 4.2). Let us see if the algorithm can find a design with a higher average efficiency.

The search algorithm has several parameters that can be set to modify the search. These are fully explained in the manual for the *Crossover* R package and in Rohmeyer and Jones (2015). For example, the optimality criterion for the standard additive model is a weighted sum of the average efficiencies of the pairwise treatment and pairwise carry-over comparisons and these weights can be specified. In this example the weights have been set to 1 and 0, respectively. Another parameter is the number of starting designs to use. For each randomly chosen starting design, the algorithm looks for a modification that will increase the efficiency of the design. The parameter that controls the maximum number of modifications (referred to as the number of steps) can also be specified. Using the standard settings for the search parameters (20 starting designs and 5000 steps), a design with an efficiency of 0.8151 was found quite quickly. To confirm that this is the best that could be found within a limited search time, the algorithm was run again with 50 starting designs and 10,000 steps. The design that was found had a higher average efficiency of 0.8171. However, the six treatments were not equally replicated in the design, with treatment 2

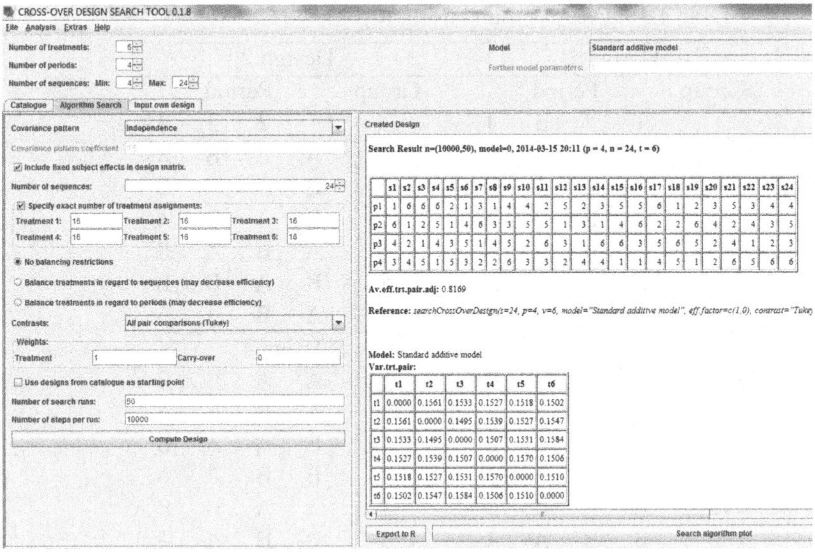
CROSS-OVER DESIGN SEARCH TOOL 0.1.8
File Analysis Extras Help
Number of treatments: 6
Number of periods: 4
Number of sequences: Min: 4 Max: 24
Model Standard additive model
Further model parameters:
Catalogue
Algorithm Search
Input own design
Covariance pattern Independence
Covariance pattern coefficient
Include fixed subject effects in design matrix.
Number of sequences: 24
Specify exact number of treatment assignments:
Treatment 1: 16 Treatment 2: 16 Treatment 3: 16
Treatment 4: 16 Treatment 5: 16 Treatment 6: 16
No balancing restrictions
Balance treatments in regard to sequences (may decrease efficiency)
Balance treatments in regard to periods (may decrease efficiency)
Contrasts: All pair comparisons (Tukey)
Weights:
Treatment 1 Carry-over 0
Use designs from catalogue as starting point
Number of search runs: 50
Number of steps per run: 10000
Compute Design
Created Design
Search Result n=(10000,50), model=0, 2014-03-15 20:11 (p = 4, n = 24, t = 6)
s1 s2 s3 s4 s5 s6 s7 s8 s9 s10 s11 s12 s13 s14 s15 s16 s17 s18 s19 s20 s21 s22 s23 s24
p1 1 6 6 6 2 1 3 1 4 4 2 5 2 3 5 5 6 1 2 3 5 3 4 4
p2 6 1 2 5 1 4 6 3 3 5 5 1 3 1 4 6 2 2 6 4 2 4 3 5
p3 4 2 1 4 3 5 1 4 5 2 6 3 1 6 6 3 5 6 5 2 4 1 2 3
p4 3 4 5 1 5 3 2 2 6 3 3 2 4 4 1 1 4 5 1 2 6 5 6 6
Av.eff.trt.pair.adj: 0.8169
Reference: searchCrossOverDesign(s=24, p=4, v=6, model="Standard additive model", eff.factor=c(1,0), contrast="Tukey
Model: Standard additive model
Var.trt.pair:
t1 t2 t3 t4 t5 t6
t1 0.0000 0.1561 0.1533 0.1527 0.1518 0.1502
t2 0.1561 0.0000 0.1495 0.1539 0.1527 0.1547
t3 0.1533 0.1495 0.0000 0.1507 0.1531 0.1584
t4 0.1527 0.1539 0.1507 0.0000 0.1570 0.1506
t5 0.1518 0.1527 0.1531 0.1570 0.0000 0.1510
t6 0.1502 0.1547 0.1584 0.1506 0.1510 0.0000
Export to R
Search algorithm plot

Figure 4.3: Screenshot from *Crossover* R package GUI: design found by search algorithm for $t = 6$, $p = 4$ and $s = 24$.

having a replication of 17, treatment 3 having a replication of 15 and the rest of the treatments a replication of 16. Therefore the algorithm was run again, but with the constraint that all treatments had to have equal replication. The design found, which is shown in Figure 4.3, had an average efficiency of 0.8169, slightly lower than the previous design found by the algorithm but slightly higher than that of PB2.94. Although not of major practical importance, this does not have such a simple (group divisible) structure as PB2.94 and its 20th sequence repeats treatment 2.

This example illustrates a feature of searching for a design, rather than using a mathematical theory to construct it. That is, the result of the search is dependent on many things which can be varied, like, for example, the number of starting designs and the desired treatment replication. By varying the values of the parameters in the algorithm and/or increasing the search time, there is always the possibility of improving on a given or found design. In practice, a difference in efficiency of one or two decimal points is unlikely to be important, as long as the chosen design is relatively efficient. Of course, there is not a mathematical theory to construct every design that will be required in practice and this is why search algorithms, such as the one we use, are so important for filling in the gaps.

Using the GUI to find designs for different models for the carry-over effects

To illustrate the use of the search algorithm for different models for the carry-over effects, we searched for designs for two treatments in four periods that

Table 4.35: Designs found using R package *Crossover*.

Design 1					Design 2				
Group	Period				Group	Period			
	1	2	3	4		1	2	3	4
1	B	A	A	B	1	A	B	B	A
2	B	A	A	B	2	B	A	A	B
3	A	B	B	A	3	B	A	B	A
4	A	B	B	A	4	A	B	A	B
5	B	B	A	A	5	B	A	B	B
6	A	A	B	B	6	A	B	A	A
Design 3					Design 4				
1	A	A	B	B	1	A	A	B	B
2	B	B	A	A	2	A	B	B	A
3	A	A	B	B	3	B	A	A	B
4	B	B	A	A	4	B	B	A	A
5	A	A	B	B	5	A	A	B	B
6	B	B	A	A	6	B	B	A	A
Design 5					Design 6				
1	A	A	B	B	1	A	A	B	A
2	B	A	A	A	2	B	B	A	B
3	B	B	A	A	3	B	A	B	A
4	A	A	B	B	4	A	B	A	B
5	A	B	B	B	5	A	B	A	B
6	B	B	A	A	6	B	A	B	A
Design 7					Design 8				
1	A	B	B	A	1	B	B	A	A
2	B	A	A	B	2	A	B	A	B
3	B	A	B	A	3	B	A	A	A
4	A	B	A	B	4	A	B	B	B
5	B	B	A	B	5	A	A	B	B
6	A	A	B	A	6	B	A	B	A

used six sequences, assuming an independent correlation structure for the within-subject errors. The designs found are given in Table 4.35, where the designs are numbered to correspond to the eight models for the carry-over effects we listed above. We note that for two treatments, the self-adjacency model and the interaction model are equivalent.

The variances of the estimated treatment parameter, adjusted for the other parameters in the model, for these designs are given in Tables 4.36 and 4.37. In addition, we have included the variances for Designs 4.6.136 and 4.6.146 from Chapter 3. These, it will be recalled, were constructed using six different sequences and were noted in Chapter 3 as being designs with good properties.

Table 4.36: Variance (in multiples of σ^2/n) of the estimated treatment parameter.

Design	Additive	Self-adjacency	Proportional	Placebo
	$\tau\|\lambda$	$\tau\|\lambda,\lambda'$	τ	$\tau\|\lambda$
1	0.042	0.231	0.038	0.042
2	0.068	0.223	0.066	0.068
3	0.046	0.250	0.029	0.046
4	0.042	0.231	0.033	0.042
5	0.049	0.262	0.032	0.049
6	0.120	0.234	0.090	0.120
7	0.068	0.223	0.066	0.068
8	0.047	0.250	0.043	0.047
4.6.136	0.046	0.251	0.037	0.046
4.6.146	0.050	0.233	0.041	0.050

Table 4.37: Variance (in multiples of σ^2/n) of treatment estimates.

Design	No carry-over into self	Decay	Interaction	2nd-order carry-over
	$\tau\|\lambda$	$\tau\|\lambda$	$\tau\|\lambda,(\tau\lambda)$	$\tau\|\lambda,\theta$
1	0.074	0.067	0.231	0.111
2	0.134	0.053	0.223	0.090
3	0.062	0.083	0.250	—
4	0.067	0.074	0.231	0.168
5	0.061	0.083	0.262	0.074
6	0.203	0.047	0.234	0.135
7	0.134	0.053	0.223	0.088
8	0.080	0.062	0.250	0.047
4.6.136	0.067	0.074	0.251	0.064
4.6.146	0.077	0.074	0.233	0.055

For Models 2 and 7 (which we have already noted are equivalent in this example) the original designs found by the algorithm had unequal replications for A and B (11,13). When the search algorithm was run again under the constraint that the replications had to be equal (i.e.,12 and 12), two equivalent designs were found and so we have included both in Table 4.35. These are given as Design 2 and Design 7 in Table 4.35.

For Model 6 (treatment decay), the design originally found by the algorithm did not include any sequences where the same treatment occurred in two successive periods, and so the treatment decay was not estimable. However, when the treatment and carry-over effects were given weights of 1 and 0.01,

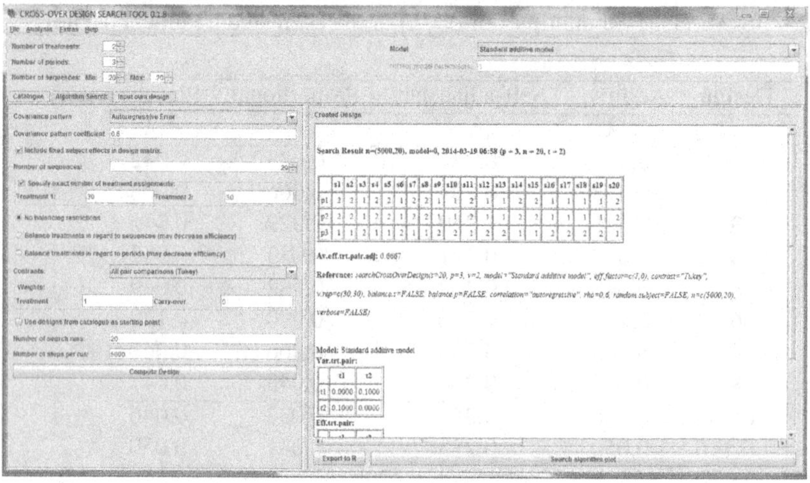

Figure 4.4: Screenshot from *Crossover* R package GUI: for a design assuming autocorrelated errors for $t = 2$.

respectively, a design that does estimate all the parameters in Model 6 was found by the algorithm. This design (Design 6) includes the sequences AABA and BBAB, in addition to two of each of sequences ABAB and BABA.

The fact that we did not always find good designs at the first attempt when using the algorithm illustrates the point made earlier about having to run the search algorithm under different options before making a final choice of the designs to use.

Using the GUI to find optimal designs for autocorrelated errors
Here we will search for the designs described by Matthews (1987), which are for $t = 2$ and $p = 3, 4$. The assumption made here is that the errors of the repeated measurements on each subject follow a first-order autoregression. That is, the covariance between the measurements in period i and j equals $\rho^{|i-j|}/(1-\rho^2)$, for $-1 < \rho < 1$.

For $p = 3$, for example, Matthews (1987) shows that the optimal design for $\rho = 0.6$ has the sequences AAB and BBA in equal proportions. For $\rho = 0.8$ the optimal design contains sequences AAB and BBA in a proportion of 0.962 times and ABA and BAB in a proportion of 0.038 times. In practice, this latter design cannot be achieved and so the alternative best design would only contain the sequences AAB and BBA in equal proportion. In Figure 4.4, we show a screenshot of the GUI, where we have specified that we want a design for $t = 2$, $p = 3$ and $s = 20$, for $\rho = 0.6$. It can be seen that the search algorithm has found the optimal design. As a further example, we repeated the search for a design when $\rho = -0.6$, although in practice we do not expect ρ to be negative. In the optimal design, sequences AAB and BBA should occur 4.286 times each and sequences ABB and BAA should occur 5.714 times each. The design found by the algorithm was the closest practical approximation to this design, with each of the aforementioned sequences occurring five times each.

Matthews (1987) also gave optimal designs for $p = 4$ and the search algorithm can also be used to search for these.

Chapter 5

Analysis of continuous data

5.1 Introduction

In this chapter we develop analyses for continuous outcomes from cross-over trials. These will largely be parametric, using conventional linear regression and analysis of variance, as introduced in Section 1.5. For particular settings these models will be extended to incorporate other random terms and other covariance structures, i.e., we will be using *linear mixed models*. We have already met simple versions of such models with fixed and random subject effects in Chapters 2 and 3. Here we provide a systematic development. Analyses will be illustrated using the SAS procedures `mixed` and `glimmix`. In addition, we will describe some methods of analysis that are robust to the covariance structure of the measurements from one individual that can be used in very small samples.

We first introduce an example which will be used to illustrate analyses for the basic multi-period cross-over trial. We then develop these analyses for more complicated settings, such as incomplete period designs, multicenter trials, experiments with many periods, trials in which repeated measurements are collected within treatment periods, and methods that can be used which are robust to the true covariance structure of the data, with a special emphasis on very small trials. We complete the chapter by looking at a case study with many periods; this allows us to further illustrate and expand on a number of issues raised in the preceding sections.

5.1.1 Example 5.1: INNOVO trial: dose–response study

The INNOVO trial was funded by the UK Medical Research Council to investigate the effect of ventilation with inhaled nitric oxide on babies with severe respiratory failure (less than 34 weeks gestation). As part of this, a dose-response study was introduced to compare four doses of nitric oxide (5 (A), 10 (B), 20 (C) and 40 (D) parts per million (ppm)) in preterm babies. Each baby received all the doses, which were of 15 minutes' duration with a minimum of 5 minutes' wash-out between treatment periods in which no nitric oxide was given. This wash-out was expected to allow the blood gases to return to baseline levels. Measurements were taken of several quantities from the arterial blood both at baseline and after treatment for each treatment period. The design is slightly unusual in that no attempt was made to balance subjects across

Table 5.1: Example 5.1: Treatment occurrence by period in the INNOVO design.

	Periods			
Treatments	1	2	3	4
A	2	3	4	3
B	1	4	4	3
C	7	3	1	1
D	2	2	3	5

sequences; rather, each of the 13 babies recruited received the treatments in a random order. The consequent design has a considerable degree of nonorthogonality between treatments and periods. Some of the lack of balance in the design can be seen from Table 5.1, which gives the numbers of times each treatment occurs in a period. For example, treatment C (dose 20) occurs seven times in Period 1, but only once in Periods 3 and 4.□□□

The data from the primary outcome measure, post-ductal arterial oxygen tension (PaO_2), are presented in Table 5.1 in units of kPa. One baby, subject 11, was withdrawn after the first period because of coagulopathy. We follow the decision of the original investigators and retain this pair of observations in the analysis. The distribution of the raw data is somewhat skewed to the right. However, the following analysis will be based on the untransformed observations. In considering the distribution of outcomes and assumptions, such as normality of response, it must be remembered in the fixed subject effects analysis that it is the behavior of *within-patient* deviations or differences that is relevant, not the raw measurements. In fact, the fixed subject effects analysis *conditions* on the overall subject levels and makes no assumptions about their distributional behavior. This is no longer the case when more sophisticated analyses are used that introduce *random* subject effects, as, for example in Section 5.3.

5.2 Fixed subject effects model

5.2.1 *Ignoring the baseline measurements*

Recall from Section 1.5 (1.1) the linear model that can be used to represent the data from a cross-over trial such as the INNOVO study,

$$Y_{ijk} = \mu + \pi_j + \tau_{d[i,j]} + s_{ik} + e_{ijk}, \tag{5.1}$$

where the terms in this model are

μ, an intercept;

π_j, an effect associated with period $j, j = 1, \ldots, p$;

Table 5.2: Example 5.1: Post-ductal arterial oxygen tension (kPa) from the INNOVO trial.

		Period							
		1		2		3		4	
Subject	Sequence	Base	Resp	Base	Resp	Base	Resp	Base	Resp
1	DCBA	6.4	6.1	4.5	6.1	3.0	5.6	5.1	7.8
2	BCAD	11.1	11.4	7.0	7.6	8.1	10.8	11.0	12.1
3	CDBA	7.0	10.7	5.9	7.6	6.7	10.1	6.8	8.0
4	ABCD	2.6	2.9	2.5	2.8	2.3	2.7	2.1	3.4
5	DCAB	8.7	9.9	8.3	8.1	8.0	6.0	5.5	12.2
6	CABD	5.8	5.9	6.8	7.2	7.1	9.0	7.3	9.0
7	CDAB	7.0	6.7	6.4	5.8	6.0	6.5	6.1	6.6
8	CBDA	7.4	9.6	6.5	7.6	6.3	12.6	6.0	7.9
9	ABDC	5.9	6.6	6.0	7.4	5.9	7.3	5.9	7.1
10	CADB	6.5	9.8	4.7	9.6	4.1	12.9	4.8	10.0
-11	ACBD	2.1	7.4	—	—	—	—	—	—
12	CABD	7.8	17.8	7.7	14.3	8.3	12.6	8.5	10.3
13	CBAD	2.6	4.6	4.8	3.4	3.9	4.1	2.5	5.1

Base: baseline measurement, Resp: post-treatment measurement.

$\tau_{d[i,j]}$, an effect associated with the treatment applied in period j of sequence i, $d[i,j] = 1,\ldots,t$;

s_{ik}, an effect associated with the kth subject on sequence $i, i = 1,\ldots,s$, $k = 1,\ldots,n_i$;

e_{ijk}, a random error term, with zero mean and variance σ^2.

In this section we assume that the subject effects are fixed, unknown constants. In the current context of the normal linear model, this is equivalent to working conditionally on their sufficient statistics. Analogous techniques can be used with categorical data, and we return to this in Chapter 6. Conditional on the subject effects, it is assumed that the observations are independent.

We illustrate the use of this model using the INNOVO data, with the natural logarithm of the post-ductal PaO_2 as the response. To begin with, the baseline measurements are ignored. Suppose that the relevant variates are labeled as follows:

subject (levels 1–13):	`subject`
period (levels 1–4):	`period`
doses (levels (1–4):	`dose`
baseline PaO_2:	`pco2base`
response PaO_2:	`pco2resp`

The following SAS `proc mixed` commands provide a basic regression analysis for model (5.1):

```
proc mixed;
  class subject period dose;
  model pco2resp = subject period dose / solution;
run;
```

The resulting overall F-tests for the model terms are then:

```
               Type 3 Tests of Fixed Effects

                 Num      Den
Effect            DF       DF     F Value     Pr > F

subject           12       30       10.66     <.0001
period             3       30        1.23     0.3177
dose               3       30        0.53     0.6655
```

There is no evidence of a dose effect. The estimated means for each dose are

Dose	Estimate	SE
5	7.6052	0.4801
10	8.2954	0.5223
20	7.8982	0.5840
40	8.4076	0.5257

with standard errors of differences ranging between 0.708 and 0.709. It would be possible to provide a more powerful test through a test for trend associated with dose. This could be done by regressing on the actual doses within the analysis, but the lack of pattern in the observed means suggests strongly that in this case there would be little evidence of consistent response to dose.

The simple analysis above might be appropriate in the absence of baseline measurements, but in the present setting it might be argued that some use should be made of these. In general, whether the baselines contribute to the efficiency of the analysis depends on the comparative sizes of various dependencies among the sequence of the $2p$ observations from a subject, including both the dependence between a response measurement and its baseline, and a response measurement and the preceding response measurement. This difference in these dependencies will vary from trial to trial, but is likely to be influenced by the time between adjacent response measurements and the time between a response measurement and its baseline. If the latter are much closer in time than the former, then it is likely that adjustment for the baseline values will make a non-negligible contribution. There are as well situations in which the primary outcome is *defined* as a change from baseline, or relative change from baseline. It turns out, however, that the appropriate use of such baseline values raises some rather subtle issues, with a real danger of constructing an invalid analysis if these are ignored. We give a simple analysis here that is valid under fairly basic assumptions, but return to the topic for a much more thorough treatment in Section 5.4.

We incorporate the baselines in a manner that mirrors their use in parallel group trials, that is, the preceding baseline is included as a covariate in the model for the following response measurement. This is, at first sight, a natural and obvious thing to do, but we note here that such an approach will be valid in general (with some mild symmetry assumptions) only when *fixed* subject effects are included in the model, as here. The reasons for this are explored below in Section 5.4. For comparison purposes we also analyze the change from baseline as dependent variable, again with baseline as covariate. For the analysis of covariance, the baseline `pco2base` is simply added to the model:

```
proc mixed;
class subject period dose;
model pco2bresp = subject pco2base period dose / solution;
run;
```

This produces the overall F-tests:

Type 3 Tests of Fixed Effects

Effect	Num DF	Den DF	F Value	Pr > F
subject	12	29	5.38	0.0001
pco2base	1	29	0.15	0.7004
period	3	29	1.24	0.3131
dose	3	29	0.55	0.6492

The introduction of the baseline as covariate has added nothing to the variation previously explained by the subject effects, as shown by the small contribution of the baseline term. This does not mean that baseline and response are not correlated (the correlation in fact exceeds 0.6), just that correction for average subject effect removes this dependency, which would anyway only help with the between-subject treatment information, of which there is little here. As we should predict from this, the adjustment for baseline has minimal effect on the dose effects estimates and their significance.

The same analysis can be repeated with `pco2diff = pco2resp - pco2base` as dependent variable:

```
...
model pco2diff = subject pco2base period dose / solution;
...
```

As should be expected, we see that the adjusted analyses using the response alone and change from baseline as dependent variable are essentially equivalent; all estimates and inferences are identical except that the coefficient of the baseline ($\hat{\beta}$) is reduced by one:

Dependent Variable	pco2resp		pco2diff	
Effect	Estimate	SE	Estimate	SE
Intercept	5.19	1.53	5.19	1.53
pco2base	–0.12	0.32	–1.12	0.32
period 1–4	0.49	0.84	0.49	0.84
...	...	...		

5.2.2 *Adjusting for carry-over effects*

In Section 1.5 the introduction of carry-over effects was briefly described. Recall that a carry-over term has the special property as a factor, or class variate, of having no level in the first period. By definition, a factor classifies *all* observations into two or more classes. We can get around this problem in practice by using the fact that carry-over effects will be adjusted for period effects (by default all effects are adjusted for all others in these analyses). As a consequence, any level can be assigned to the carry-over variate in the first period, provided the same level is always used. Adjustment for periods then "removes" this part of the carry-over term. For example, consider the period, treatment and first-order carry-over variate for the first three subjects of the INNOVO trial:

Subject	Period	Treatment	Carry-over
1	1	4	1
1	2	3	4
1	3	2	3
1	4	1	2
2	1	2	1
2	2	3	2
2	3	1	3
2	4	4	1
3	1	3	1
3	2	4	3
3	3	2	4
3	4	1	2

Here the value 1 has been assigned to the carry-over variate in the first period. Similar reasoning can be used to construct higher-order carry-over factors. Although the wash-out period in the INNOVO trial can be used to justify the absence of carry-over effect, we will introduce first-order additive carry-over into the model as an illustration of the use of such a term. With a carry-over variate `carry1` defined as above, we have the model:

```
...
class subject period dose carry1;
model pco2resp = subject period dose carry1 / solution;
...
```

Note the absence of the baseline covariate from the model. If we did believe that previous treatment administration were affecting later results, then, in this setting, we would also expect these baseline measurements to be affected. Indeed, an alternative approach to adjustment through an explicit carry-over term would be to use these baselines as covariates. The two approaches, however, imply different models for the carry-over effect.

The model above produces the following F-tests with the PaO_2 data:

Type 3 Tests of Fixed Effects

Effect	Num DF	Den DF	F Value	Pr > F
subject	12	27	10.77	<.0001
period	2	27	0.63	0.5415
dose	3	27	0.22	0.8785
carry1	3	27	1.06	0.3804

The carry-over effects are far from statistical significance.

5.3 Random subject effects model

5.3.1 *Random subject effects*

One consequence of using fixed subjects effects, as done in the previous section, is that all treatment information contained in the subject totals is discarded. For the typical well-designed higher-order trial there will be little information lost and so this is usually a sensible route to take, especially as it avoids the need to make explicit assumptions about the distribution of the subject effects.

To recover the information in the subject totals we need to introduce random subject effects. Because such analyses introduce extra assumptions and, as will be seen below, the use of approximations in the inference procedures as well, we need to be sure that this extra step is worthwhile, that is, it should be considered only when a substantial amount of information is contained in the subject totals, and this will be true for some incomplete designs, such as those described in Chapter 4. The 2×2 design is an extreme example of this in which *all* the information on carry-over effects is contained in the subject totals.

The model for random subject effects is identical to that introduced earlier (5.1).

$$Y_{ijk} = \mu + \pi_j + \tau_{d[i,j]} + s_{ik} + e_{ijk},$$

with the exception that the subject effects s_{ik} are now assumed to be random draws from some distribution. In practice this is almost always assumed to be a normal distribution,

$$s_{ik} \sim \mathrm{N}[0, \sigma_s^2],$$

where σ_s^2 is called the **between-subject variance**. For this random subjects model

$$\mathrm{V}(Y_{ijk}) = \sigma^2 + \sigma_s^2$$

and

$$\mathrm{Cov}(Y_{ijk}, Y_{ij'k}) = \sigma_s^2, \text{ for all } j \neq j'.$$

In other words, assuming a random subjects model is equivalent to imposing a specific covariance structure on the set of measurements from one subject:

$$\mathrm{V}\begin{bmatrix} Y_{i1k} \\ Y_{i2k} \\ \vdots \\ Y_{ipk} \end{bmatrix} = \begin{bmatrix} \sigma^2+\sigma_s^2 & \sigma_s^2 & \cdots & \sigma_s^2 \\ \sigma_s^2 & \sigma^2+\sigma_s^2 & \cdots & \sigma_s^2 \\ \vdots & \vdots & \ddots & \vdots \\ \sigma_s^2 & \sigma_s^2 & \cdots & \sigma^2+\sigma_s^2 \end{bmatrix}.$$

This is an **exchangeable** or **compound symmetry** structure.

The introduction of the random effects means that this is no longer an example of a simple linear regression model, and ordinary least squares estimation and standard least squares theory no longer apply. Instead, a modified version of maximum likelihood is used for estimation, called **restricted maximum likelihood (REML)**. This can be thought of as a two stage procedure in which the variance components (σ^2 and σ_s^2) are first estimated from a marginal likelihood that does not depend on the fixed effects (period and treatment). The fixed effects are then estimated using generalized least squares with a covariance matrix constructed from the estimated variance components. In matrix terms, if $\mathbf{Y}$ is the vector of observations, with covariance matrix Σ and expectation

$$\mathrm{E}(\mathbf{Y}) = \mathbf{X}\beta$$

for $\mathbf{X}$ the design matrix and β the vector of fixed effects, then the REML estimator of β is

$$\tilde{\beta} = (\mathbf{X}^T\hat{\Sigma}^{-1}\mathbf{X})^{-1}\mathbf{X}^T\hat{\Sigma}^{-1}\mathbf{Y}$$

where $\hat{\Sigma} = \Sigma(\hat{\sigma}^2, \hat{\sigma}_s^2)$, for $\hat{\sigma}^2$ and $\hat{\sigma}_s^2$, the REML estimators of σ^2 and σ_s^2. Asymptotically, as the number of subjects increases,

$$\tilde{\beta} \sim \mathrm{N}\left[\beta, \, (\mathbf{X}^T\Sigma^{-1}\mathbf{X})^{-1}\right].$$

However, cross-over trials are often small in size, and it is not obvious that in the current setting this will always provide an adequate approximation. We return to this point in Section 5.3.3.

REML is the default method for linear mixed models in `proc mixed`. To fit this simple random subject effects model, the `subject` indicator is simply moved from the `model` statement to the `random` statement, i.e., change

```
...
model y = subject period treatment;
...
```

for fixed subject effects to

```
...
model y = period treatment;
random subject;
...
```

5.3.2 *Recovery of between-subject information*

When a design has low efficiency for the within-subject estimates, there will be information on the treatment comparisons in the subject totals. The introduction of random subject effects into the model allows this information to be incorporated in the analysis. Such random subject analyses are examples of the **recovery of interblock information**. In such an analysis a weighted average is implicitly used that combines between- and within-subject estimates. The weights are equal to the inverse of the variances of the two estimates. If there is little information in the subject totals, recovery of this information is not worth the effort, and the amount of such information will depend on two things: the size of the between-subject variance (σ_s^2) relative to the within-subject variance (σ^2), often measured by the **intra-class correlation**,

$$\frac{\sigma_s^2}{\sigma^2 + \sigma_s^2},$$

and the efficiency of the design. We need an inefficient design, a moderately small intra-class correlation and a sufficiently large number of subjects to make the procedure worthwhile. Otherwise it may even be counterproductive because the need to estimate the weights introduces extra variation into the combined estimate. In a very small trial these weights will be poorly estimated. Also, as mentioned earlier, the simpler fixed subjects analysis is more robust, and, as will be seen in the next section, moving to the random effects analysis means moving from small sample inference based on exact distribution theory to methods of inference based on distributional approximations. In conclusion, recovery of interblock information should be considered only when there is likely to be a worthwhile benefit.

5.3.2.1 Example 5.2

We illustrate this procedure using data from a three-treatment two-period design, in which the response is a measure of efficacy. For the purposes of confidentiality, the actual data have been disguised. The design consists of three complete replicates of all possible two-treatment sequences. The design and outcomes are given in Table 5.3. □□□

To show the process of the recovery of between-subject information we first analyze separately the subject sums and differences. The latter is identical to the conventional analysis with fixed subject effects. In this way we obtain separate estimates from the within- and between-subject strata. Estimating

Table 5.3: Example 5.2: Data from the three-treatment two-period design.

	Treatment		Outcome	
Subject	Period 1	Period 2	Period 1	Period 2
1	C	B	5.15	5.97
2	B	C	3.19	4.74
3	A	B	6.59	6.28
4	C	A	2.26	4.12
5	B	A	5.87	2.99
6	A	C	4.94	3.71
7	C	A	3.81	1.54
8	A	C	6.18	5.56
9	A	B	2.37	5.76
10	C	B	5.15	5.87
11	B	A	3.09	1.44
12	B	C	3.91	4.32
13	A	B	4.32	6.07
14	B	A	4.94	0.62
15	C	A	2.68	5.76
16	B	C	3.60	1.85
17	C	B	4.43	5.15
18	A	C	0.82	0.62

treatment comparisons in terms of the A–C and B–C differences, and using a model *without* carry-over effects, gives

	Within-subject		Between-subject	
Comparison	Estimate	SE	Estimate	SE
A–C	–0.122	0.614	–0.498	1.711
B–C	1.250	0.614	1.390	1.711

The standard errors of the between-subject estimates are much larger, indicating that most of the information on the treatment effects is contained in the within-subject stratum. We would not expect to gain much by adding the between-subject information. The estimates are combined using an average weighted by the inverse of the variance. For example, for the A–C comparison,

$$\text{combined estimate} = \frac{-0.122/0.614^2 - 0.498/1.711^2}{1/0.614^2 + 1/1.711^2} = -0.165.$$

An approximate standard error for this estimate is given by

$$\sqrt{\frac{1}{1/0.614^2 + 1/1.711^2}} = 0.578.$$

As expected, neither the estimate nor its standard error are far from the corresponding within-subject values (–0.122 and 0.614). The combined estimate of the B–C comparison is similarly 1.266 with the same SE. It may appear that we have nothing to lose by combining the information in this way: although the change in standard error is small, it has been reduced, and in a purely arithmetical sense, this will always happen. However, as we show in the next section, this can be misleading, as the standard error is only an approximation, and it can be shown that it is always an underestimate of the true standard error.

If carry-over is now included in the model, then the design becomes much less efficient for direct treatment effects and we expect to see a greater proportion of information in the between-subject stratum. The estimates for both treatment and carry-over effects are as follows.

	Within-subject		Between-subject	
Comparison	Estimate	SE	Estimate	SE
Treatment adjusted for carry-over				
A–C	–1.203	1.270	–0.812	1.739
B–C	0.477	1.270	3.112	1.739
Carry-over adjusted for treatment				
A–C	–2.163	2.200	0.628	1.739
B–C	–1.547	2.200	–3.444	1.739

The within- and between-subject standard errors have indeed moved closer together, indicating a more equal distribution of information. The recovery of between-subject information is much more likely to be worthwhile in this setting. Note that there appears to be great inconsistency in some estimates from the two strata. The differences are in fact not large given the size of the corresponding standard errors. Applying the combination formula to these four effects, we get

Comparison	Combined Estimate	SE
Treatment adjusted for carry-over		
A–C	−1.067	0.689
B–C	1.393	0.689
Carry-over adjusted for treatment		
A–C	−0.446	1.047
B–C	−2.715	1.047

This explicit estimation of separate effects and their standard errors allows us to see how the procedure of recovery of between-subject information operates, but is not the approach that would now normally be used in practice. It is inefficient because the variance components are obtained under the assumption that the fixed effects estimates are different in the two strata. It would be possible to re-estimate these variance components given the combined effects estimate, and then recalculate the weights. This process could then be repeated until the estimates converge. This is effectively what the REML analysis does with random subject effects. We now apply this to the same models, first without carry-over effects. Assuming a conventionally arranged data set, we have the following `proc mixed` statements:

```
proc mixed;
  class subject period treatment;
  model response = period treatment / solution;
  random subject;
run;
```

This analysis provides explicit estimates of the two variance components:

```
Cov Parm      Estimate

SUBJECT         1.1400
Residual        1.6709
```

The estimate of the intra-class correlation is then

$$\frac{1.140}{1.671+1.14} = 0.41.$$

This is small enough to make it likely that the recovery of between-subject information will be worthwhile for a sufficiently inefficient design. The effects estimates can be compared with those obtained earlier:

	Weighted combination		REML	
Comparison	Estimate	SE	Estimate	SE
A–C	–0.165	0.578	–0.168	0.571
B–C	1.266	0.578	1.267	0.571

The estimates and standard errors are very similar. We can then repeat this with carry-over included in the model:

```
proc mixed;
  class subject period treatment carry-over;
  model response = period treatment carry-over/ solution;
  random subject;
run;
```

The results from this analysis are compared with the earlier results in Table 5.4. The SEs obtained by the two approaches are very similar, and the differences in the estimates are small in light of these SEs. Finally, we need to make inferences about these effects. For this we need to consider how these estimates and their precision behave in small samples. We consider this in the next section.

5.3.3 *Small sample inference with random effects*

We have already seen in Section 5.3.1 that the introduction of random subject effects implies that estimates of precision and subsequent inferences are no longer based on exact small sample results. Recall that the REML estimate of the fixed effects parameters can be written as a generalized least squares estimator:

$$\tilde{\beta} = (\mathbf{X}^T\hat{\Sigma}^{-1}\mathbf{X})^{-1}\mathbf{X}^T\hat{\Sigma}^{-1}\mathbf{Y}.$$

Table 5.4: Example 5.2: Recovery of between-subject information using simple weighted and REML estimates, with carry-over effects in the model.

	Weighted combination		REML	
Comparison	Estimate	SE	Estimate	SE
Treatment adjusted for carry-over				
A–C	–1.067	0.689	–0.351	0.702
B–C	1.393	0.689	0.704	0.702
Carry-over adjusted for treatment				
A–C	–0.446	1.047	–0.486	1.083
B–C	–2.715	1.047	–1.527	1.083

In large samples the covariance matrix of $\tilde{\beta}$ tends to

$$\Phi = (\mathbf{X}^T \Sigma^{-1} \mathbf{X})^{-1}.$$

A natural estimator of this quantity is

$$\hat{\Phi} = (\mathbf{X}^T \hat{\Sigma}^{-1} \mathbf{X})^{-1}.$$

In small samples $\hat{\Phi}$ will be biased for $V(\tilde{\beta})$, for two reasons. First, it takes no account of the uncertainty in the estimate of Σ used in the generalized least squares formula for $\tilde{\beta}$. Second, it ignores the fact that we are anyway using a biased estimator of Φ. It turns out that both the sources of bias act in the same direction, causing the estimated standard errors to be too small.

To illustrate this, we use the same three-treatment two-period six-sequence design met in the previous section:

A	B
B	A
A	C
C	A
B	C
C	B

This is balanced for treatments. For a single treatment comparison $\eta = \mathbf{c}^T\beta$ consider the ratio

$$R(\eta) = 100 \times \frac{V[\tilde{\eta}]}{\mathrm{E}\left[\mathbf{c}^T\hat{\Phi}\mathbf{c}\right]}.$$

This compares the expected value of the estimated variance of η with the true variance. We can use simple simulations to get a good approximation to $R(\eta)$ and from the balance in the design this will take the same value for any treatment contrast and the same value for any carry-over contrast. In the following table we give the value of this ratio for sequence replications equal to 2 and 4, i.e., for designs with 12 and 24 subjects, respectively. First-order carry-over is included in the model and the intra-class (or within-subject) correlation is set equal to 1/3.

Replication	$R(\eta)$	
per sequence	Direct	Carry-over
2	122	126
4	110	111

The bias in the variance estimators is approximately 20% in the smaller design and 10% with the larger.

A second issue surrounding small sample approximation concerns the procedures for inference. Conventionally, inferences about a set of effects

$$\mathbf{C}\beta,$$

where $\mathbf{C}$ has c rows, are based on Wald statistics of the form

$$W = c^{-1}(\tilde{\beta} - \beta)^T \mathbf{C}^T (\mathbf{C}\hat{\Phi}\mathbf{C}^T)^{-1} \mathbf{C}(\tilde{\beta} - \beta).$$

Standard F (and t, when $c = 1$) tests and confidence intervals can be constructed under the assumption that W follows an $F_{c,v}$ distribution. With conventional regression this will hold exactly, and v will be equal to the residual degrees of freedom. With a linear mixed model, the F-distribution is only an approximating one and an appropriate value for v must be calculated. Several suggestions have been made for this. A comprehensive solution is given by Kenward and Roger (1997, 2009) which describes both how $\hat{\Phi}$ can be modified for small samples and how v should then be calculated when the modified form of $\hat{\Phi}$ is used in W. This procedure is implemented in SAS procs `mixed` and `glimmix` with the `ddfm=kenwardroger` and `ddfm=kenwardroger2` (`glimmix` only) options to the `model` statement. The adjustment will only have a notable effect in very small, unbalanced settings, but has the advantage of producing the exact result when this exists and otherwise, when little small sample correction is needed, the procedure will make a negligible adjustment. Hence there is no loss in using it routinely.

We can apply this to the random effects analysis used in Section 5.3.2. The same `proc mixed` commands are used with

```
ddfm=kenwardroger
```

added as an option to the `model` statement. The parameter estimates are the same as before; only the standard errors are affected. The modification also provides degrees of freedom for the t- and F-tests. The corrected results are compared with the unadjusted in Table 5.5 for the model with carry-over included. It can be seen how the standard errors have been increased to account for the estimation of the variation components.

Table 5.5: Example 5.2: Small sample adjusted standard errors and degrees of freedom.

	Standard Error		
Comparison	Unadjusted	Adjusted	DF
Treatment adjusted for carry-over			
A–C	0.702	0.728	30
B–C	0.702	0.728	30
Carry-over adjusted for treatment			
A–C	1.083	1.133	26.4
B–C	1.083	1.133	26.4

5.3.4 Missing values

Missing values raise two main issues with cross-over trials. The first is that of accommodating the subsequent lack of balance in the data. The modeling tools that we now have available mean that this is today much less of a difficulty than in the past. The second is concerned with the impact of the missing data on the conclusions that can reasonably be drawn from the trial. When intended data are missing, ambiguity is almost inevitably introduced into the inferences that can be drawn that goes beyond familiar ideas of statistical uncertainty. This is a difficult problem that reaches beyond the scope of this book. For further reading on this, see Molenberghs and Kenward (2007) for a general treatment of the problem in clinical trials, and Matthews and Henderson (2013), Matthews et al. (2013), Ho et al. (2013) and Rosenkranz (2014) for considerations specific to cross-over trials.

In this section we briefly consider the first issue. We assume that the probability of an observation being missing does not depend on any of the actual missing observations themselves, once we have allowed for information provided by the observed data and the design.

When subjects have missing values in a cross-over trial, a fixed subject effects analysis can be applied as before with no modification. There are two consequences, however: (1) subjects with a single remaining observation will contribute nothing to the analysis, and (2) typically nonorthogonality will be increased between subjects and treatments. These two points imply that it may be worth considering the use of a random subjects model when there are more than very few missing observations. An extreme case is the 2×2 design, where the conventional analysis would discard any subject with a single missing observation. Here, a random effects model might be considered to recover the information in the singleton observations. As with the recovery of between-subject information, the analysis implicitly uses a weighted average to estimate the treatment effect, one estimate coming from the complete pairs, the other from the singletons. To illustrate this, a random set of values has been deleted from Example 2.1, the trial on chronic obstructive pulmonary disease (COPD). The modified data set is shown in Table 5.6.

We fit the same random subject effects model as used earlier in this chapter, with `pefr` the response variable:

```
proc mixed;
  class subject period treatment;
  model pefr = period treatment / s ddfm=kenwardroger;
  random subject;
run;
```

Table 5.6: Morning PEFR from the COPD trial, with created missing values.

AB Group			BA Group		
Subject Label	Period 1	Period 2	Subject Label	Period 1	Period 2
7	121.905	116.667	3	138.333	138.571
8	218.500	—	10	225.000	256.250
9	235.000	217.143	11	392.857	381.429
13	250.000	196.429	16	190.000	—
14	—	185.500	18	191.429	228.000
15	231.563	221.842	23	226.190	—
17	443.250	—	24	201.905	193.500
21	198.421	207.692	26	134.286	128.947
22	270.500	213.158	27	—	248.500
28	360.476	384.000	29	—	140.000
35	—	188.250	30	232.750	276.563
36	—	221.905	32	172.308	170.000
37	255.882	253.571	33	266.000	305.000
38	—	267.619	39	171.333	186.333
41	160.556	163.000	43	—	191.429
44	172.105	182.381	47	200.000	222.619
58	267.000	313.000	51	146.667	183.810
66	230.750	211.111	52	208.000	—
71	271.190	—	55	208.750	218.810
76	276.250	222.105	59	271.429	225.000
79	398.750	404.000	68	143.810	—
80	67.778	70.278	70	104.444	135.238
81	195.000	—	74	145.238	152.857
82	325.000	306.667	77	215.385	240.476
86	368.077	362.500	78	306.000	—
89	—	227.895	83	160.526	150.476
90	236.667	220.000	84	—	369.048
			85	293.889	308.095
			99	371.190	—

First we note the estimates of the variance components:

Cov Parm	Estimate
subject	5823.00
Residual	307.90

The corresponding within-subject correlation is

$$\frac{5823.0}{307.90 + 5823.0} = 0.95.$$

This is very high and implies that the information contained in the singleton observations will be negligible compared with that in the within-subject differences. In this case we should therefore expect very little gain over the analysis of those subjects only with complete pairs. For comparison we give the estimates from both analyses:

	Completers only			Random effects analysis		
Comparison	Estimate	SE	DF	Estimate	SE	DF
A–B	10.706	4.060	35	10.514	4.081	35.9

As expected, the two analyses give almost identical results. This reinforces the message that the recovery of between-subject information will be worthwhile only under certain conditions.

5.4 Use of baseline measurements

5.4.1 Introduction and examples

We have seen earlier that baseline covariates may be measured either at the beginning of the study (prior to randomization), which we here call *pre-randomization*, or at the beginning of each treatment period, which we call *period-dependent.* It has recently been shown by Kenward and Roger (2010) that one common way of incorporating period-dependent baselines into cross-over analyses in the presence of random subject effects is in fact wrong. Following the development in Kenward and Roger (2010), we identify the source of this error and set out some alternative analyses that do not suffer from the same problem.

To illustrate fully the use of such baselines we need to use cross-over designs for which their incorporation is advantageous. For many commonly used designs, especially those based on Williams square and related complete designs, this is not the case, so to make the contrast between the two situations we introduce two new examples, the first a simple balanced complete design, the second a highly unbalanced design with missing data.

Example 5.3: Systolic blood pressures

These data are from a three-treatment cross-over trial involving 12 subjects. The effects of the three treatments on blood pressure are to be compared. Treatments A and B consist of the trial drug at 20 mg and 40 mg doses, respectively, while treatment C is a placebo. Two complete replicates of the Williams arrangement were used in which all six possible sequences occur. The measurements are of systolic blood pressure (in mm Hg), measured under each treatment at 10 successive times: 30 and 15 minutes before treatment, and 13, 30, 45, 60, 75, 90, 120 and 240 minutes after treatment. These data are presented in Table 5.7 and the mean profiles are plotted in Figure 5.1. Here we use the

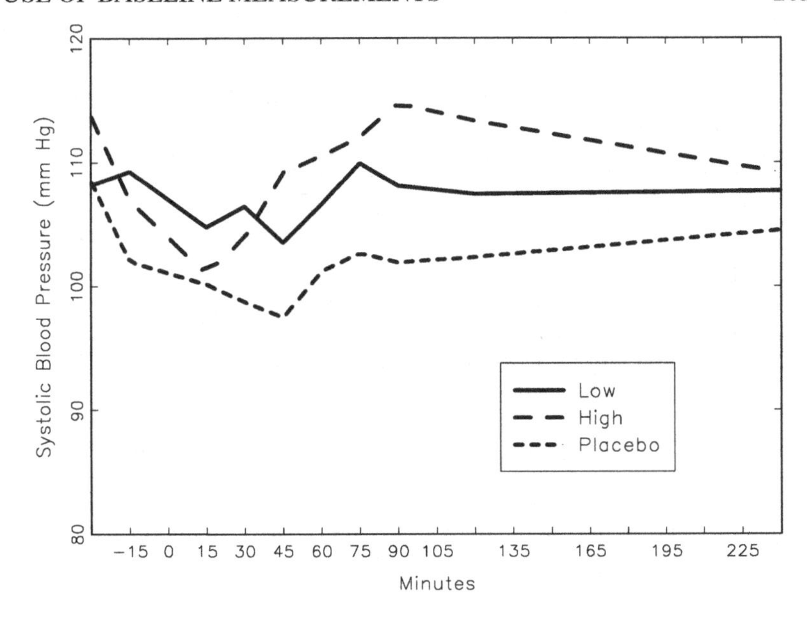

Figure 5.1: Example 5.3: Mean treatment profiles.

average of the two pre-treatment measurements as the period-dependent baselines and the measurement at 90 minutes as the response. For the analyses we will focus on the high versus low dose treatment comparison.□□□

Example 5.4 An increasing dose cohort design

The second example is taken from a first-in-human single dose study organized as a five-period cross-over in two cohorts, with ten healthy volunteers in each cohort. This data set appeared in a plenary data analysis session at the 2006 conference of Statisticians in the Pharmaceutical Industry (PSI) and has been made available as Supplementary Material on the *Biostatistics* website. It was one of the examples used in Kenward and Roger (2010). The trial has eight treatments: a negative control (P), a positive control (G) and six increasing doses (A, B, C, D, E and F), three in each cohort organized as ascending doses within each subject, alternating between cohorts. The doses are 10, 30, 60, 150, 250 and 400 μg of an inhaled substance. The design has two replicates of five sequences within each cohort of ten subjects. Three subjects, on the sequences ACPEG, GBDFP and BDPFG, respectively, withdrew after one period and three replacement subjects were added using the same three sequences. These subjects completed all five periods. One subject, on GBDFP, withdrew after three periods and was not replaced. Doses, A, C and E only appear in cohort 1,

Table 5.7: Example 5.3: Systolic blood pressures (in mm Hg) from a three-period cross-over trial.

S	P	T	Time of measurement (minutes relative to treatment)									
			–30	–15	15	30	45	60	75	90	120	240
1	1	C	112	114	86	86	93	90	106	91	84	102
1	2	B	108	103	100	100	97	103	92	106	106	96
1	3	A	107	108	102	111	100	105	113	109	84	99
2	1	B	101	100	99	81	106	100	100	111	110	96
2	2	A	96	101	101	100	99	101	98	99	102	101
2	3	C	111	99	90	93	81	91	89	95	99	97
3	1	A	105	113	109	104	102	102	111	106	104	101
3	2	C	104	96	84	84	100	91	109	94	108	108
3	3	B	96	92	88	89	91	121	122	135	121	107
4	1	A	112	109	108	92	102	101	101	98	102	106
4	2	B	105	116	105	108	141	103	110	109	113	112
4	3	C	110	112	111	102	99	104	108	102	112	101
5	1	C	96	93	94	96	83	95	88	93	88	93
5	2	A	103	98	97	108	93	101	108	105	104	101
5	3	B	114	97	96	109	102	99	110	105	104	106
6	1	B	115	117	91	102	126	122	128	125	119	117
6	2	C	104	84	88	95	97	115	93	102	90	101
6	3	A	103	97	84	97	102	115	108	114	113	107
7	1	C	82	88	85	87	81	91	87	78	85	81
7	2	B	133	89	93	98	92	94	90	90	94	100
7	3	A	87	83	78	92	80	83	88	88	93	98
8	1	A	124	131	115	119	115	110	108	103	116	109
8	2	C	116	113	109	93	112	89	108	111	107	111
8	3	B	121	120	87	93	94	100	95	100	114	117
9	1	B	118	107	105	111	105	115	137	128	115	114
9	2	A	111	104	112	109	108	114	116	127	117	117
9	3	C	113	107	115	117	105	117	104	110	105	117
10	1	B	111	112	102	111	107	113	105	111	113	101
10	2	C	115	91	111	114	104	105	112	112	102	105
10	3	A	112	110	109	112	110	103	116	106	110	110
11	1	C	120	117	110	110	110	116	115	118	125	125
11	2	A	104	123	119	115	120	120	127	122	125	128
11	3	B	117	113	117	120	125	130	123	128	126	123
12	1	A	134	134	123	118	111	124	125	120	119	115
12	2	B	125	117	129	125	124	126	132	129	125	121
12	3	C	118	110	119	108	105	110	113	117	123	113

S: subject, P: period, T: treatment.

while doses B, D and F only appear in cohort 2. Both the negative and positive controls appear in every sequence. The design is as follows:

Cohort 1					
Period	1	2	3	4	5
N=2	P	A	G	C	E
N=2	G	A	C	E	P
N=2+	A	C	P	E	G
N=2	A	P	C	G	E
N=2	A	G	C	P	E

Cohort 2					
Period	1	2	3	4	5
N=2	P	B	G	D	F
N=1++	G	B	D	F	P
N=2+	B	D	P	F	G
N=2	B	P	D	G	F
N=2	B	G	D	P	F

There was a one week interval between each test day, meaning that subjects in each cohort had a 14 day wash-out period. Within each period, lung function was measured using Forced Expiratory Volume in 1 second (FEV_1 liters) seven times, at baseline (0), 2, 6, 9, 12, 22 and 24 hours. All subjects were dosed at time zero, just after their baseline measurement had been taken. This start time was standardized across periods within subject. The actual start time varied by up to an hour from subject to subject. Here, as the outcome variable, we consider only the FEV_1 measurement taken at 12 hours. The design is highly unbalanced, so we will focus on two treatment contrasts that reflect very different sources of information: (1) the difference between the positive and negative controls, both of which all subjects received (except those who withdrew), with a design efficiency of 97%, and (2) the difference between the high and low doses, for which *no* subject received both, with a design efficiency of 46%. We expect within-subject information to dominate in estimating the former, and between-subject information to be relatively more important for the latter.□□□

We first set out a general modeling framework for the cross-over setting with baselines and briefly review the use of baseline covariates in parallel group studies and we see how these ideas carry over to the particular case of pre-randomization baselines in cross-over studies. We then explore the role of period-dependent baselines, in terms of change-from-baseline analyses, their use as covariates (conditional) and as outcomes (unconditional). We also touch on the relevance of missing data from a modeling (not inferential) perspective.

5.4.2 Notation and basic results

Denote by $\mathbf{Y}_{ik}$ the vector of p response measurements from the periods under active treatment from the kth subject in sequence i, $i = 1, \ldots, s$. We assume that both period and direct treatment effects are included in the model, but not other effects, such as carry-over. Similarly, denote by $\mathbf{X}_{ik}$ the corresponding set of baseline measurements. Denote the individual measurements by X_{ijk} and Y_{ijk} for $j = 1, \ldots, p$. We assume in the following that these have a joint multivariate normal distribution, although, strictly, when using analysis of covariance we require only that the Ys have the appropriate conditional joint normal distribution given the Xs.

We further assume that $\mathrm{E}(\mathbf{Y}_{ik}) = \mathbf{A}_i\beta$ for design matrix $\mathbf{A}_i$ associated with the ith sequence and β the corresponding set of parameters, and $\mathrm{E}(\mathbf{X}_{ik}) = \phi$, a $(p \times 1)$ vector of means corresponding to the p times of the baseline measurements. Then

$$\begin{pmatrix} \mathbf{X}_{ik} \\ \mathbf{Y}_{ik} \end{pmatrix} \sim \mathrm{N}\left\{ \begin{pmatrix} \phi \\ \mathbf{A}_i\beta \end{pmatrix}; \begin{pmatrix} \Sigma_{XX} & \Sigma_{XY} \\ \Sigma_{XY}^T & \Sigma_{YY} \end{pmatrix} \right\}. \tag{5.2}$$

Three important expressions immediately follow from this. First, the marginal distribution of the Ys alone:

$$\mathbf{Y}_{ik} \sim \mathrm{N}(\mathbf{A}_i\beta;\ \Sigma_{YY}). \tag{5.3}$$

Second, the marginal distribution of the p changes from baseline:

$$\mathbf{Y}_{ik} - \mathbf{X}_{ik} \sim \mathrm{N}\left(\mathbf{A}_i\beta - \phi;\ \Sigma_{YY} + \Sigma_{XX} - \Sigma_{XY} - \Sigma_{XY}^T\right). \tag{5.4}$$

Third, the conditional distribution of $\mathbf{Y}_{ik}$ given $\mathbf{X}_{ik}$:

$$\mathbf{Y}_{ik} \mid \mathbf{X}_{ik} \sim \mathrm{N}\left\{\mathbf{A}_i\beta - \Theta(\phi - \mathbf{X}_{ik});\ \Sigma_{YY} - \Sigma_{XY}^T {\Sigma_{XX}}^{-1}\Sigma_{XY}\right\}, \tag{5.5}$$

for $\Theta = \Sigma_{XY}^T {\Sigma_{XX}}^{-1}$. The conditional distribution of the differences $\mathbf{Y}_{ik} - \mathbf{X}_{ik}$ given the baselines $\mathbf{X}_{ik}$ is identical to (5.4), except that the mean is shifted by $\Theta\mathbf{X}_{ik}$.

The comparative behavior of the three analyses that can be derived from these representations, (1) analysis of the outcome Y only, (2) analysis of change from baseline $Y - X$ and (3) analysis of Y conditional on X, depends on the model chosen and on the size and form of the covariance matrices Σ_{XX} and Σ_{YY}, and the covariances in Σ_{XY}. We explore the relevance of particular forms for these in the following. In particular, we begin by making the assumption of variance and covariance homogeneity within the Xs, and within the Ys, and between the Xs and the Ys. In other words, we assume an exchangeable, or compound symmetry, structure for each of three matrices:

$$\begin{aligned} \Sigma_{XX} &= \sigma_{xx}\mathbf{I}_p + \eta_{xx}\mathbf{J}_p \\ \Sigma_{YY} &= \sigma_{yy}\mathbf{I}_p + \eta_{yy}\mathbf{J}_p \\ \Sigma_{XY} &= \sigma_{xy}\mathbf{I}_p + \eta_{xy}\mathbf{J}_p = \Sigma_{XY}^T, \end{aligned} \tag{5.6}$$

where $\mathbf{I}_p$ and $\mathbf{J}_p$ denote the $p \times p$ identity matrix and matrix of ones, respectively. We regard these as the least constrained forms for these matrices that are compatible with the stability assumption inherent in most analyses for cross-over trials. Note that these expressions do not constrain the baseline and response variables to have the same variances, although they are each assumed to be constant across periods. Nor is the correlation between an adjacent baseline and a response measurement assumed to be the same as that between a baseline and a response from a different period. To see this more precisely consider the following variances and covariances implied by (5.6):

$$\begin{aligned} V(Y_{ijk}) &= \sigma_{yy} + \eta_{yy},\ V(X_{ijk}) = \sigma_{xx} + \eta_{xx}, \\ \text{Cov}(Y_{ijk}, X_{ijk}) &= \sigma_{xy} + \eta_{xy},\ \text{Cov}(Y_{ijk}, X_{ij'k}) = \eta_{xy}. \end{aligned}$$

From this it can be seen that σ_{xy} determines the additional covariance due to a baseline and response being from the same period; we will call these the *associated* baseline and response measurements, indicating they come from the same period.

We can get additional insight into this structure through the reformulation of the joint model for the Ys and Xs in (5.2), imposing the structure in (5.6) on Σ_{XX}, Σ_{XY} and Σ_{YY}. This is conveniently done in terms of two 2×2 unstructured covariance matrices, Σ_W and Σ_B, where

$$\Sigma_W = \begin{pmatrix} \sigma_{xx} & \sigma_{xy} \\ \sigma_{xy} & \sigma_{yy} \end{pmatrix} \text{ and } \Sigma_B = \begin{pmatrix} \eta_{xx} & \eta_{xy} \\ \eta_{xy} & \eta_{yy} \end{pmatrix}. \tag{5.7}$$

If the observations from a subject, $\mathbf{Z}_{ik}$ say, are then ordered by time, i.e., $\mathbf{Z}_{ik} = (X_{ik1}, Y_{ik1}, X_{ik2}, \ldots, X_{ikp}, Y_{ikp})^T$, then, in terms of these two covariance matrices,

$$V(\mathbf{Z}_{ik}) = \mathbf{I}_p \otimes \Sigma_W + \mathbf{J}_p \otimes \Sigma_B. \tag{5.8}$$

In this way Σ_W represents the covariance matrix for X and Y within a full treatment period, and Σ_B the covariance matrix between baseline and response at the subject level. To fit the model in (5.2) with this covariance structure, a fixed effects model is then constructed with a categorical time effect with $2p$ levels, one for each element of $\mathbf{Z}$, and a categorical treatment term which applies to the Ys only.

The following SAS `proc mixed` code will fit the model in (5.2) using the covariance structure given by (5.6) expressed in the form (5.7). We define the following variates: `subject`, the subject identifier; `per`, the period label, with baseline and outcome sharing the same period; `treat`, the treatment identifier associated with the outcome variable with a separate level (zero, say) for baseline; `type`, an indicator variable taking the value 1 for outcome (Y) and 0 for baseline (X). The data, `z`, consist of the baselines and outcomes in time order.

```
proc mixed;
  class subject per treat type;
  model z = per*type treat*type / solution ddfm=kenwardroger;
  random type /subject=subject type=un;
  repeated type / subject=subject*per type=un;
run;
```

The same code can be used for `proc glimmix`, with the `repeated` statement replaced by the following `random` statement:

```
proc glimmix;
  ...
  random type / subject=subject*per type=un residual;
  ...
```

Many of the conclusions below will depend on the actual values taken by the six covariance parameters in (5.6). It is therefore of interest to examine estimates of these. Kenward and Roger (2010) present estimates of these parameters from a range of examples representing very different types of design and endpoint, and from these several broad conclusions can be drawn. The subject-level correlations (ρ_B) are consistently very high indeed, often approaching one. Also, they do not vary across time for the endpoints measured repeatedly. By contrast, the within-period correlations are very much smaller, in some cases negligible. This represents dependency that exists locally in time, once the overall subject-level dependency has been accounted for. These correlations tend to decay with time as we move away from baseline measurement. But also the correlation roughly a day later (18 or 24 hours) can sometimes increase again. This commonly observed feature might be due to some personalized diurnal rhythm. The variability of the Xs and of the Ys within a trial can be very similar, or quite different, depending on the setting. We return to a detailed discussion of the values of these parameters estimated for our two examples, as given in Table 5.8, when we consider the analysis of these trials in more detail below.

To simplify the essential discussion we focus on designs that are variance balanced with respect to treatment, so in considering the precision of different approaches to the estimation of treatment effects, we need consider only a single treatment contrast, τ say, whose exact form is irrelevant to the comparisons of efficiency. We have seen above that, depending on the particular design used, and in the absence of period-dependent covariates, information on τ may be present only in the within-subject stratum, or in both the within-subject and between-subject strata. Recall that we refer to designs that lead to the former

Table 5.8: Covariance parameters and correlations estimated from Examples 5.3 and 5.4.

	Estimated Covariance Parameter						XY Correlation	
Source	$\hat{\sigma}_{xx}$	$\hat{\eta}_{xx}$	$\hat{\sigma}_{yy}$	$\hat{\eta}_{yy}$	$\hat{\sigma}_{xy}$	$\hat{\eta}_{xy}$	W-P	B-P
Example 5.3: Systolic BP ($N = 12$)	51.79	59.31	55.77	101.45	-12.14	64.06	-0.2260	0.8259
Example 5.4: FEV_1 ($N = 21$)	0.0276	0.4534	0.0233	0.4992	0.0109	0.4756	0.4298	0.9997

as orthogonal and to the latter as nonorthogonal. The first illustrative example is both variance balanced and orthogonal, the second neither of these.

We assume that τ is estimated using generalized least squares (GLS) with the appropriate *known* covariance matrix. In practice, a consistent estimator of this covariance matrix would be used, implying that the given measures of precision only hold asymptotically. This is acceptable for our goal of making *comparisons* of precision of different estimators. When these methods are applied in practice, however, some small sample adjustment will be needed in some settings for the estimated variances and associated inferences; the appropriate corrections are discussed above in Section 5.3.3.

5.4.3 Pre-randomization covariates

In the context of parallel group studies two main roles for adjustment for baseline covariates have been widely discussed, e.g., Pocock et al. (2002), namely, reducing variability and adjusting for baseline imbalance. In the current cross-over context of pre-randomization covariates, we are concerned only with the former, i.e., we assume that the role is to explain variability in the outcome measurements and so increase precision in the treatment estimators. In the cross-over setting a pre-randomization covariate can influence only between-subject information, and so has strictly limited value. This is in contrast to the situation we meet below with period level baselines, which can influence both between- and within-subject information. In an orthogonal design, such as a complete Williams square, all information on the treatment effects is wholly within-subject, and so a pre-randomization covariate will have no effect at all on the treatment estimators and their precision.

Adjustment for pre-randomization covariates will therefore make a worthwhile improvement to precision when there exists a nontrivial amount of information on the treatment effect in the between-subjects stratum, which requires a highly nonorthogonal design, such as the *incomplete* designs for which $p < t$ considered in Section 4.2.2, or when there is a very high proportion of dropouts from an originally orthogonal one. Consider, as an illustration, the three-treatment Williams design consisting of all six possible sequences. With a single replicate of this design, and using the model introduced above, the generalized least squares estimator of any treatment difference has variance

$$\frac{\sigma_{yy}(\sigma_{yy}+2\eta_{yy})}{2\sigma_{yy}+3\eta_{yy}} = \sigma_{yy}\left(\frac{1+\rho_Y}{2+\rho_Y}\right) \tag{5.9}$$

for $\rho_Y = \eta_{yy}/(\sigma_{yy}+\eta_{yy})$. Even in the impossibly extreme case in which the covariate removes the between-subject variability *altogether*, the ratio of variances of the unadjusted and adjusted estimators is still only

$$1+\frac{\rho_Y}{2+\rho_Y}.$$

which, with a correlation of 0.8, for example, is less than 1.3. For the trials considered by Kenward and Roger (2010) this quantity is remarkably stable, ranging from 1.19 to 1.33. In practice, adjustment will be less effective than this, possibly much less so. Thus we do not usually expect a large gain in precision in such settings, but adjustment may still be considered worthwhile in some cases. The problem is that the variability that is being explained, i.e., the between-subject component, is usually the far less important part of the information contributing to the treatment estimator, even in nonorthogonal designs. On the other hand, such adjustment should have a negligible effect as well on power, so it can be regarded as a relatively safe, if pointless, exercise.

5.4.4 *Period-dependent baseline covariates*

5.4.4.1 *What we mean by a baseline*

We now consider the use of period-dependent baselines. In contrast to the previous section, we are now considering the impact of these with respect to information at the between-subject and within-subject level; hence both variance reduction and baseline imbalance between treatments are potentially important.

We also need at this point to clarify the use of baseline as a term. It is sometimes used to refer to a measurement made in a trial (parallel or cross-over) as part of the measurement process, but following treatment. Examples are measurements made at the start of exercise tests, and before challenges. Such baselines should never be used as covariates, and we exclude them from the current development. Although the period-dependent baselines we consider here are made following randomization of the subject to sequence, we are assuming that they are made before treatment is given within each period and that the wash-out periods are sufficient to ensure that these baselines are not influenced by previous treatment, that is, they are not affected by carry-over. There are situations in which the wash-out is insufficiently long to firmly rule out the possibility of baseline contamination through carry-over effects. Such contamination obviously makes such baselines unsuitable as covariates. Although one might test for this formally before deciding whether even to consider incorporating the baseline measurements in the analysis, such a sequential procedure raises many of the issues associated with prior testing in the two-period two-treatment design as discussed in Section 2.7 and should generally be avoided.

5.4.4.2 *Change from baseline*

We begin by considering a conventional analysis of the change from baseline, $D = Y - X$. It follows immediately from (5.4) that any least squares estimator of the direct treatment effect will be unbiased, as the impact of ϕ in the expectation will be only to modify the intercept and period effects. Hence the design matrices for both approaches here coincide. The consequence on the analysis, in comparison with that of the Ys only, will therefore only be in terms of precision. Under the covariance assumptions in (5.6) we see that the p changes $\mathbf{D}_{ik}$ for one subject have the compound symmetry covariance structure:

$$\mathrm{V}(\mathbf{D}_{ik}) = \mathrm{V}(\mathbf{Y}_{ik} - \mathbf{X}_{ik}) = (\sigma_{xx} + \sigma_{yy} - 2\sigma_{xy})\mathbf{I}_p + (\eta_{xx} + \eta_{yy} - 2\eta_{xy})\mathbf{J}_p,$$

compared with that of the original Ys:

$$\mathrm{V}(\mathbf{Y}_{ik}) = \sigma_{yy}\mathbf{I}_p + \eta_{yy}\mathbf{J}_p.$$

It follows that in any given setting, depending on the relative sizes of these parameters, and on the particular design, either an analysis of the Ys or of the changes from baseline $Y - X$ may lead to more precise estimators of the treatment effects. We need to consider what is likely to occur in common settings. Suppose first that the design is orthogonal in the sense introduced in Section 5.4.2. In such designs the treatment estimators do not depend on the variance parameters. Let $\widehat{\tau}_Y$ and $\widehat{\tau}_D$ denote, respectively, the GLS estimators from the response data alone and the changes from baseline. It follows immediately that

$$R = \frac{\mathrm{V}(\widehat{\tau}_D)}{\mathrm{V}(\widehat{\tau}_Y)} = \frac{\sigma_{yy} + \sigma_{xx} - 2\sigma_{xy}}{\sigma_{yy}}.$$

The analysis of the changes D will be more precise only when $\sigma_{xx} < 2\sigma_{xy}$. Recall that σ_{xx} is the within-subject, or residual, variance of the baselines, and σ_{xy} represents the amount by which the covariance of an associated baseline and response exceeds that of a response and baseline from different periods. This inequality holds for only three of the examples considered by Kenward and Roger (2010), and in these this feature has decayed by later time points within periods. Both parameters relate to the within-subject distribution and the property is generally about the size of the local rather than long-term (or between-subject) correlation. If the variance of baseline is the same as that of the response, then this is equivalent to the within-subject correlation of response with baseline being greater than a half.

Suppose that we have an exchangeable covariance structure across all eight measurements, as would be implied by a simple random subject effects model. This might be appropriate when the time interval between baseline and associated response is of the same order as between a response and a baseline from the following period, or both long enough although of different lengths, and the variance is stable across all measurements. This would imply that $\sigma_{yy} = \sigma_{xx}$, $\eta_{yy} = \eta_{xx} = \eta_{xy}$ and $\sigma_{xy} = 0$. We call this the *uniform assumption*. Under this we have the ratio

$$R = \frac{\mathrm{V}(\widehat{\tau}_D)}{\mathrm{V}(\widehat{\tau}_Y)} = \frac{\sigma_{yy} + \sigma_{xx} - 2\sigma_{xy}}{\sigma_{yy}} = \frac{\sigma_{yy} + \sigma_{yy} - 2 \times 0}{\sigma_{yy}} = 2;$$

the estimator from the differences D would have twice the variance of that based on the simple responses Y alone.

In conclusion, the analysis of the differences will only be worth considering in those settings in which $\sigma_{xx} < 2\sigma_{xy}$. This is most likely to happen if baselines are relatively close in time to that of the associated responses, compared to the gap between treatment periods, implying that σ_{xy} may plausibly be non-negligible. This highlights the importance of the local (or serial) nature of the correlation, for an analysis of difference from baseline to be appropriate. In addition to this, the inequality is also more likely to hold if the baseline variables are considerably less variable than the response measurements. This can happen when there is large heterogeneity of response to treatment among a group of carefully selected subjects, or the baseline measurement has been averaged over several baseline measurements. Empirical examples of the former are given in Kenward and Jones (1987). Although the results given here depend on exact balance and orthogonality, mild departures from this due to dropout and incomplete replication of sequences would not be expected to greatly change this overall picture.

As an illustration we consider Example 5.3, the three-treatment Williams design which is balanced and orthogonal. The six covariance parameter estimates are presented in Table 5.8. Note that $\hat{\sigma}_{xy}$, the additional within-subject covariance for associated X and Y, is negative but comparatively small. Consequently we would expect the analysis of change from baseline ($D = Y - X$) to be far less precise than the analysis of Y alone, and this is indeed what is found. Using REML to fit a random subject effects model with categorical period and direct treatment fixed effects, the high-low dose comparison is estimated (with accompanying SE) for Y and D, as 6.67 (3.04) and 5.08 (4.61), respectively, showing a 52% increase in SE in the latter. Using Y alone the effect is statistically significant at 5% ($P = 0.04$), while using D it is far from significance ($P = 0.28$). The use of change from baseline is, for this example, clearly counterproductive.

When designs are used in which treatments and periods are highly non-orthogonal, such as Example 5.4, then it is harder to provide broad guidelines. In such settings we have seen that the GLS estimators consist of weighted combinations of within-subject and between-subject information, with the weights depending directly on the parameters of the covariance structure. It is possible that the changes from baseline may remove considerable variability from the subject sums component, and hence markedly increase the contribution of the between-subject information to the overall precision. However, this may well be counterbalanced by the potential loss in precision of the within-subject differences, as seen above in orthogonal designs. How these two contributions balance out in practice depends both on the covariance parameters and the particular design. Consider again, as an example, the three-treatment Williams design. From (5.9) it can be seen that the ratio of the variances from the estimators using the differences $Y - D$, and Y alone, respectively, is in terms of the original covariance parameters,

$$R = \frac{(2\sigma_{yy}+3\eta_{yy})(\sigma_{yy}+\sigma_{xx}-2\sigma_{xy})(\sigma_{yy}+\sigma_{xx}-2\sigma_{xy}+2\eta_{xx}+2\eta_{yy}-4\eta_{xy})}{\sigma_{yy}(\sigma_{yy}+2\eta_{yy})(2\sigma_{yy}+2\sigma_{xx}-4\sigma_{xy}+3\eta_{xx}+3\eta_{yy}-6\eta_{xy})}$$

$$= \frac{(\sigma_{yy}+\sigma_{xx}-2\sigma_{xy})}{\sigma_{yy}} \frac{(1+\rho_D)}{(2+\rho_D)} \frac{(2+\rho_Y)}{(1+\rho_Y)} \tag{5.10}$$

where

$$\rho_D = \frac{\eta_{yy}+\eta_{xx}-2\eta_{xy}}{\sigma_{yy}+\sigma_{xx}-2\sigma_{xy}+\eta_{yy}+\eta_{xx}-2\eta_{xy}}$$

is the within-subject correlation of the differences $Y-X$. Suppose now that the uniform assumption holds, i.e., as before, $\sigma_{yy}=\sigma_{xx}$, $\eta_{yy}=\eta_{xx}=\eta_{xy}$ and $\sigma_{xy}=0$. Under these assumptions, R in (5.10) is equal to $(2+\rho_Y)/(1+\rho_Y)$, which, for $0<\rho_Y<1$, is in the range $1.5<R<2$. Again, we see that the use of the changes from baseline increases the variance compared with the use of the Ys alone. The reduction in between-subject variability makes some contribution, and so R is smaller than the value 2 seen above for the orthogonal cross-over designs, but never enough to counterbalance the increase in within-subject variability. This is an inefficient design, with considerable between-subject information. Even in this setting we see that the use of change from baseline, under the uniform assumption, increases the variability. Given this, we conjecture that only with the most extreme inefficient designs would the use of change from baseline improve the precision relative to the use of Y alone, and our recommendation, if the uniform assumption approximately holds, is to use the latter, not the former, even with nonorthogonal designs.

In the general covariance setting (5.6) it is harder to draw broad conclusions because of the relative complexity of (5.10). However, if we again assume that $\sigma_{xx}<2\sigma_{xy}$, the condition under which the differences lead to more precise estimates than Y alone for orthogonal designs, then a sufficient condition for greater precision from the analysis of the differences is that $\rho_D<\rho_Y$, which in turn implies

$$\left(\frac{1-\rho_Y}{\rho_Y}\right)(\eta_{xx}-2\eta_{xy}) < \sigma_{xx}-2\sigma_{xy} < 0.$$

The first term on the left hand side, $(1-\rho_Y)/\rho_Y$, will always be less than one for $\rho_Y>0.5$, and this implies that, depending on the size of ρ_Y, η_{xy}, the covariance between any nonassociated X and Y must not be much smaller than η_{xx}, the covariance between any two Xs. Given that an X must be measured in the interval between any other X and a nonassociated Y, and given the symmetry in the assumed covariance structure, it is plausible that η_{xy} will typically be less than η_{xx}, so this condition is not one which might automatically be assumed to hold.

We now consider Example 5.4 in the light of these results. A random subject effects model with categorical period and direct treatment fixed effects has again been fitted using REML. We note first that the estimated residual and between-subject variance estimates are 0.023 and 0.503 for the raw outcomes Y, and 0.030 and 0.001 for the differences D, respectively. There is very high correlation between the baselines X and outcomes Y, and virtually all random between-subject variability has been removed from the differences. The covariance parameter estimates are given in Table 5.8. Note the size of $\hat{\sigma}_{xy}$: this strongly suggests that the uniform assumption does not hold here. The key quantity $\sigma_{xx} - 2\sigma_{xy}$ is here estimated as 0.0057, which would suggest, for an orthogonal design, that subtracting the baseline would have very little effect on precision. Here we would expect this to apply to the first (efficiently estimated) contrast. For the second contrast it is harder to predict the effect of subtracting X. From the analyses of Y and D, respectively, we get, for contrast (1), the estimates (and SEs) 0.126 (0.049) and 0.224 (0.055). Although these estimates are rather different, the use of change from baseline has increased the variance only very slightly. For the second contrast, the estimates from Y and D are, respectively, 0.055 (0.100) and −0.014 (0.099). Again the estimates are somewhat different but there is very little difference in precision. The differences we see between the treatment estimates (with and without change from baseline) represent the differences between the baseline scores for these contrasts (−0.081 and 0.072). In conclusion, analyzing change from baseline has had little effect on precision compared with the analysis of response alone. The consequences for the estimates are not negligible, however, and this is probably due to the exceptionally high correlation between baseline and response at the subject level, estimated here as 0.997. This very high value has other implications for the analysis of these data, which we will explore below.

The appropriate route therefore is to introduce the baselines as covariates, whether for the raw responses (Y) or the differences ($Y - X$). In this way any baseline imbalance is accommodated, but the data are being allowed to select between absolute and difference from baseline. This, however, introduces new issues that need to be addressed, as we see below.

5.4.4.3 Baselines as covariates

Without particular constraints on the covariance structure, *all* p observed baselines appear in the expectations of each element of $\mathbf{Y}_{ik}$ in the conditional distribution of $\mathbf{Y}_{ik}$ given $\mathbf{X}_{ik}$. This implies an analysis of covariance in which all p baselines appear as covariates for all p response variables. Such an analysis is rarely, if ever, done in practice, however. Conventionally, only the associated baseline is used to adjust the corresponding response. We therefore begin, for the covariance structure introduced in Section 5.4.2, by considering what constraints on this structure would lead to this conventional analysis. From (5.5) we see that the regression coefficients of $\mathbf{Y}_{ik}$ on $\mathbf{X}_{ik}$ are given by the elements of $\Theta = \Sigma_{XY}^T \Sigma_{XX}{}^{-1}$, or in terms of the expressions for the covariance components in (5.6).

$$\begin{aligned} \Theta &= (\sigma_{xy}\mathbf{I}_p + \eta_{xy}\mathbf{J}_p)(\sigma_{xx}\mathbf{I}_p + \eta_{xx}\mathbf{J}_p)^{-1} \\ &= \frac{\sigma_{xy}}{\sigma_{xx}}\mathbf{I}_p + \frac{\eta_{xy}\sigma_{xx} - \eta_{xx}\sigma_{xy}}{\sigma_{xx}(\sigma_{xx} + p\eta_{xx})}\mathbf{J}_p. \end{aligned} \tag{5.11}$$

For the conventional analysis of covariance model to hold, θ must be diagonal because each element of $\mathbf{Y}_{ik}$ is regressed only on the element of $\mathbf{X}_{ik}$ from the same period, which in turn implies that $\eta_{xy}\sigma_{xx} - \eta_{xx}\sigma_{xy} = 0$. First we note that this cannot hold under the uniform assumption, for which $\sigma_{xy} = 0$, unless all measurements are mutually independent. More generally, this requirement implies that Σ_{XY} is proportional to Σ_{XX}, and it is difficult to find a practical justification for this rather contrived assumption.

We consider next the behavior of the conventional analysis of covariance under the covariance structure of Section 5.4.2, Equation (5.6). To explore potential bias we again examine separately the within-subject and between-subject information. Let the fixed matrix $\mathbf{K}$ be any $p \times (p-1)$ matrix satisfying $\mathbf{K}^T\mathbf{K} = \mathbf{I}_{p-1}$ and $\mathbf{K}^T\mathbf{j}_p = \mathbf{0}$, for $\mathbf{j}_p$ a p dimensional vector of ones. The within-subject information for the ikth subject can be represented by $\mathbf{K}^T\mathbf{Y}_{ik}$, which has regression model

$$\mathrm{E}(\mathbf{K}^T\mathbf{Y}_{ik} \mid \mathbf{X}_{ik}) = \mathbf{K}^T\mathbf{A}_i\beta - \mathbf{K}^T\Theta\phi + \mathbf{K}^T\Theta\mathbf{X}_{ik}.$$

Using (5.11) we see that the regression coefficient for the covariates reduces to a constant for the appropriate functions of the covariates:

$$\begin{aligned} \mathbf{K}^T\Theta\mathbf{X}_{ik} &= \frac{\sigma_{xy}}{\sigma_{xx}}\mathbf{K}^T\mathbf{I}_p\mathbf{X}_{ik} + \frac{\eta_{xy}\sigma_{xx} - \eta_{xx}\sigma_{xy}}{\sigma_{xx}(\sigma_{xx} + p\eta_{xx})}\mathbf{K}^T\mathbf{J}_p\mathbf{X}_{ik} \\ &= \frac{\sigma_{xy}}{\sigma_{xx}}\mathbf{K}^T\mathbf{X}_{ik} \\ &= \theta_W\mathbf{X}_{ik}^W, \text{ say.} \end{aligned} \tag{5.12}$$

This implies that a conventional (i.e., each response adjusted by its associated covariate only) within-subject analysis of covariance will be unbiased for the treatment effects. Such an analysis would be produced, for example, by using fixed subject effects with the original data.

We now consider the between-subject information, which can be represented by $\mathbf{j}_p^T\mathbf{Y}_{ik}$. This has regression model

$$\mathrm{E}(\mathbf{j}_p^T\mathbf{Y}_{ik} \mid \mathbf{X}_{ik}) = \mathbf{j}_p^T\mathbf{A}_i\beta - \mathbf{j}_p^T\Theta\phi + \mathbf{j}_p^T\Theta\mathbf{X}_{ik},$$

and the regression coefficient of the covariates reduces to

$$\begin{aligned}
\mathbf{j}_p^T \Theta \mathbf{X}_{ik} &= \frac{\sigma_{xy}}{\sigma_{xx}} \mathbf{j}_p^T \mathbf{I}_p \mathbf{X}_{ik} + \frac{\eta_{xy}\sigma_{xx} - \eta_{xx}\sigma_{xy}}{\sigma_{xx}(\sigma_{xx} + p\eta_{xx})} \mathbf{j}_p^T \mathbf{J}_p \mathbf{X}_{ik} \\
&= \frac{\sigma_{xy} + p\eta_{xy}}{\sigma_{xx} + p\eta_{xx}} \mathbf{j}^T \mathbf{X}_{ik} \\
&= \theta_B X_{ik}^B, \text{ say.} \qquad (5.13)
\end{aligned}$$

This implies that, for designs in which treatments can be estimated using between-subject information only, such as the main plot treatment in a split-plot design, these treatment estimators will be unbiased.

However, when both between-subject and within-subject information is combined in the conventional REML analysis of covariance, the assumption is implicitly made that both the within-subject covariate functions $\mathbf{X}_{ik}^W$ and between-subject function X_{ik}^B have the same regression coefficient, i.e., $\theta_W = \theta_B$, and it is clear from (5.12) and (5.13) that this can never be true unless the very artificial constraint $\sigma_{xy} = \eta_{xy} = 0$ holds. Thus, in general, the conventional analysis of covariance will be biased for the treatment effects. This is an example of so-called *cross-level bias* (Sheppard (2003)).

This bias can be avoided in two ways. In the first, the analysis is restricted to within-subject information, that is, by using fixed subject effects. This is anyway the appropriate approach when there is little or no relevant between-subject information in the data, such as with a Williams design. Second, if random subject effects are used, then different coefficients *must* be allowed for the between- and within-subject covariate regressions. This can be done simply by adding to the model the variate that consists of the value of the covariate averaged over each subject. An alternative solution under the random subject effects model is to introduce fixed *sequence* effects, but as this anyway removes all between-subject information from the treatment estimators, and it is a rather pointless exercise; it is then more logical to use fixed subject effects, or use the baselines as outcomes.

We now return to the two Examples 5.3 and 5.4. First we consider the Williams design from the study on blood pressure. In the absence of covariates, treatment effects are, in this design, completely orthogonal to periods and subjects. The introduction of covariates will introduce some nonorthogonality, but in a design like this it would not be expected to be great. Consequently, within-subject information will still dominate the treatment estimates and so it is the size of the within-subject covariate coefficient that will be critical when considering the impact of wrongly omitting the separation of within-subject and between-subject covariate regressions. When a common covariate is fitted (we label this coefficient θ_C), the estimated coefficient will be a weighted combination of the within-subject and between-subject coefficients (labeled θ_W and θ_B, respectively, in (5.12) and (5.13)) and the greater the relative precision of the former, the smaller the difference will be between the $\hat{\theta}_C$ and $\hat{\theta}_W$, which in turn will reduce the resulting bias of the common covariate analysis. For this example, fitting a single overall covariate results in an estimate (SE) of $\hat{\theta}_C = 0.08$ (0.23), which is close to zero. However, the within-subject and between-subject estimates are, respectively, $\hat{\theta}_W = -0.23$ (0.24) and $\hat{\theta}_B = 0.78$ (0.31). In terms of precision, the within-subject estimate remains negligible, but the between-subject coefficient is comparatively large and statistically significant. The consequences for the high-low treatment comparison are as follows. For the common and separate covariate analyses the estimated comparisons (SEs) are, respectively, 6.53 (3.18) and 7.04 (3.07). The impact of the difference in covariate coefficient is, in the present example, not great, being equivalent to an increase in sample size of 7%. This is partly because the analysis largely involves only within-subject information; it would typically be considerably greater in a highly nonorthogonal design. The impact is, however, sufficient in this example to change the associated P-value from $P = 0.06$ to $P = 0.03$ using for the analyses common and separate covariates, respectively. The impact also depends, however, on the imbalance of the covariates between the treatments within periods: if they are perfectly balanced, the covariate has no effect on the adjusted means. Here the imbalance is comparatively small.

For the second illustrative example it is much harder to predict the impact of inappropriately using the common covariate. Within-subject and between-subject information is combined in a complex way both in estimating the effects of interest and in estimating the covariate coefficients, and the lack of balance means that, in principle, the consequences can be quite different for different treatment effects. In this particular example the very large subject-level correlation between baseline and response noted earlier (0.997) will have a large impact. Fitting a common covariate produces an estimated coefficient of $\hat{\theta}_C = 1.01$ (0.03), while fitting the covariate separately at the within-subject and between-subject levels produces estimated coefficients of $\hat{\theta}_W = 0.42$ (0.10) and $\hat{\theta}_B = 1.04$ (0.03), respectively. The latter coefficient is very close to one and is far more precise than the within-subject coefficient, and the combined estimate $\hat{\theta}_C$ is, as seen, also close to one, implying that adjustment by the single covariate and change from baseline will, in this very particular setting, be numerically very similar, implying in turn that the bias should not be great using the single covariate in spite of the large difference between $\hat{\theta}_W$ and $\hat{\theta}_B$. This is indeed what is seen. For comparison between the positive and negative controls, the use of the single covariate produces an estimate (SE) of 0.225 (0.055), which is almost identical to that seen earlier in the analysis of change from baseline D: 0.224 (0.055). Adjustment using both within-subject and between-subject covariates produces by comparison an estimate (SE) of 0.173 (0.046). There is an increase in precision associated with the smaller estimated within-subject residual, and the change in estimated coefficient is of the order of one SE. For the comparison between high dose and low dose, the corresponding three estimates (SEs) are 0.011 (0.100), 0.014 (0.099), and 0.040 (0.084). The relative decrease in the size of the standard error is the same for the two comparisons. But the change in estimated value is less extreme in the second case than in the first because this comparison makes more use of the between-subject information. The gain in precision through using the two baseline covariates is equivalent to an increase in sample size of 40%.

5.4.5 *Baselines as response variables*

An alternative approach to inclusion of the baseline variables in the analysis is to treat them as additional response variables without accompanying fixed treatment effects. Such an approach is well established in the analysis of parallel group longitudinal studies; see, for example, Kenward et al. (2010). One important result is that in particular balanced orthogonal settings under certain models, the treatment estimates obtained through the use of baselines as covariates or as responses are *identical*, with very similar standard errors and a difference of one in degrees of freedom. A proof of this is given in Appendix 4.4 of Carpenter and Kenward (2008). In other settings, such as with unbalanced and/or nonorthogonal designs, we typically expect very similar estimates and inferences that converge asymptotically. There will be systematic differences between the two approaches, typically still small, however, when numbers of observations differ among subjects. We return to this issue below. Here we assume that there are no missing values and that numbers of periods are the same for all subjects.

The model we use is precisely the joint one for the time-ordered data $\mathbf{Z}_{ik}$ described in Section 5.4.2, and can be fitted using the generic SAS `mixed` code given there. Note that we do not in general constrain the period effects associated with baseline and response to be the same, hence the presence of the type-by-period interaction in the MIXED model statement.

Applying this analysis to Example 5.3, we obtain an estimated high versus low dose comparison (SE, DF) of −0.949 (1.793, 20), compared with that from the analysis of covariance in the previous section with separate within-subject and between-subject covariates of −0.949 (1.763, 19). In this very special balanced/orthogonal setting we see, as predicted, that the estimates are identical, the SEs are very similar, and the d.f. differ by one. With such a design, and complete data, both analyses are, for practical purposes, identical.

Example 5.4 is neither balanced nor orthogonal. We begin with the first contrast, positive versus negative control. Applying the above approach to the joint analysis of the the baselines and outcomes, we get a contrast estimate (SE, d.f.) of 0.170 (0.045, 67.6), compared with the analysis of covariance from the previous section: 0.173 (0.046, 66.1). The estimates and associated SEs are similar but the difference in d.f. suggests that more is different between these two analyses than in the balanced/orthogonal case. This is indeed the case, and the difference is partly due to the missing data. We return to this point below. A similar picture is seen with the second treatment contrast, the high versus low dose comparison. The estimates (SE, d.f.) from the joint and covariance based analyses are 0.0343 (0.0825, 82) and 0.0270 (0.0830, 83.4), respectively. Here the estimates show a greater difference. The patterns in these two sets of comparisons reflect the range of influences on differences between these two types of analysis: lack of balance, nonorthogonality, incompleteness and estimated variance parameters. In spite of these, however, the differences remain small and are negligible from a practical perspective.

We note finally that, strictly, the sample space is different in the two types of analysis, respectively marginal and conditional, for the joint-model and covariate-based analysis. This implies that we should be careful in comparing, for example, precision from the two approaches. We see, however, both from theory and empirically, that in such settings the practical differences between the analyses in terms of estimates, precision and inferences are usually negligible, and so we do not regard this distinction as an important issue in the current setting.

5.4.6 *Incomplete data*

As pointed out in the introduction to Section 5.4.2, without specific constraints on the covariance structure of the $2p$ repeated measurements, all p baselines $\mathbf{X}_{ik}$ will appear as covariates in the analysis of covariance of $\mathbf{Y}_{ik}$, and the coefficients of these may be different among the Ys within a subject. The reduction of these to just two common coefficients for the within-subject baselines ($\mathbf{X}_{ik}^W$) and for the average baseline (X_{ik}^B) depends on the particular form of covariance structure specified in (5.6), with the relevant coefficients presented in (5.12) and (5.13), respectively. For the derivation of these, and the consequences on the analysis, it was assumed in Section 5.4.2 that p is a constant, that is, all subjects have a complete set of measurements. When data are missing, which is a common occurrence in practice, this will no longer be the case and we examine here the implications of this for the results presented so far. Because of the symmetry of our covariance structure, the implication of missing data will be the same (in terms of the covariate structure of the analysis of covariance) whichever periods the data are missing from. So it is only the total number of periods observed for a particular subject, p_{ik} say, that is relevant, not the pattern of missingness, and we can apply the arguments leading to (5.12) and (5.13) subject by subject, replacing p by p_{ik} in each case. It follows immediately that the reduction to the within-subject and between-baseline covariates, ($\mathbf{X}_{ik}^W$ and X_{ik}^B), still holds. Next we note that the coefficient for $\mathbf{X}_{ik}^W$ does not depend on p, so this remains the same irrespective of missing data, and therefore holds across all subjects. In contrast, we see that the coefficient of X_{ik}^B *does* depend on p. The coefficient of this covariate therefore depends on the number of missing data and, strictly, in the analysis of covariance θ_B should be allowed to take different values for each of the possible values of p. Holding this to a constant value, as we have done above in the analysis of the second example, introduces bias into the estimates which does not disappear with increasing sample size if the proportion and pattern of missing data are maintained. We conjecture, however, that in practice such bias will be very small indeed, and the simpler analysis presented earlier will provide a perfectly acceptable approximation. There are two main reasons for this. First, in the simpler analysis the bias only comes from the contribution of the between-subject information, which is typically the much less important component. Second, unless an unusually high proportion of subjects have missing data, the estimate of the common covariate coefficient will anyway be dominated by subjects with complete data, and so be close to the required coefficient for these subjects. Finally, in the approach of the previous section in which the baselines are treated as responses, this modification of the between-subject covariate coefficient is (implicitly) done correctly and this source of bias does not arise.

Of the two examples used in this section, only the second, 5.4, has missing data, but there are two main reasons why we expect the bias discussed here to be negligible in this case. First, only four subjects have missing data. Second, the between-subject covariance parameters $(\eta_{xx}, \eta_{yy}, \eta_{xy})$ dominate the within-subject parameters $(\sigma_{xx}, \sigma_{yy}, \sigma_{xy})$ and, if the coefficient (5.13) is re-written as

$$\theta_B = \frac{\eta_{xy} + \sigma_{xy}/p}{\eta_{xx} + \sigma_{xx}/p},$$

it is clear that in such circumstances the coefficient is almost independent of p. We see this reflected in the analysis. Looking at the first treatment comparison, positive versus negative control, the previous analysis of covariance gave an estimate (SE, d.f.) of 0.173 (0.046, 66.1). Allowing θ_B to differ for the subject with incomplete data gives, by comparison, 0.170 (0.045, 67.6), which is very similar.

In conclusion: strictly, when there are missing data, the between-subject covariate coefficient should be allowed to differ according to the size of p_{ik}. We suggest, however, that, in practice, the simpler analysis with common coefficient will provide a very good approximation to such an approach. If there are concerns about such bias, the coefficient can be allowed to differ in the analysis, or the marginal analysis of Section 5.4.5 can be used.

Finally, we note that when baselines are missing but their associated response variables are observed, the joint analysis of Section 5.4.5 does have an advantage over the analysis of covariance. The analysis of covariance will discard the associated responses, while the joint approach will lead to their inclusion.

5.5 Analyses for higher-order two-treatment designs

5.5.1 Analysis for Balaam's design

5.5.1.1 Example 5.5: Amantadine in Parkinsonism

We will illustrate the analysis of Balaam's design by using some data from a trial described by Hunter et al. (1970). The aim of the trial was to determine

Table 5.9: Example 5.5: Average scores for amantadine trial.

Group	Subject	Baseline	Period 1	Period 2
1 AA	1	14	12.50	14.00
	2	27	24.25	22.50
	3	19	17.25	16.25
	4	30	28.25	29.75
2 BB	1	21	20.00	19.51
	2	11	10.50	10.00
	3	20	19.50	20.75
	4	25	22.50	23.50
3 AB	1	9	8.75	8.75
	2	12	10.50	9.75
	3	17	15.00	18.50
	4	21	21.00	21.50
4 BA	1	23	22.00	18.00
	2	15	15.00	13.00
	3	13	14.00	13.75
	4	24	22.75	21.50
	5	18	17.75	16.75

if amantadine hydrochloride produced a beneficial effect on subjects suffering from Parkinsonism. Amantadine (treatment A) was compared to a matching placebo (treatment B) on 17 subjects over a period of 9 weeks. Each subject's physical signs were evaluated in week 1, prior to receiving A or B, and then at weekly intervals. There were no wash-out periods. Necessarily the sequence groups are of different sizes. Each treatment was administered, in a double-blind fashion, for a period of 4 consecutive weeks. Subjects were evaluated by using a scoring system. Each of 11 physical signs (drooling saliva, finger dexterity, walking, rising from chair, balance, speech, rigidity, posture, tremor, sweating and facial masking) were scored on a 0 to 4 point scale.

For our analysis we will consider a period to be made up of the 4 weeks on each treatment and we will use the average score over the 4 weeks as our response measurement. The total of these 11 scores then gives the final score. These summary scores observed are presented in Table 5.9, along with the baseline scores taken in week 1. It should be noted that Groups 3 and 4, as presented in this table, correspond to Groups 4 and 3, respectively, as given by Hunter et al. (1970).□□□

We begin our analysis of these data by looking at the subject profiles given in Figure 5.2. For each subject in each group we have plotted the baseline score, the scores for Periods 1 and 2, and joined them up. Apart from noticing that most subjects respond with a lower score in Period 1 as compared to their

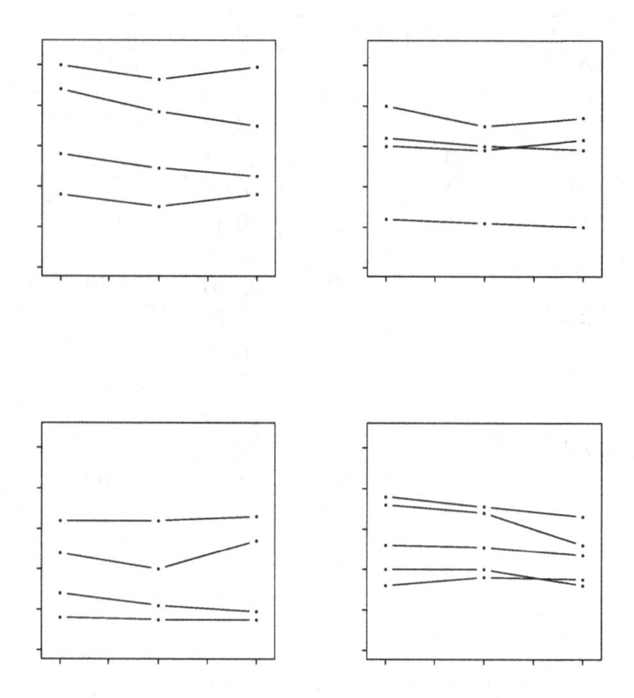

Figure 5.2: Example 5.5: Subject profiles for each group.

baseline and that there does not appear to be a period effect, there is nothing else striking about these plots.

Additional information can be obtained from the baseline and period means in each group. These are given in Table 5.10. The means are more informative than the plots and suggest that (a) within Groups 3 and 4, A gives a lower score than B, (b) the difference between A and B is greater when the baseline score is high and (c) in Groups 1 and 2 there is no period effect. One of the

Table 5.10: Example 5.5: Group-by-period means.

Group	Size	Baseline	Period 1	Period 2
1 AA	$n_1 = 4$	22.50	$\bar{y}_{11.} = 20.56$	$\bar{y}_{12.} = 20.63$
2 BB	$n_2 = 4$	19.25	$\bar{y}_{21.} = 18.13$	$\bar{y}_{22.} = 18.44$
3 AB	$n_3 = 4$	14.75	$\bar{y}_{31.} = 13.81$	$\bar{y}_{32.} = 14.63$
4 BA	$n_4 = 5$	18.60	$\bar{y}_{41.} = 18.30$	$\bar{y}_{42.} = 16.60$

points made about Balaam's design when it was described in Chapter 3 was that it provided within-subject information on the carry-over effect, but that the real benefit depended on the assumption that there was no treatment-by-carry-over interaction. In the following we show how these two terms can be examined in this design, but we again emphasize that in small trials, like the current example, tests for such effects will have low power.

We now investigate these suggestions more formally by fitting the following model:

$$Y_{ijk} = \mu + \pi_j + \tau_{d[i,j]} + \lambda_{d[i,j-1]} + (\tau\lambda)_{d[i,j]} + s_{ik} + e_{ijk}, \quad i = 1,2,3,4, \quad j = 1,2,$$

for $\{\lambda_{d[i,j-1]}\}$, the additive carry-over effects, and $\{(\tau\lambda)_{d[i,j]}\}$, the treatment-by-carry-over interaction effects. In Balaam's design there is no within-subject information on direct treatment effect in the AA and BB sequences; hence it is important in this setting to consider the recovery of between-subject information. Following the steps in Section 5.3, we do this by introducing random subject effects into the model:

```
proc mixed;
  class  patient period treatment carry;
  model score = period treatment carry carry*treatment / s
                                         ddfm=kenwardroger;
  random patient;
run;
```

The estimates of the within- and between-subject variances are as follows:

Cov Parm	Estimate
patient	29.7409
Residual	1.1374

The between-subject component of the variance is almost 30 times larger than the within-subject component. This means that in this particular trial the between-subject totals contain very little useful information and this has implications for the value of this particular design in this setting. This produces the following Wald tests:

Type 3 Tests of Fixed Effects				
Effect	Num DF	Den DF	F Value	Pr > F
period	1	14.1	0.00	0.9898
treatment	1	14	5.13	0.0398
carry	1	15	0.17	0.6891
treatment*carry	1	14	1.15	0.3010

These are very close to those that would be obtained using *fixed* subject effects:

Type 3 Tests of Fixed Effects				
	Num	Den		
Effect	DF	DF	F Value	Pr > F
patient	16	13	50.78	<.0001
period	1	13	0.01	0.9133
treatment	1	13	5.49	0.0358
carry	1	13	0.05	0.8256
treatment*carry	1	13	0.83	0.3797

This similarity is a consequence of the very large between-subject variation. We can think of the fixed subject effects analysis as a limiting case of the random subjects analysis in which this variance tends to infinity.

From either analysis there is little evidence of an interaction between carry-over and treatment. However, the power for this test is not high compared with that for the direct treatment effect: the SEs are 1.31 and 0.49, respectively, for the interaction and the *unadjusted* direct treatment effect. Hence we should not read too much into this lack of significance. However, to make progress we need to assume that this interaction is negligible. Dropping it from the model (and for simplicity keeping fixed subject effects, because we know the choice is relatively unimportant here), we get the following Wald tests from the reduced model:

Type 3 Tests of Fixed Effects				
	Num	Den		
Effect	DF	DF	F Value	Pr > F
patient	16	14	53.09	<.0001
period	1	14	0.13	0.7241
treatment	1	14	4.74	0.0472
carry	1	14	0.02	0.9008

We can see that when adjusted for carry-over effects the direct treatment difference is not significant (P = 0.05). If we wish to adjust for carry-over and avoid the problems associated with sequential testing, at least with respect to the carry-over term, then we have to stay with this estimator. Adjusting for carry-over has roughly doubled the variance of the estimated direct treatment effect. In the absence of carry-over, the test for the direct treatment effect would have had a *P*-value of 0.02. In this reduced model the point estimate of $\tau_2 - \tau_1$ is 1.29 with a standard error of 0.486 on 15 d.f. A 95% confidence interval is (0.25, 2.32). When adjusted for carry-over it is 1.33 with an SE of 0.61 and 95% confidence interval (0.02, 2.64). Once again, with respect to the analysis strategy in simple two-period designs, to avoid loss of power and complications caused by prior testing, we conclude that it is probably best to rely on prior information and assume that carry-over is negligible. The additional sequences in Balaam's design have not really helped the basic problem. This comparison does depend to some extent, however, on the relative sizes of the between-subject and within-subject variances.

We have not yet made use of the run-in baseline measurements, and in a setting where there is very large between-subject variability (and poor efficiency with respect to within-subject information) inclusion of a run-in baseline can make a substantial contribution in terms of precision. To use the baseline as a simple covariate we need to use *random* subject effects , otherwise the contribution of the covariate will be absorbed into the subject term. Note that we are here using a run-in baseline, not a period-dependent baseline, so the issues identified in Section 5.4 that occur with random subject effects do not arise here.

We use the following, with all other terms in the model:

```
proc mixed;
  class  patient period treatment carry;
  model score = baseline period treatment carry
                     carry*treatment / s ddfm=kenwardroger;
  random patient;
```

The estimates of the within- and between-subject variances are now:

Cov Parm	Estimate
patient	0.6689
Residual	1.0803

The between-subject variance has been reduced from nearly 30 to less than 1. The baseline covariate has explained 98% of the between-subject variability. This will have a great impact on any estimates that have a nontrivial dependence on between-subject information. The covariate adjusted Wald tests are:

Type 3 Tests of Fixed Effects

Effect	Num DF	Den DF	F Value	Pr > F
base	1	14.5	372.64	<.0001
period	1	19	0.00	0.9449
treatment	1	25.3	5.69	0.0249
carry	1	27.8	0.20	0.6592
treatment*carry	1	25	0.40	0.5316

Although the coverall conclusions are very similar, the standard error of the carry-over treatment-by-carry-over interaction has been reduced from 0.93 and 1.29 to 0.78 and 1.06, respectively. These are worthwhile reductions, but not exceptional. This reflects the fact that the marked increase in precision of the between-subject component of the information that follows from the use of this highly predictive run-in baseline is still of only limited value, given the important role of the within-subject information which is unaffected by this. We refer back to the discussion in Section 5.4.

Example 5.6: A two-treatment three-period design.

Ebbutt (1984) describes the analysis of data from a two-treatment three-period design from a trial on hypertension. Subjects were randomly assigned to the four sequence groups ABB, BAA, ABA and BAB. There was a pre-trial run-in period followed by three 6-week treatment periods. For ethical reasons there were no wash-out periods. Among other variates, the systolic blood pressure of each subject was measured at the end of each period. Ebbutt used the data from only ten subjects in each group. Tables 5.11 and 5.12 contain the systolic blood pressure in each period for all the subjects who completed the trial.□□□

We note that in Table 5.11, Groups 1 and 2 make up Design 3.2.1 and in Table 5.12, Groups 3 and 4 make up Design 3.2.2. Here we will consider the data only from Groups 1 and 2 in order to illustrate the analysis for Design 3.2.1.

The period means for Groups 1 and 2 are given in Table 5.13. We note that the groups are not of equal size. These means suggest that blood pressure is lower on treatment B. Ignoring the baseline responses for the moment, the `proc mixed` commands to fit a model that includes fixed effects for subjects, periods, direct treatments and carry-over are as follows:

```
proc mixed;
  class patient period treatment carry;
  model sbp = patient period treatment carry / s;
run;
```

and the corresponding F- (Wald) tests are

Type 3 Tests of Fixed Effects

Effect	Num DF	Den DF	F Value	Pr > F
patient	48	94	3.75	<.0001
period	2	94	0.67	0.5134
treatment	1	94	6.58	0.0119
carry	1	94	1.00	0.3188

There is no evidence of a carry-over difference but there is fairly strong evidence of a direct treatment effect. After refitting the model with carry-over omitted, the estimate of the (B–A) treatment difference is –5.92 with a standard

Table 5.11: Example 5.6: Systolic blood pressures from a three-period design with four groups – sequence groups ABB and BAA.

Group	Subject	Period			
		Run-in	1	2	3
1 ABB	1	173	159	140	137
	2	168	153	172	155
	3	200	160	156	140
	4	180	160	200	132
	5	190	170	170	160
	6	170	174	132	130
	7	185	175	155	155
	8	180	154	138	150
	9	160	160	170	168
	10	170	160	160	170
	11	165	145	140	140
	12	168	148	154	138
	13	190	170	170	150
	14	160	125	130	130
	15	190	140	112	95
	16	170	125	140	125
	17	170	150	150	145
	18	158	136	130	140
	19	210	150	140	160
	20	175	150	140	150
	21	186	202	181	170
	22	190	190	150	170
2 BAA	1	168	165	154	173
	2	200	160	165	140
	3	130	140	150	180
	4	170	140	125	130
	5	190	158	160	180
	6	180	180	165	160
	7	200	170	160	160
	8	166	140	158	148
	9	188	126	170	200
	10	175	130	125	150
	11	186	144	140	120
	12	160	140	160	140
	13	135	120	145	120
	14	175	145	150	150
	15	150	155	130	140
	16	178	168	168	168
	17	170	150	160	180
	18	160	120	120	140
	19	190	150	150	160
	20	160	150	140	130
	21	200	175	180	160
	22	160	140	170	150
	23	180	150	160	130
	24	170	150	130	125
	25	165	140	150	160
	26	200	140	140	130
	27	142	126	140	138

Table 5.12: Example 5.6: Systolic blood pressures from a three-period design with four groups – sequence groups ABA and BAB.

Group	Subject	Period			
		Run-in	1	2	3
3 ABA	1	184	154	145	150
	2	210	160	140	140
	3	250	210	190	190
	4	180	110	112	130
	5	165	130	140	130
	6	210	180	190	160
	7	175	155	120	160
	8	186	170	164	158
	9	178	170	140	180
	10	150	155	130	135
	11	130	115	110	120
	12	155	180	136	150
	13	140	130	120	126
	14	180	135	140	155
	15	162	148	148	162
	16	185	180	180	190
	17	220	190	155	160
	18	170	178	152	174
	19	220	172	178	180
	20	172	164	150	160
	21	200	170	140	140
	22	154	168	176	148
	23	150	130	120	130
4 BAB	1	140	160	145	112
	2	156	156	152	140
	3	215	195	195	180
	4	150	130	126	122
	5	170	130	136	130
	6	170	140	140	150
	7	198	160	160	160
	8	210	140	180	165
	9	170	140	135	125
	10	160	100	129	120
	11	168	148	164	148
	12	200	150	170	134
	13	240	205	240	150
	14	155	140	140	140
	15	180	154	180	156
	16	160	150	130	160
	17	150	140	130	130

Table 5.13: Example 5.6: Period means for each sequence group.

Group	Size	Period		
		1	2	3
1 ABB	$n_1 = 22$	$\bar{y}_{11.} = 157.09$	$\bar{y}_{12.} = 151.36$	$\bar{y}_{13.} = 145.91$
1 BAA	$n_2 = 27$	$\bar{y}_{21.} = 147.11$	$\bar{y}_{22.} = 150.56$	$\bar{y}_{13.} = 150.44$

error of 2.28 and a corresponding 95% confidence interval of (–10.50, –1.34). This confirms the impression given by the simple means in Table 5.13.

We might consider using the run-in baseline measurement as a covariate in the analysis. For a design like the current one, in which most of the information is within-subject, a baseline covariate will make only a minimal contribution to the precision of the effects estimates. Hence we would only consider its use further if we wanted to investigate possible treatment-by-covariate interaction. For the same reasons we would not consider using random subject effects in this design.

5.6 General linear mixed model

Cross-over designs are used in more complex settings than those considered so far in this chapter. For example, the same basic cross-over design may be used in several centers or repeated measurements may be collected within treatment periods. In Section 5.8 we consider cross-over data themselves as repeated measurements, and in Chapter 7 we need to accommodate a variety of random effects structures for examining bioequivalence.

To accommodate the full range of possible model settings, the simple random subject effects model introduced above needs to be generalized. We now introduce the *general linear mixed model*.

- There is a set of p **fixed** effects, represented by β. This will contain treatment, period and other relevant effects.
- There is also a set of r **random** effects, $\mathbf{U}$, with

$$\mathrm{E}(\mathbf{U}) = \mathbf{0} \quad \text{and} \quad \mathrm{V}(\mathbf{U}) = \mathbf{G}.$$

  In the simple random effects model, $\mathbf{U}$ consists of just the random subject effects, and $\mathbf{G} = \sigma_s^2\mathbf{I}$.
- Conditionally, on the values of $\mathbf{U}$,

$$\begin{aligned} \mathrm{E}(\mathbf{Y} \mid \mathbf{U}) &= \mathbf{X}\beta + \mathbf{Z}\mathbf{U} \\ \mathrm{V}(\mathbf{Y} \mid \mathbf{U}) &= \mathbf{R} \end{aligned}$$

  for the design/covariate matrices $\mathbf{X}$ and $\mathbf{Z}$. $\mathbf{R}$ is the covariance matrix of the errors around the conditional means.

- Finally, assuming that the observations and random effects have a joint multivariate normal distribution, the marginal distribution of $\mathbf{Y}$ can be written:

$$\mathbf{Y} \sim \mathrm{N}\left[\mathbf{X}\beta,\ \mathbf{R}+\mathbf{ZGZ}^T\right]. \tag{5.14}$$

This can be seen to be a conventional multivariate linear model, with a very particular structure for the covariance matrix. Very commonly (but not necessarily) it is assumed that

$$\mathbf{R} = \sigma^2\mathbf{I}.$$

The model in (5.14) can be fitted using REML with the same procedures for inference used as in the simple random subjects model. For a more thorough treatment of the linear mixed model in the repeated measurements context, see Diggle et al. (2002) and Verbeke and Molenberghs (2000).

The use of SAS procs `mixed` and `glimmix` to fit (5.14) can be summarized as follows :

- $\mathbf{X}$ (hence β) is determined by the right hand side of the `model` statement.
- The structure of $\mathbf{R}$ is determined by `type=` option in the `repeated` statement in `proc mixed`, and in a random statement in `proc glimmix` (together with the `residual` option).
- $\mathbf{Z}$ is determined in the `random` statement.
- The structure of $\mathbf{G}$ is determined by `type=` option in the `random` statement.

In the repeated measurements setting (which includes cross-over trials) the subject structure is an essential part of the model. This is indicated in both the `random` and `repeated` (`mixed` only) statements by the `subject=` option. Usually this is set equal to the class variate that identifies the subjects. Note that more than one `random` statement is permitted. This allows quite complex random structures to be fitted. We now illustrate the use of the general modeling approach with two different settings.

5.7 Analysis of repeated measurements within periods

It is common practice in trials and experiments to collect a sequence of observations from each subject. The cross-over trial is an example of this. We shall use the term *repeated measurements* in the present setting to refer to the situation in which a sequence of observations is collected under the same treatment in each treatment period. In most trials and experiments an attempt is made to ensure that all measurements are made at equivalent times on each subject, and we shall assume that this has been done in the following. There may be missing values, but this does not affect the basic structure of common times of measurement. Such balance, which is often absent in observational studies, brings some simplification to the analysis.

There are many reasons for collecting repeated measurements and naturally these will determine in any given situation how we approach the statistical analysis. Each subject produces a set of profiles of repeated measurements, one from each treatment period, and the aim of the analysis is usually to examine the effect of treatments on these profiles. One simple and useful approach is to reduce each profile of repeated measurements to a small number of summary statistics that each represent aspects of the individual profiles that are relevant to the trial under analysis. Three commonly used summary statistics are (1) a particular end point, (2) the area under the profile and (3) the average slope of the profile. Many others might be considered. The advantages of such an approach are that once the summary statistics have been extracted, the analysis can proceed as for a single outcome variable; the conclusions will be expressed in terms of quantities that have already been identified as relevant to the trial; and the approach is robust in that it makes few modeling assumptions about the joint behavior of the repeated measurements. When applicable, it is to be recommended. However, the approach does require the assumption that each subject provides roughly equivalent information on the summary statistics in each period, and this will not be true if there are more than a few missing values; it may not be possible in some settings to identify appropriate statistics. In this section we consider how such data might be modeled when the summary statistics approach is not thought appropriate. First we consider two sequence designs, because these allow one particular and valuable simplification. Then we turn to more general multisequence designs.

5.7.1 *Example 5.7: Insulin mixtures*

This trial was used as an example by Ciminera and Wolfe (1953). Its purpose was to compare the effect on blood sugar level of two insulin mixtures (A and B). The following two-sequence design was used:

$$\begin{array}{cccc} A & B & A & B \\ B & A & B & A \end{array}$$

This is the design labeled (4.2.2) in Chapter 3. Twenty-two female rabbits were divided equally, at random, between the two sequence groups. The insulin mixtures were administered by injection at weekly intervals and, for each rabbit, blood samples were obtained at 0, $1\frac{1}{2}$, 3, $4\frac{1}{2}$ and 6 hours after injection. The full data set is given in Table 5.14 (after Ciminera and Wolfe (1953), Table II). The simple treatment means are plotted for each time point in Figure 5.3.□□□

One of the issues in modeling cross-over data with repeated measurements is how best to handle both the between-period and within-period covariance structure. We shall later use a nested arrangement for this. However, in two-sequence designs, in particular the 2×2, we can avoid the need to introduce a between-period structure by exploiting the fact that all estimators take the

Table 5.14: Example 5.7: Blood sugar levels (mg%).

Group 1												
	Hours	Rabbit										
Period (treatment)	after injection	1	2	3	4	5	6	7	8	9	10	11
1 (A)	0.0	77	77	77	81	90	103	99	90	90	90	85
	1.5	52	56	43	56	73	47	47	35	64	35	68
	3.0	35	43	64	22	52	22	52	22	47	12	56
	4.5	56	56	39	35	60	60	47	26	47	26	68
	6.0	64	64	64	39	64	99	81	22	60	68	73
2 (B)	0.0	90	85	90	107	94	90	99	94	81	81	94
	1.5	47	52	30	47	60	47	26	8	39	26	56
	3.0	52	60	30	47	60	30	64	30	47	35	68
	4.5	68	81	47	47	77	43	52	26	77	30	73
	6.0	90	94	60	73	90	68	90	43	94	85	90
3 (A)	0.0	85	103	99	77	90	85	90	103	77	81	105
	1.5	52	26	39	26	60	56	43	39	56	56	73
	3.0	35	68	39	56	18	56	18	22	26	60	47
	4.5	39	30	73	64	35	77	30	39	64	81	77
	6.0	60	30	90	64	64	94	39	94	94	103	90
4 (B)	0.0	94	107	103	116	94	111	111	90	94	90	97
	1.5	60	60	60	52	56	73	56	18	52	22	73
	3.0	60	68	60	26	47	85	43	26	47	52	52
	4.5	77	90	90	68	81	103	90	18	81	85	81
	6.0	94	94	99	120	99	111	111	22	90	90	94

Group 2												
	Hours	Rabbit										
Period (treatment)	after injection	1	2	3	4	5	6	7	8	9	10	11
1 (B)	0.0	103	85	85	85	85	103	90	81	85	85	94
	1.5	26	68	35	35	35	56	52	22	30	47	39
	3.0	22	56	8	47	39	47	35	12	22	33	35
	4.5	39	64	64	77	85	64	35	22	52	77	52
	6.0	68	81	99	68	77	56	39	77	94	107	85
2 (A)	0.0	90	94	90	85	85	103	90	81	90	85	94
	1.5	35	52	35	39	47	35	43	12	30	39	26
	3.0	30	43	30	52	56	39	30	2	26	39	30
	4.5	39	47	43	52	77	68	47	30	52	43	39
	6.0	94	56	99	64	81	99	77	77	90	60	81
3 (B)	0.0	103	85	73	90	90	90	77	68	85	85	90
	1.5	56	43	22	12	43	35	56	12	39	35	22
	3.0	26	22	12	43	35	18	64	8	22	26	26
	4.5	56	68	56	85	64	64	81	8	56	43	73
	6.0	103	103	103	99	81	94	99	39	90	73	99
4 (A)	0.0	111	111	94	92	85	107	111	85	105	90	103
	1.5	68	52	52	52	52	47	60	26	68	43	47
	3.0	52	99	47	73	52	43	68	12	64	35	35
	4.5	77	103	73	99	77	85	107	18	81	81	64
	6.0	103	120	101	101	99	101	111	39	81	90	94

Reproduced with permission from Ciminera and Wolfe (1953).

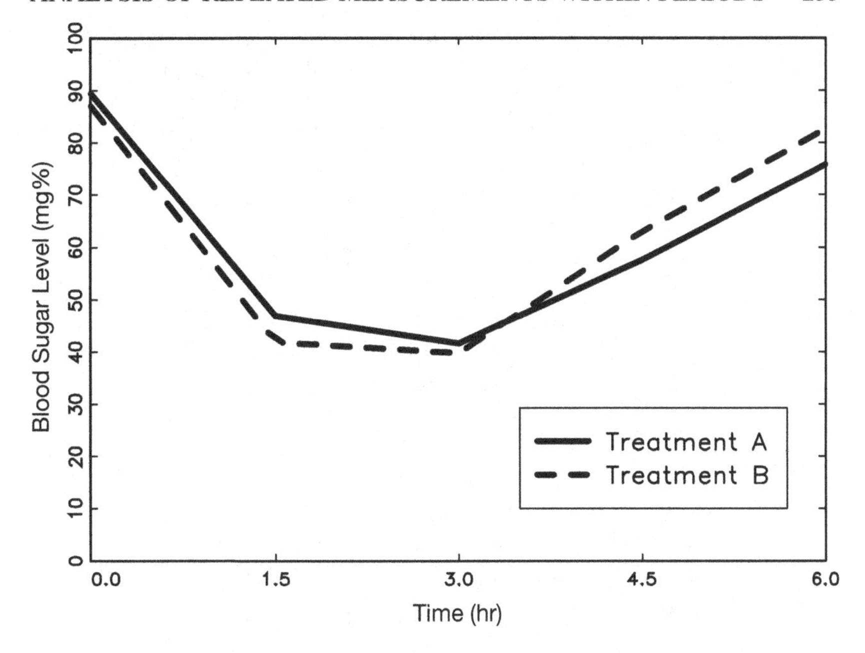

Figure 5.3: Example 5.5: Mean treatment profiles.

form

$$\bar{A}_1 - \bar{A}_2$$

for

$$\bar{A}_i = \sum_{j=1}^{p} a_j \bar{Y}_{ij\cdot},$$

and for within-subject estimators

$$\sum_{j=1}^{p} a_j = 0.$$

Conventional repeated measurements methods can then be applied to the derived subject contrasts:

$$C_{ij} = \sum_{j=1}^{p} a_j Y_{ijk}.$$

For the insulin example, the coefficients of the contrasts are

treatment (unadjusted):	$\frac{1}{4}(-1,1,-1,1)$
treatment adjusted for carry-over:	$\frac{1}{4}(-4,1,2,1)$
carry-over:	$(-1,0,1,0)$.

These linear combinations are calculated for each individual and each time point. For example, suppose that the data set has the following structure:

```
sub seq  hrs    y1    y2    y3    y4

  1   1  0.0    77    90    85    94
  1   1  1.5    52    47    52    60
  1   1  3.0    35    52    35    60
  1   1  4.5    56    68    39    77
  1   1  6.0    64    90    60    94
  2   1  0.0    77    85   103   107
  2   1  1.5    56    52    26    60
...
 21   2  6.0   107    60    73    90
 22   2  0.0    94    94    90   103
 22   2  1.5    39    26    22    47
 22   2  3.0    35    30    26    35
 22   2  4.5    52    39    73    64
 22   2  6.0    85    81    99    94
```

Then the contrasts can be calculated simply as follows:

```
data insulin;
...
tru = 0.25*(-y1+y2_y3+y4);
tra = 0.25*(-4*y1+y2+2*y3+y4);
cr1 = (-y1+y3);
...
```

This produces the contrasts for each subject, as shown in Table 5.15. These can be plotted against time of measurement, either individually, as in Figure 5.4, or as sequence group means, as in Figure 5.5. The difference of the two profiles in Figure 5.5 gives a plot of the estimated treatment difference over time, as shown in Figure 5.6. There is a clear suggestion here of a downward trend in the treatment effect.

As an illustration, we consider the analysis of the unadjusted treatment effect. The same approach can be used for the other contrasts. The treatment effect is represented by the difference in the mean values of the two sequence group contrasts, so the setup is formally the same as a conventional repeated measurements analysis with two treatment groups. We have no reason to expect a particular form for the treatment effect over time, so we will build a model around a saturated means model, that is, a full factorial structure is used to represent treatment and time effects. Similarly, we have no reason to suppose any particular structure for the covariance matrix, so an unstructured form is used, implying no constraints on the variances and covariances other than the

Table 5.15: Example 5.7: Calculated treatment contrasts.

OBS	SUB	SEQ	HRS	tru	tra	cr1
1	1	1	0.0	5.50	11.50	8
2	1	1	1.5	0.75	0.75	0
3	1	1	3.0	10.50	10.50	0
4	1	1	4.5	12.50	–0.25	–17
5	1	1	6.0	15.00	12.00	–4
6	2	1	0.0	3.00	22.50	26
7	2	1	1.5	7.50	–15.00	–30
...						
101	21	2	0.0	1.25	1.25	0
102	21	2	1.5	0.00	–9.00	–12
103	21	2	3.0	3.75	–1.50	–7
104	21	2	4.5	1.00	–24.50	–34
105	21	2	6.0	–7.50	–33.00	–34
106	22	2	0.0	3.25	0.25	–4
107	22	2	1.5	3.00	–9.75	–17
108	22	2	3.0	1.00	–5.75	–9
109	22	2	4.5	–5.50	10.25	21
110	22	2	6.0	–2.25	8.25	14

matrix should be positive definite. The following `proc mixed` commands can be used for this model, where the variates have obvious labels:

```
proc mixed
class rabbit sequence hours;
model tru = sequence hours sequence*hour
                              / solution ddfm=kenwardroger;
repeated hours / type = un subject = rabbit;
run;
```

This leads to the following Wald tests for the overall effects:

```
                    Num      Den
Effect               DF       DF     F Value     Pr > F

sequence              1       20        0.35     0.5619
hours                 4       17        3.43     0.0314
sequence*hours        4       17        2.39     0.0920
```

There is at best borderline evidence of a treatment effect, and this is associated with an interaction with time. It can be argued that this is an inefficient

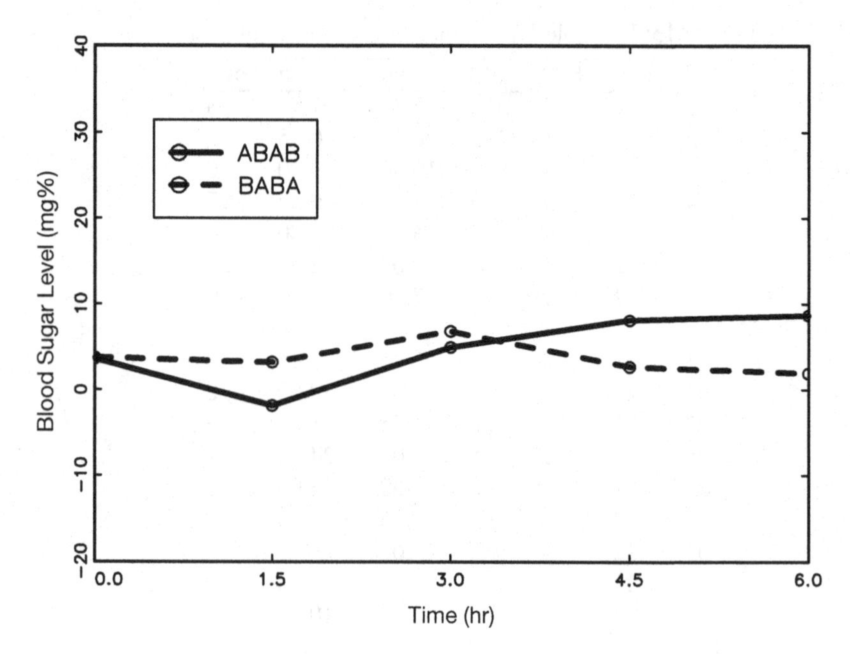

Figure 5.4: Example 5.7: Individual treatment contrast profiles.

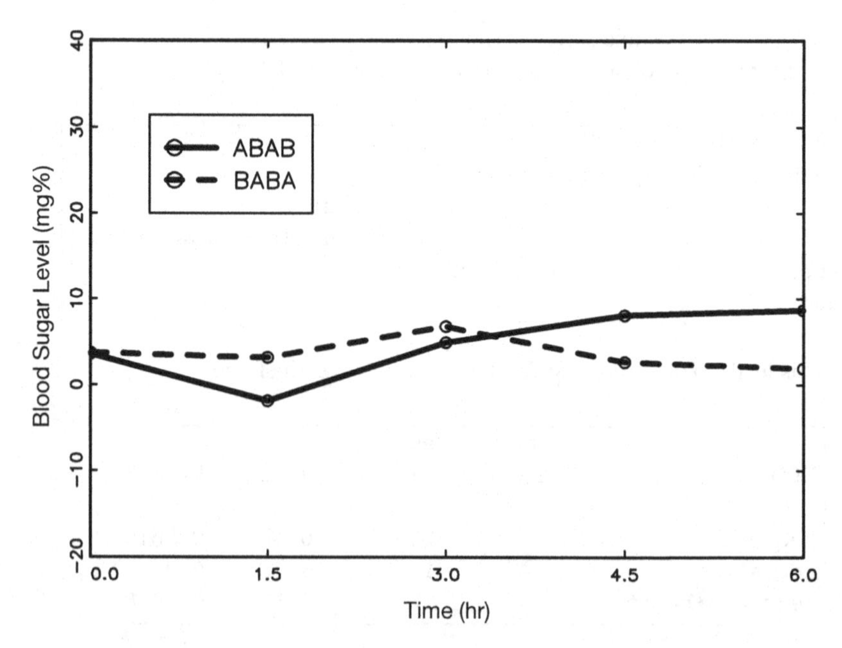

Figure 5.5: Example 5.7: Mean treatment contrast profiles.

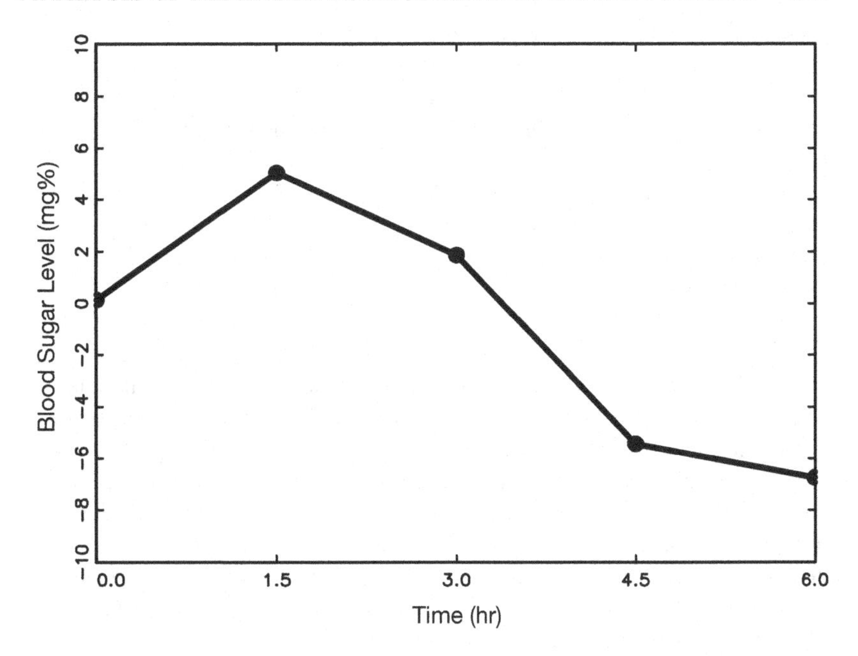

Figure 5.6: Example 5.7: Difference in mean treatment contrast profiles.

analysis, however. Possibly a more parsimonious covariance structure could be found, and the use of a saturated means model implies that specific treatment effects, such as those associated with a trend, may be hidden in the overall test. A more refined analysis could be developed. As a first step we separate out a linear component for the time effect. For this a variate `hx` is introduced which is equal numerically to `hours` but not defined as a class variate. Also, the *type 3* tests must be replaced by sequential *type 1* tests, to allow the separation of the one degree of freedom associated with the linear trend in time:

```
proc mixed
class rabbit sequence hours;
model tru = sequence hx hours sequence*hx
  sequence*hours / solution htype=1 ddfm=kenwardroger;
repeated hours / type = un subject = rabbit;
run;
```

This produces the following type 1 Wald tests:

Effect	Num DF	Den DF	F Value	Pr > F
sequence	1	20	0.35	0.5619
hx	1	20	3.06	0.0955
hours	3	18	3.71	0.0307
hx*sequence	1	20	7.09	0.0149
sequence*hours	3	18	2.59	0.0847

The suggestive slope observed in Figure 5.6 is supported by the significant `hx*sequence` effect. This points to a B–A treatment difference that decreases over time. However, this should be interpreted with caution. This particular comparison has been chosen following an inspection of the plot of the data, and the significance probability therefore cannot carry its full weight. It does illustrate, however, the importance of identifying in advance features that are of interest. If it were known before the trial that overall trends in treatment effect were likely to be important, this contrast could have been pre-defined, and its interpretation would have been less equivocal. Alternatively, a summary statistic analysis could have been constructed from the within-subject slopes.

Further refinement of the analysis is possible, but we do not pursue this here. The key point is that by reducing the sets of repeated measurements to a single set of between-period contrasts, we are able to apply conventional tools for repeated measurements analysis without additional hierarchical modeling of the repeated measurements within periods. The next example is a multi-sequence trial for which this reduction is not possible.

5.7.1.1 Example 5.6 continued

Systolic Blood Pressures.

These data, which are from a trial on the effects of three treatments, were introduced in Section 5.4, where our interest was in the use of the within-period baselines. Although repeated measurements were collected within each period, we earlier used only the last of these as our dependent variable. Now we consider an analysis in which all of the repeated measurements are modeled. To recap, the design consists of two complete replicates of a three treatment Williams design; hence there are 12 subjects in total. The treatments are the trial drug at 20 mg and 40 mg doses, respectively (treatments A and B), and a placebo (treatment C). The measurements are of systolic blood pressure (in mm Hg), measured under each treatment at 10 successive times: 30 and 15 minutes before treatment, and 13, 30, 45, 60, 75, 90, 120 and 240 minutes

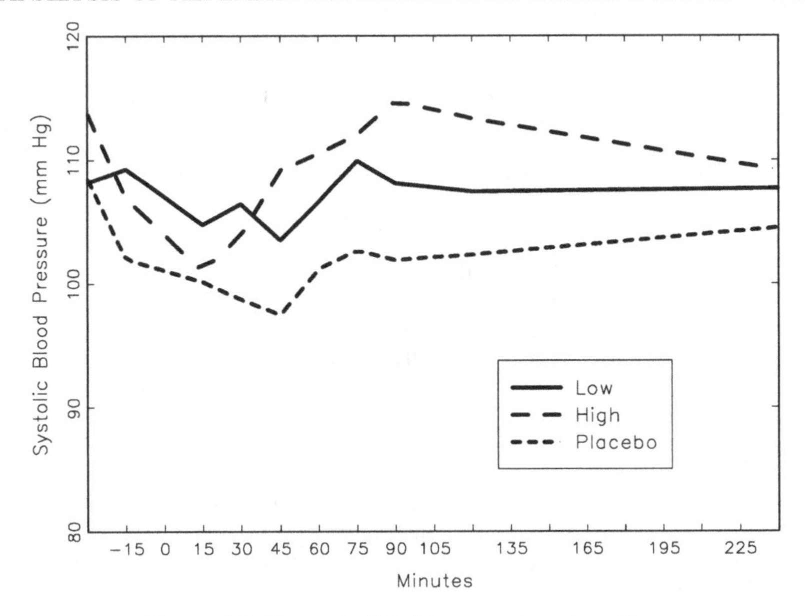

Figure 5.7: Example 5.6: Mean treatment profiles.

after treatment. These data are presented in Table 5.16 and the mean profiles are plotted in Figure 5.7.□□□

In modeling these data we need to take into account two types of covariance pattern among measurements from the same subject: there are dependencies among measurements in the same treatment period and among measurements from different treatment periods. There is no guarantee that these should take a particularly simple form, but we might reasonably expect the stability of a conventional cross-over trial to imply that the patterns of variances and correlations that we observed in one treatment period will be similar to those in another. This implies that the between- and within-period covariance structures are separable. This is the type of structure implied by a proper hierarchical sampling scheme, i.e., one in which random sampling (or randomization) is used at the higher level. Here we hope that a similar structure applies, albeit without the usual justification. To accommodate between-period dependencies we take the same route as with the ordinary cross-over trial without repeated measurements and introduce subject effects. The same arguments developed in Section 5.3.2 about the use of random or fixed effects applies equally here. The present Williams design suggests strongly that fixed subjects effects would be the more appropriate. We will, however, use both fixed and random effects to illustrate the use of both approaches. The baseline measurements will also be incorporated (the average of the two will be used), and this should be expected to reduce the contribution of the subject effects. With

Table 5.16: Example 5.6 (continued): Systolic blood pressures (in mm Hg) from a three-period cross-over trial.

S	P	T	Time of measurement (minutes relative to treatment)									
			–30	–15	15	30	45	60	75	90	120	240
1	1	C	112	114	86	86	93	90	106	91	84	102
1	2	B	108	103	100	100	97	103	92	106	106	96
1	3	A	107	108	102	111	100	105	113	109	84	99
2	1	B	101	100	99	81	106	100	100	111	110	96
2	2	A	96	101	101	100	99	101	98	99	102	101
2	3	C	111	99	90	93	81	91	89	95	99	97
3	1	A	105	113	109	104	102	102	111	106	104	101
3	2	C	104	96	84	84	100	91	109	94	108	108
3	3	B	96	92	88	89	91	121	122	135	121	107
4	1	A	112	109	108	92	102	101	101	98	102	106
4	2	B	105	116	105	108	141	103	110	109	113	112
4	3	C	110	112	111	102	99	104	108	102	112	101
5	1	C	96	93	94	96	83	95	88	93	88	93
5	2	A	103	98	97	108	93	101	108	105	104	101
5	3	B	114	97	96	109	102	99	110	105	104	106
6	1	B	115	117	91	102	126	122	128	125	119	117
6	2	C	104	84	88	95	97	115	93	102	90	101
6	3	A	103	97	84	97	102	115	108	114	113	107
7	1	C	82	88	85	87	81	91	87	78	85	81
7	2	B	133	89	93	98	92	94	90	90	94	100
7	3	A	87	83	78	92	80	83	88	88	93	98
8	1	A	124	131	115	119	115	110	108	103	116	109
8	2	C	116	113	109	93	112	89	108	111	107	111
8	3	B	121	120	87	93	94	100	95	100	114	117
9	1	B	118	107	105	111	105	115	137	128	115	114
9	2	A	111	104	112	109	108	114	116	127	117	117
9	3	C	113	107	115	117	105	117	104	110	105	117
10	1	B	111	112	102	111	107	113	105	111	113	101
10	2	C	115	91	111	114	104	105	112	112	102	105
10	3	A	112	110	109	112	110	103	116	106	110	110
11	1	C	120	117	110	110	110	116	115	118	125	125
11	2	A	104	123	119	115	120	120	127	122	125	128
11	3	B	117	113	117	120	125	130	123	128	126	123
12	1	A	134	134	123	118	111	124	125	120	119	115
12	2	B	125	117	129	125	124	126	132	129	125	121
12	3	C	118	110	119	108	105	110	113	117	123	113

S: subject, P: period, T: treatment.

overall subject effects in the model, the remaining within-period dependencies will be accommodated using conventional models for repeated measurements covariance structures. Note that there will be settings in which the overall subject effects remove much of the overall within-subject dependence, for example, when differences in subject levels persist throughout the trial, and then the repeated measurements covariance structure will account for fluctuations in variability and shorter term correlations.

As with Example 5.7, we start with a factorial structure for time and treatment and an unstructured covariance matrix within periods. The two sets of `proc mixed` statements are as follows for the analyses with fixed subject effects:

```
proc mixed;
class subject period time treatment carry1;
model sbp = subject base period treatment time
  period*time treatment*time / solution ddfm=kenwardroger;
repeated time / type = un subject = subject*period;
run;
```

and random subject effects:

```
proc mixed;
class subject period time treatment carry1;
model sbp = base period treatment time period*time
            treatment*time / solution ddfm=kenwardroger;
random subject;
repeated time / type = un subject = subject*period;
run;
```

Note the use of the `subject*period` identifier for the within-period covariance structure. The output resulting from these two analyses is presented in Table 5.17. As expected, both analyses give very similar overall conclusions. In fact, it can be seen that the tests are *identical* for within-period effects (those involving time). This is a consequence of the subject-period orthogonality in the design in the absence of carry-over effects. There is some evidence of average treatment effects, but not of an interaction with time. As with the previous example, this analysis could be refined both through modeling of the response over time and through imposition of structure on the covariance matrix.

5.8 Cross-over data as repeated measurements

5.8.1 Allowing more general covariance structures

In the previous section we considered the problem of modeling the covariance structure of repeated measurements within treatment periods. Up to now we

Table 5.17: Example 5.6: Wald tests from analyses with fixed and random subject effects.

Effect	Num DF	Den DF	F Value	Pr > F
subject	11	19	11.18	<.0001
base	1	19	7.51	0.0130
period	2	21.8	1.32	0.2865
treatment	2	21.8	8.19	0.0022
time	7	25	1.83	0.1251
period*time	14	37.3	0.92	0.5509
time*treatment	14	37.3	1.32	0.2421
base	1	21.1	13.68	0.0013
period	2	19	1.55	0.2376
treatment	2	19	6.64	0.0065
time	7	25	1.83	0.1251
period*time	14	37.3	0.92	0.5509
time*treatment	14	37.3	1.32	0.2421

have largely ignored the fact that the observations from a subject in a conventional cross-over trial themselves constitute a sequence of repeated measurements, and in principle the question of appropriate covariance structure also applies to these. Let Σ now represent the covariance matrix for the set of p measurements from one individual, i.e.,

$$\Sigma = \text{Cov}\begin{bmatrix} Y_{i1k} \\ \vdots \\ Y_{ipk} \end{bmatrix}.$$

We are assuming that there is only a single response measurement from each treatment period. The analyses based on fixed or random subject effects that have been used up to now are consistent with **exchangeability** of errors within a subject, which is justified under other experimental designs through within-subject randomization. This is clearly impossible when time is involved: time points cannot be randomly allocated. Hence the justification for the simple subject effects models with repeated measurements is empirical. It can be shown that the randomization of subjects to sequences in balanced cross-over designs can place restrictions on the form of possible covariance structures that need to be considered for the analysis (Kunert, 1987) but this is of very little practical help. However, in most cross-over trials the exchangeability assumption is probably a reasonable working approximation; sequences are typically short and the response is comparatively stable over time. For designs with very many periods, such as used in psychology, the approximation is less likely to work well and we explore this in the next section in a case study. Here we briefly consider some alternatives that might be applied if we are concerned that the usual covariance assumptions are inappropriate in a conventional trial with few periods.

To begin with we note that formal selection of the covariance structure through test statistics will not be very informative in small trials. Such tests have low power and are very sensitive to departures from normality. Similarly, methods based on information criteria such as AIC and BIC are not reliable. An illustration of both points is given in Table II of Skene and Kenward (2010b).

We therefore do not advocate a two-stage procedure of first testing the adequacy of the covariance assumption and attempting to select an appropriate structure before the fixed effects analysis. Instead we consider two alternative routes. To avoid making assumptions about the covariance structure we can (1) use an unstructured covariance matrix with conventional REML or (2) consider alternative methods that avoid the direct use of the covariance matrix but that are, in one way or another, robust to the true structure. We will see that there are several ways of approaching this. Two-treatment designs have special properties that lend them to simple robust analyses and we consider this in the next section. We then explore how approaches (1) and (2) might be used for general higher-order designs.

5.8.2 Robust analyses for two-treatment designs

5.8.2.1 Single dual pair designs

If a two-treatment design is made up of a pair of dual sequences, as defined in Section 3.5, then an analysis that is valid under any covariance structure is simple to construct. The analysis uses two-sample t-tests or, if the data are very non-normal, Wilcoxon rank-sum tests. The analysis is robust in the sense that the only assumptions made are (a) the responses from different subjects are independent, (b) the two groups of subjects are a random sample from the same statistical population and (c) period, treatment and other effects act additively. The method of analysis is similar to that described in Sections 2.10 and 5.7. That is, we express the estimator of the parameter of interest as a difference between the groups of a particular contrast between the period means. To illustrate the method we will consider Design 3.2.1 and the data from Example 5.6. We first define the contrast for carry-over adjusted for treatment ($\lambda \mid \tau$ for short) and show how a t-test can be constructed; then we do the same for treatment adjusted for carry-over ($\tau \mid \lambda$).

For the kth subject in Group 1, $k = 1, 2, \ldots, n_1$, we define $d_{11k} = -y_{12k} + y_{13k}$ and for the kth subject in Group 2, $k = 1, 2, \ldots, n_2$, we define $d_{21k} = -y_{22k} + y_{23k}$. We then let $\bar{d}_{11.} = -\bar{y}_{12.} + \bar{y}_{13.}$ and $\bar{d}_{21.} = -\bar{y}_{22.} + \bar{y}_{23.}$.

We can then, using the formula for $\hat{\lambda} \mid \tau$ given in Section 3.5, write

$$\hat{\lambda}|\tau = \frac{1}{4}(\bar{d}_{11.} - \bar{d}_{12.}).$$

If $\sigma_1{}^2 = \mathrm{V}[d_{11k}] = \mathrm{V}[d_{21k}]$, then

$$\mathrm{V}[\hat{\lambda} \mid \tau] = \frac{\sigma_1{}^2}{16}\left[\frac{1}{n_1} + \frac{1}{n_2}\right].$$

To estimate $\sigma_1{}^2$ we use the usual pooled estimator

$$s_1{}^2 = \frac{(n_1 - 1)s_{11}^2 + (n_2 - 1)s_{21}^2}{(n_1 + n_2 - 2)},$$

where s_{11}^2 is the sample variance of d_{11k} and $s_{21}{}^2$ is the sample variance of d_{21k}.

To test the null hypothesis that $\lambda = 0$ we calculate

$$t = \frac{\bar{d}_{11.} - \bar{d}_{12.}}{\left[\frac{s_1^2}{16}\left(\frac{1}{n_1} + \frac{1}{n_2}\right)\right]^{\frac{1}{2}}}$$

which, on the null hypothesis, has the t-distribution with $(n_1 + n_2 - 2)$ d.f.

The d.f. for the above t-statistic are half those for the conventional F-test used for Example 5.6. This loss in d.f. is the price to be paid for making less stringent assumptions. The price, however, as here, is not usually a high one.

To test the null hypothesis that $\tau = 0$ we proceed in exactly the same way, except now the contrasts are $d_{12k} = -2y_{11k} + y_{12k} + y_{13k}$ in Group 1 and $d_{22k} = -2y_{21k} + y_{22k} + y_{23k}$ in Group 2.

The estimator of $\tau \mid \lambda$, which equals the estimator of τ in Design 3.2.1, can be written as

$$\hat{\tau} = \frac{1}{8}[\bar{d}_{12.} - \bar{d}_{22.}]$$

and has variance

$$\mathrm{V}[\hat{\tau}] = \frac{\sigma_2^2}{64}\left[\frac{1}{n_1 + \frac{1}{n_2}}\right],$$

where σ_2^2 is the variance of the subject contrast for τ.

The values of the two contrasts for each subject are given in Tables 5.18 and 5.19, along with the corresponding sample means and variances.

If the data are arranged by subject (as opposed to observation), then the necessary contrasts are very straightforward to calculate in the SAS `data` step:

```
data ex54;
input group pat base per1 per2 per3;
datalines;
1   1  173  159  140  137
1   2  168  153  172  155
.   .   .    .    .    .
.   .   .    .    .    .
2  26  200  140  140  130
2  27  142  126  140  138
;
run;
data ex54;
  set ex54;
  d1 = -per2+per3;
  d2 = -2*per1+per2+per3;
run;
```

The required t-statistics are then easy to calculate. We have $\hat{\lambda} \mid \tau = (-5.45 + 0.11)/4 = -1.33$, as in the analysis in Example 5.6. The pooled estimate of σ_1^2 is 332.045 on 47 d.f. giving a pooled variance of $\hat{\lambda} \mid \tau$ of 1.712, giving a t-statistic of –1.02 on 47 d.f. Clearly, there is no evidence of a difference in carry-over effects (P = 0.313).

Repeating the above for τ gives $\hat{\tau} = (-16.91 - 6.78)/8 = -2.96$ and a pooled estimate of σ_2^2 equal to 1070.95. The pooled variance of $\hat{\tau}$ is 1.380, giving a t-statistic for testing $\tau = 0$ of –2.52 on 47 d.f. This is significant at the 5% level, giving good evidence to reject the null hypothesis of equal direct effects ($P = 0.015$).

5.8.2.2 *Multiple dual pair designs*

We can extend the simple analysis described above in an obvious way to more than two groups. To illustrate this, consider again Example 5.6, this time considering all four sequence groups. The full set of data is given in Tables 5.11 and 5.12. Recall that the design is a mixture of Designs 3.2.1 and 3.2.2: Groups 1 and 2 were on sequences ABB and BAA, and Groups 3 and 4 on sequences ABA and BAB, respectively. The group sizes are $n_1 = 22$, $n_2 = 27$, $n_3 = 23$ and $n_4 = 16$ (with an outlier removed).

We first consider the estimation and testing of $\lambda \mid \tau$. The OLS estimator of $\lambda \mid \tau$, obtained from Design 3.2.1, is labeled as $[\hat{\lambda} \mid \tau]_1$, and can be written

$$[\hat{\lambda} \mid \tau]_1 = \frac{1}{4}(-\bar{y}_{12.} + \bar{y}_{13.} + \bar{y}_{22.} - \bar{y}_{23.}).$$

Table 5.18: Example 5.6: Subject contrasts for $\lambda \mid \tau$ and τ – group ABB.

Group	Subject	Contrast d_{11k}	Contrast d_{12k}
1 ABB	1	–3	–41
	2	–17	21
	3	–16	–24
	4	–68	12
	5	–10	–10
	6	–2	–86
	7	0	–40
	8	12	–20
	9	–2	18
	10	10	10
	11	0	–10
	12	–16	–4
	13	–20	–20
	14	0	10
	15	–17	–73
	16	–15	15
	17	–5	–5
	18	10	–2
	19	20	0
	20	10	–10
	21	–11	–53
	22	20	–60
	Mean	–5.45	–16.91
	Variance	342.45	913.33

The estimator in Design 3.2.2, which we label as $[\hat{\lambda} \mid \tau]_2$, is

$$[\hat{\lambda} \mid \tau]_2 = \frac{1}{2}(-\bar{y}_{31.} + \bar{y}_{33.} + \bar{y}_{41.} - \bar{y}_{43.}).$$

Let

$$d_{11k} = -y_{12k} + y_{13k}$$

$$d_{21k} = -y_{22k} + y_{23k}$$

$$d_{31k} = -y_{31k} + y_{33k}$$

$$d_{41k} = -y_{41k} + y_{43k}$$

be contrasts, respectively, for the kth subject in Groups 1, 2, 3 and 4.

The values of contrasts d_{11k} and d_{21k} were given earlier in Tables 5.18 and 5.19 and the values of d_{31k} and d_{41k} are given in Tables 5.20 and 5.21. Also given in these tables are the contrast means and variances.

Table 5.19: Example 5.6: Subject contrasts for $\lambda \mid \tau$ and τ – group BAA.

Group	Subject	Contrast d_{21k}	Contrast d_{22k}
2 BAA	1	19	–3
	2	–25	–15
	3	30	50
	4	5	–25
	5	20	24
	6	–5	–35
	7	0	–20
	8	–10	26
	9	30	118
	10	25	15
	11	–20	–28
	12	–20	20
	13	–25	25
	14	0	10
	15	10	–40
	16	0	0
	17	20	40
	18	20	20
	19	10	10
	20	–10	–30
	21	–20	–10
	22	–20	40
	23	–30	–10
	24	–5	–45
	25	10	30
	26	–10	–10
	27	–2	26
	Mean	–0.11	6.78
	Variance	323.64	1198.26

We note that

$$[\hat{\lambda} \mid \tau]_1 = \frac{1}{4}(\bar{d}_{11.} - \bar{d}_{21.})$$

and

$$[\hat{\lambda} \mid \tau]_2 = \frac{1}{2}(\bar{d}_{31.} - \bar{d}_{41.}).$$

The variances of these estimators are

$$\mathrm{V}([\hat{\lambda} \mid \tau]_1) = \frac{\sigma_1^2}{16}\left[\frac{1}{n_1} + \frac{1}{n_2}\right]$$

Table 5.20: Example 5.6: Subject contrasts for group 3 (ABA).

Group	Subject	Contrast d_{31k}	Contrast d_{32k}
3 ABA	1	–4	–14
	2	–20	–20
	3	–20	–20
	4	20	–16
	5	0	20
	6	–20	40
	7	5	–75
	8	–12	0
	9	10	–70
	10	–20	–30
	11	5	–15
	12	–30	–58
	13	–4	–16
	14	20	–10
	15	14	–14
	16	10	–10
	17	–30	–40
	18	–4	–48
	19	8	4
	20	–4	–24
	21	–30	–30
	22	–20	36
	23	0	–20
Mean		–5.48	–18.70
Variance		251.26	816.86

and

$$V([\hat{\lambda} \mid \tau]_2) = \frac{\sigma_2^2}{4}\left[\frac{1}{n_3} + \frac{1}{n_4}\right]$$

where σ_1^2 is the variance of each of the contrasts d_{11k} and d_{21k}, and σ_2^2 is the variance of each of the contrasts d_{31k} and d_{41k}.

Using the values given in Tables 5.18 to 5.21, we obtain

$$[\hat{\lambda} \mid \tau]_1 = -1.336$$

and

$$[\hat{\lambda} \mid \tau]_2 = -0.833.$$

The pooled sample variance of $[\hat{\lambda} \mid \tau]_1$, is 1.712 on 47 d.f. and the pooled sample variance of $[\hat{\lambda} \mid \tau]_2$ is 7.128 on 37 d.f. The extra precision obtained by using Design 3.2.1 is clearly evident here.

Table 5.21: Example 5.6: Subject contrasts for group 4 (BAB).

Group	Subject	Contrast d_{41k}	Contrast d_{42k}
4 BAB	1	–48	18
	2	–16	8
	3	–15	15
	4	–8	0
	5	0	12
	6	10	-10
	7	0	0
	8	25	55
	9	–15	5
	10	20	38
	11	0	32
	12	–16	56
	14	0	0
	15	2	50
	16	10	–50
	17	–10	–10
	Mean	–3.81	13.69
	Variance	295.10	774.23

A combined estimator, $[\hat{\lambda} \mid \tau]_w$, can be obtained by taking a weighted average of our two estimators, where the weights are taken to be inversely proportional to the variances of the estimators. That is,

$$W_1 = \frac{1}{\mathrm{V}([\hat{\lambda} \mid \tau]_1)}$$

and

$$W_2 = \frac{1}{\mathrm{V}([\hat{\lambda} \mid \tau]_2)}.$$

Then

$$[\hat{\lambda} \mid \tau]_w = \frac{W_1[\hat{\lambda} \mid \tau]_1 + W_2[\hat{\lambda} \mid \tau]_2}{W_1 + W_2}.$$

We do not know W_1 and W_2 and so we replace them with their estimates, $\hat{W}_1 = 1/1.712$ and $\hat{W}_2 = 1/7.128$. This gives

$$[\hat{\lambda} \mid \tau]_w = 0.81(-1.336) + 0.19(-0.833) = -1.240.$$

The estimate of the variance of the combined estimator, again obtained using our estimated weights, is

$$(0.81)^2(1.712) + (0.19)^2(7.128) = 1.381.$$

Recall, however, from the discussion in Section 5.3.3 that if the sample sizes are small, the weights may be poorly estimated and introduce extra variability into the estimator. This may then make the combined estimator less precise than a simple average.

A simple approximation to the d.f. of the estimated variance of our combined estimator can be obtained using the result given by Satterthwaite (1946). (See also Kenward and Roger (1997).) We let

$$a_1 = \frac{W_1}{W_1 + W_2}$$

$$a_2 = \frac{W_2}{W_1 + W_2},$$

$$V_1 = \mathrm{V}([\hat{\lambda} \mid \tau]_1),$$

$$V_2 = \mathrm{V}([\hat{\lambda} \mid \tau]_2),$$

$$V_w = \mathrm{V}([\hat{\lambda} \mid \tau]_w)$$

and let f_1, f_2 and f_w be the degrees of freedom, respectively, of $\hat{V}_1$, $\hat{V}_2$ and $\hat{V}_w$. Then

$$f_w = \frac{[a_1\hat{V}_1 + a_2\hat{V}_2]^2}{\frac{[a_1\hat{V}_1]^2}{f_1} + \frac{[a_2\hat{V}_2]^2}{f_2}}.$$

Putting our values into this formula gives $f_w = 83.03$. Rounding this up we have 83 degrees of freedom for $\hat{V}_w$. The t-statistic for testing the null hypothesis that $\lambda = 0$ is then $-1.240/1.175 = -1.06$ on 83 degrees of freedom. Hence there is insufficient evidence to reject the null hypothesis of equal carry-over effects.

To estimate the direct treatment effect τ and to test the null hypothesis that $\tau = 0$ (given that $\lambda = 0$) we repeat the steps described above but with the following contrasts:

$$d_{12k} = -2y_{11k} + y_{12k} + y_{13k},$$

$$d_{22k} = -2y_{21k} + y_{22k} + y_{23k},$$

$$d_{32k} = -y_{31k} + 2y_{32k} - y_{33k}$$

and

$$d_{42k} = -y_{41k} + 2y_{42k} - y_{43k}.$$

Then

$$[\hat{\tau}]_1 = \frac{1}{8}(\bar{d}_{12.} - \bar{d}_{22.})$$

and

$$[\hat{\tau}]_2 = \frac{1}{8}(\bar{d}_{32.} - \bar{d}_{42.}).$$

The variances of these estimators are

$$\mathrm{V}([\hat{\tau}]_1) = \frac{\sigma_3^2}{64}\left[\frac{1}{n_1}+\frac{1}{n_2}\right]$$

and

$$\mathrm{V}([\hat{\tau}]_2) = \frac{\sigma_4^2}{64}\left[\frac{1}{n_3}+\frac{1}{n_4}\right]$$

where σ_3^2 is the variance of each of the contrasts d_{12k} and d_{22k} and σ_4^2 is the variance of each of the contrasts d_{32k} and d_{42k}.

The values of d_{12k} and d_{22k} were given in Tables 5.18 and 5.19, respectively, and the values of d_{32k} and d_{42k} are given in Tables 5.20 and 5.21. Using their means and variances, we obtain

$$[\hat{\tau}]_1 = -2.961, \ \hat{V}([\hat{\tau}]_1) = 1.380 \ \text{on} \ 47 \ \text{degrees of freedom},$$

$$[\hat{\tau}]_2 = -4.048 \ \text{and} \ \hat{V}([\hat{\tau}]_2) = 1.324 \ \text{on} \ 37 \ \text{degrees of freedom}.$$

Therefore,

$$[\hat{\tau}]_w = 0.49(-2.961) + 0.51(-4.048) = -3.515.$$

The estimated variance of $[\hat{\tau}]_w$ is 0.676 on 83 degrees of freedom, where again we have used the approximation to the degrees of freedom.

The upper 2.5% point of the t-distribution on 83 degrees of freedom is 2.00 and our calculated t-statistic is –3.515/0.822 = –4.276. There is strong evidence to reject the null hypothesis of equal treatment effects. A 95% confidence interval for $\tau_1 - \tau_2$ is (3.74, 10.32).

5.8.3 Higher-order designs

5.8.3.1 Example 5.8

We shall use as an illustration a trial whose objectives were to compare the effects of three active drugs A, B, C and a placebo P on blood flow, cardiac output and an exercise test on subjects with intermittent claudication. The trial was a single-center, double-blind trial in which each treatment period lasted a week and there was a 1-week wash-out period between the active periods. There was no run-in period. One of the observations taken at the end of each treatment period was left ventricular ejection time (LVET) measured in milliseconds (ms). The treatment sequences used in the trial and the LVET values recorded on each subject are given in Table 5.22. Note that no sequence occurs more than once.□□□

For comparison with later analyses we present the F-tests and direct treatment effects (in differences from placebo) obtained using a conventional fixed subject effects model (5.1). These are presented in Table 5.23.

Table 5.22: Example 5.8: Trial on intermittent claudication, design and LVET measurements (ms).

Subject	Sequence	Period			
		1	2	3	4
1	PBCA	590	440	500	443
2	ACPB	490	290	250	260
3	CABP	507	385	320	380
4	BPAC	323	300	440	340
5	PABC	250	330	300	290
6	ABCP	400	260	310	380
7	CPAB	460	365	350	300
8	BCPA	317	315	307	370
9	PBCA	430	330	300	370
10	CBAP	410	320	380	290
11	CAPB	390	393	280	280
12	ACBP	430	323	375	310
13	PBAC	365	333	340	350
14	APBC	355	310	295	330

Table 5.23: Example 5.8: Conventional analysis with fixed subject effects.

Effect	Estimate	SE	d.f.	t	P
A–P	47.56	16.84	36	2.82	0.008
B–P	-16.28	17.01	36	-0.96	0.345
C–P	22.00	16.79	36	1.31	0.199

Source of variation	Num. d.f.	Den. d.f.	F-test	P
Subjects	13	36	4.65	< 0.001
Period	3	36	7.87	< 0.001
Treatment	3	36	6.02	0.002

5.8.3.2 Using an unstructured covariance matrix

The difference between the simple analysis above and the use of REML with an unstructured covariance matrix is essentially that between ordinary least squares and generalized least squares (GLS). We refer back to Section 5.3.3 for the expression for the GLS form of the REML estimator. Fitting an unstructured covariance matrix to the errors is straightforward using REML, and the following `proc mixed` commands can be used:

```
proc mixed;
  class subject period treatment;
  model lvet = period treatment
                        / solution ddfm=kenwardroger;
  repeated time / type = un subject = subject r rcorr;
run;
```

where for `proc glimmix` the `repeated` statement is replaced by

```
random time / type = un subject = subject v vcorr residual;
```

There are some points to note.

- There are no subject effects in the model, random or fixed. Any within-subject dependence associated with random subject effects is absorbed into the unstructured covariance matrix. If fixed subject effects are included, then the full unstructured matrix cannot be estimated. If an unstructured matrix is required with fixed subject effects, then a modification is required to the analysis to reflect the loss of rank of the covariance structure from p to $p-1$. This can be done in several ways.
- The options `v` and `vcorr` in the `random` statement print the fitted covariance and correlation matrices, respectively. By default these are given for the first subject. In this setting the matrices are the same for all subjects.

In this example it is interesting to look at the covariance structure. This is conveniently summarized through the variance-correlation representation: variances on the diagonal, and correlations below:

$$\begin{array}{cccc} 7549 & & & \\ 0.76 & 2034 & & \\ 0.43 & 0.58 & 3705 & \\ 0.39 & 0.36 & 0.51 & 1439 \end{array}$$

The large differences in variance among periods suggests that the simple subject-effects model is not appropriate here, but it must be remembered that these variances are calculated on relatively few degrees of freedom and are poorly estimated.

Before considering the results further from this analysis, we need to consider its likely validity. Although the Kenward–Roger small sample correction has been made, we are dealing with a very small sample indeed for such a full multivariate analysis, and it is clear that at some point, as the sample size decreases, such an approximation will break down. This question has been considered in Skene and Kenward (2010a,b) for a range of repeated measurements setups, including two cross-over designs. The first uses a pair of five-period Williams designs:

	Period				
Sequence	1	2	3	4	5
1	A	B	C	D	E
2	B	D	A	E	C
3	D	E	B	C	A
4	E	C	D	A	B
5	C	A	E	B	D
6	E	D	C	B	A
7	C	E	A	D	B
8	A	C	B	E	D
9	B	A	D	C	E
10	D	B	E	A	C

with a single replicate ($n = 10$) and two replicates ($n = 20$).

Consider first the behavior of the nominal 5% test for the overall treatment effect (on 4 d.f.) from the single replicate of the ten-sequence five-period design, using conventional REML with an unstructured covariance matrix and the Kenward–Roger adjustment. The fixed effects model includes period and treatment effects but no carry-over. Skene and Kenward (2010b) presented results from a simulation study in which the actual size of this test was estimated from 1000 simulations, generated under a multivariate Gaussian model with the same fixed effects structure as fitted, and with several different alternative true covariance structures. Here we present the results from four of these structures: (1) exchangeable (EXCH), (2) first-order autoregressive with correlation 0.1 (AR(1)), (3) first-order antedependence with increasing variance (ANTE(1)) and (4) a quadratic random effects structure (QRE). For full details of these, see Appendix A of Skene and Kenward (2010b). Two test statistics are considered, the unadjusted Wald test compared with an $F_{4,32}$ distribution (32 is the residual d.f.) and the Kenward–Roger adjusted Wald test compared with an $F_{4,v}$ distribution, where v is calculated according to the formula given in Kenward and Roger (1997). The following test sizes were obtained (as percentages):

True covariance	Wald test	
structure	Unadjusted	KR adjusted
EXCH	91.2	69.0
AR(1)	90.1	67.1
ANTE(1)	93.8	71.2
QRE	93.0	69.8

Although the Kenward–Roger adjustment improves the behavior a little, these test procedures are completely unacceptable. The behavior of the individual treatment comparisons on a single d.f. are less extreme than these overall comparisons, but still too poor to be used in practice. Hence we do not pursue the interpretation of the results from the REML analysis of Example 5.8 with unstructured covariance matrix.

The problem with REML (or GLS) in such circumstances is that the very poorly estimated covariance matrix is undermining the Taylor series approximation on which the Kenward–Roger adjustment is based. An additional, and related, problem, which is not apparent from these results, is that in such very small samples the reduction in variability obtained from weighting with respect to a consistent estimator of the covariance matrix is swamped by the uncertainty introduced through the imprecision in this estimator and, as a consequence, the resulting fixed effects estimators are less precise than unweighted ones. Such small trials are simply not well suited to estimating (or selecting) covariance matrices. As a rough rule of thumb, our experience is that with more than about 30 subjects, and no more than 5 periods, the loss of gain in precision (and hence power) through use of GLS with an unstructured matrix outweighs the loss through uncertainty in the matrix estimate. However, when faced, as here, with smaller trials, then unless we take a Bayesian route and introduce strong prior information on the covariance matrix, we need to consider approaches that rely less on having a good estimator of this matrix. We consider such approaches now, beginning with simple estimating equations and the so-called sandwich estimator of error.

5.8.3.3 Estimating equations and the empirical/sandwich estimate of error

We have seen that in very small trials is probably better to avoid the use of the estimated covariance matrix when estimating the fixed effects, and instead use ordinary least squares. It is of course necessary to then ensure that the subsequent inferences are corrected for the use of the "wrong" covariance structure. One possible route for this is to use a so-called **empirical** or **sandwich** estimate of error, which has become familiar in the context of generalized estimating equations (Zeger and Liang, 1986; Zeger et al., 1988). Essentially the variance and covariance of the simple residuals are used to correct the standard errors produced by a misspecified covariance matrix, although other variations on this basic theme exist. Such an approach is commonly used when modeling repeated measurements of non-normal data, and we meet this use of the empirical/sandwich estimator in the next chapter. Here we apply it using ordinary least squares with a linear model. We use SAS `proc glimmix` for this; other options also exist, such as SAS `proc genmod`. One advantage of `proc glimmix` is that it includes small sample adjustments for the sandwich estimator; the unadjusted estimator can behave poorly if the number of subjects or clusters is small. Various alternative adjustments exist; here we use the one proposed by Mancl and DeRouen (2001), which we also use below when exploring the behavior of the GEE approach in the current setting.

The following `glimmix` statements calculate the ordinary least squares estimators of the fixed effects, with standard errors derived from the sandwich covariance estimator:

```
proc glimmix data=lvet empirical=firores;
  class subid period treat;
  model lvet = period treat / s;
  random period / subject=subid type=vc residual;
  estimate 'A-P' treat 1 0 0 -1;
  estimate 'B-P' treat 0 1 0 -1;
  estimate 'C-P' treat 0 0 1 -1;
run;
```

Two points to note:

- We need to indicate the clustering in the data without having this affect the estimates of the fixed effects. This is done through the use of the random statement, which, with the `vc` covariance structure, implies uncorrelated equally variable errors, but includes a reference to the clustering variable, `subid`.
- The `empirical` option of the `glimmix` statement requests the empirical covariance estimator, and the selection of `firores` corresponds to the Mancl–DeRouen adjustment. A plain `empirical` implies use of the unadjusted empirical estimator.

The results of this analysis for the differences from placebo are presented in Table 5.24, together with two alternative sets of SEs, those from the OLS analysis without the empirical estimator, called the model-based estimator, and with the simple unadjusted empirical estimator. First, note that the fixed effects estimates are identical to those from the fixed subject effects analysis given earlier, Table 5.23. This will always be the case for such models when both periods and treatments are orthogonal to subjects. Second, it can be seen that the model-based SEs that ignore within-subject dependence are consistently larger than the empirical estimators. We expect this when all, or most, of the information on treatments is within subject. Third, the Mancl–DeRouen adjustment increases the simple empirical SEs. Although consistent, the simple SEs tend to be biased downwards in small samples. Finally, we note the variability of the empirical SEs across the three comparisons. This suggests that the SEs themselves may not be well estimated.

We now examine the performance of test statistics based on the empirical estimator. As with the REML approach, Skene and Kenward (2010a,b) present a range of simulation results for different covariance structures and different designs. We present a selection of these here for cross-over designs

Table 5.24: Example 5.8: OLS estimates with empirical estimates of error.

		Standard Errors		
Effect	Estimate	Model based	Simple empirical	Adjusted empirical*
A–P	47.56	23.35	19.80	23.10
B–P	-16.28	23.60	15.44	17.95
C–P	22.00	23.29	12.61	14.68

* Mancl–DeRouen adjustment.

Table 5.25: Nine-period, nine-treatment 18-sequence cross-over design used in the simulations.

	Period								
Sequence	1	2	3	4	5	6	7	8	9
1	A	B	C	D	E	F	G	H	I
2	B	D	A	F	C	I	H	G	E
3	C	F	E	G	D	B	I	A	H
4	D	G	F	I	B	H	E	C	A
5	E	A	I	C	H	D	F	B	G
6	F	H	B	E	I	G	A	D	C
7	G	I	D	H	F	A	C	E	B
8	H	C	G	B	A	E	D	I	F
9	I	E	H	A	G	C	B	F	D
10	I	H	G	F	E	D	C	B	A
11	E	G	H	I	C	F	A	D	B
12	H	A	I	B	D	G	E	F	C
13	A	C	E	H	B	I	F	G	D
14	G	B	F	D	H	C	I	A	E
15	C	D	A	G	I	E	B	H	F
16	B	E	C	A	F	H	D	I	G
17	F	I	D	E	A	B	G	C	H
18	D	F	B	C	G	A	H	E	I

and a couple of covariance structures, the exchangeable and a nonstationary antedependence structure. The results seen for these settings are representative of the overall patterns observed. To the 10-sequence five-period design seen earlier, we add a second cross-over, a nine-period, nine-treatment 18-sequence design, presented in Table 5.25, with one replicate ($n = 18$) and two replicates ($n = 36$), giving four designs in total, with $n = 10, 20, 18$ and 36 subjects, respectively. To obtain reasonably acceptable test sizes in these small trials, the Mancl–DeRouen small sample adjustment has been combined with a modification due to Pan and Wall (2002).

Table 5.26: OLS-based tests, simulated test sizes (nominal 5%) and power for methods based on (1) a small sample adjusted empirical estimator,* (2) the original Box method and (3) a modified Box method (p: no. periods, n: no. subjects).

True Covariance			Actual Size			Power		
Structure	p	n	(1)	(2)	(3)	(1)	(2)	(3)
Exchangeable	5	10	3.4	3.2	4.6	56.4	95.8	97.7
		20	4.5	4.9	6.2	90.0	98.1	98.3
	9	18	3.7	3.3	4.0	53.1	99.1	99.4
		36	2.9	4.1	4.7	94.1	99.7	99.7
Antedependence	5	10	2.8	2.4	3.7	20.6	61.8	69.8
		20	2.8	4.8	5.4	39.8	68.8	69.8
	9	18	1.8	2.9	2.3	12.6	51.5	40.3
		36	1.6	4.4	5.9	24.2	57.9	59.2

* Mancl–DeRouen adjustment combined with the Pan–Wall modification.

The observed sizes of the empirical estimator based tests for the four designs and two covariance structures are presented in column 4 of Table 5.26. These are moderately close to 5%, if a little conservative for the smaller samples. One might conclude from this that such an approach is potentially acceptable for practical use. However, although an approximately correct test size is often regarded as the key property of a useable test procedure, it is only a necessary property, not a sufficient one. The potential problem here is that the empirical estimator is imprecise in small samples, for essentially the same reasons as for the unstructured covariance estimator obtained via REML. All we have done is remove this covariance matrix from the estimation of the fixed effects; it is still present in the Wald statistic, and one would expect the impact of this to be to reduce power. We need therefore to ensure that our test procedure has good comparative power among the acceptable alternatives. At the moment, however, we do not have an alternative procedure with acceptable size. We do know from Skene and Kenward (2010a,b) that the power of the empirical based test is greatly inferior to that obtained from the *known* covariance matrix of the data — but this is an unfair comparison; we cannot calculate the latter in practice. We return to the comparative power of the empirical based test when we have a suitable alternative test procedure.

5.8.3.4 *Box and modified Box procedures*

The next step is to consider an alternative approach to constructing a test statistic from the OLS fixed effects estimators, the key feature of which is the removal of the estimated covariance structure from the test statistic as well as the estimator. The estimated covariance structure will be used only in approximating the null distribution of this statistic. Such a method has a long history and goes back to Box (1954a,b). Here it was shown how any statistic that is the ratio of two quadratic forms in normal variables has a distribution that can be approximated by an F-distribution. This is obtained as follows. Let $\mathbf{Y}$, $n \times 1$, be the vector of response variables from the whole trial with covariance matrix Σ, which will be block diagonal. Let $\mathbf{X}$, $(n \times a)$, be the design matrix (of full rank) and $\mathbf{X}_R$, $n \times (a-c)$, the design matrix with the term to be tested omitted (on c degrees of freedom). Define

$$\mathbf{A} = \mathbf{I} - \mathbf{X}(\mathbf{X}^T\mathbf{X})^{-1}\mathbf{X}^T$$

and

$$\mathbf{B} = \mathbf{X}(\mathbf{X}^T\mathbf{X})^{-1}\mathbf{X}^T - \mathbf{X}_R(\mathbf{X}_R^T\mathbf{X}_R)^{-1}\mathbf{X}_R^T.$$

Then the F-statistic for the omitted term can be written

$$F = \frac{(n-a)\mathbf{Y}^T\mathbf{B}\mathbf{Y}}{c\mathbf{Y}^T\mathbf{A}\mathbf{Y}}. \tag{5.15}$$

The scaled statistic

$$\psi^{-1}F$$

has an approximate F_{v_1,v_2} distribution where

$$\psi = \frac{(n-a)\mathrm{tr}(\mathbf{B}\Sigma)}{c\,\mathrm{tr}(\mathbf{A}\Sigma)}, \quad v_1 = \frac{\{\mathrm{tr}(\mathbf{B}\Sigma)\}^2}{\mathrm{tr}(\mathbf{B}\Sigma\mathbf{B}\Sigma)} \text{ and } v_2 = \frac{\{\mathrm{tr}(\mathbf{A}\Sigma)\}^2}{\mathrm{tr}(\mathbf{A}\Sigma\mathbf{A}\Sigma)}.$$

In practice, an estimate needs to be substituted for Σ.

In simulations Bellavance et al. (1996) show that this approximation appears to work well in small cross-over trials, in the sense that it produces actual test sizes that are close to the nominal values. However, further simulations in Skene and Kenward (2010a) show that the method tends to be overly conservative in some settings, including those considered here. Some of these results are given in column 5 of Table 5.26. In light of this, Skene and Kenward (2010a) developed a modified Box procedure as follows.

Rather than approximating the distribution of the quadratic form in the ratio in (5.15)

$$\frac{Q_1}{Q_2} = \frac{\mathbf{Y}^T\mathbf{B}\mathbf{Y}}{\mathbf{Y}^T\mathbf{A}\mathbf{Y}}$$

as a ratio of independent scaled chi-squared distributions, it is instead approximated directly using a scaled F-distribution, $\lambda \mathrm{F}_{v_1,v_2}$, by matching the first two moments. Approximately

$$\mathrm{E}\left[\frac{Q_1}{Q_2}\right] \approx \frac{\mathrm{E}(Q_1)}{\mathrm{E}(Q_2)}$$

and

$$\text{Var}\left[\frac{Q_1}{Q_2}\right] = \frac{\text{E}(Q_1)^2}{\text{E}(Q_2)^2}\left\{\frac{\text{Var}(Q_1)}{\text{E}(Q_1)^2} + \frac{\text{Var}(Q_2)}{\text{E}(Q_2)^2} - \frac{2\text{Cov}(Q_1,Q_2)}{\text{E}(Q_1)\text{E}(Q_2)}\right\}.$$

Assuming, as in the Box correction, that the numerator and denominator terms in the F-statistic are independent, we then have, equating these moments with those of the scaled F-distribution,

$$\frac{1}{\lambda}\frac{\text{tr}(\mathbf{B}\Sigma)}{\text{tr}(\mathbf{A}\Sigma)} = \frac{v_2}{v_2-2}$$

and

$$\frac{1}{\lambda^2}\frac{\{\text{tr}(\mathbf{B}\Sigma)\}^2}{\{\text{tr}(\mathbf{A}\Sigma)\}^2}\left[\frac{2\text{tr}\{(\mathbf{B}\Sigma)^2\}}{\{\text{tr}(\mathbf{B}\Sigma)\}^2} + \frac{2\text{tr}\{(\mathbf{A}\Sigma)^2\}}{\{\text{tr}(\mathbf{A}\Sigma)\}^2}\right]\frac{2v_2^2(v_2+v_1-2)}{v_1(v_2-2)^2(v_2-4)}.$$

Fixing $v_1 = c$, the dimension of the test (similarly to the Kenward–Roger and small-sample empirical adjustments), these final two equations can be used to obtain expressions for the scale factor λ and the denominator degrees of freedom v_2 for the approximating distribution. This gives

$$\text{F} = \frac{(n-r)\lambda}{c}\frac{\mathbf{Y}^T\mathbf{B}\mathbf{Y}}{\mathbf{Y}^T\mathbf{A}\mathbf{Y}} \overset{\text{approx}}{\sim} \text{F}_{c,v_2}$$

where

$$\lambda^{-1} = \frac{(n-r)}{c}\left(\frac{v_2-2}{v_2}\right)\frac{\text{tr}(\mathbf{B}\Sigma)}{\text{tr}(\mathbf{A}\Sigma)}$$

$$v_2 = \frac{c(4\text{V}+1)-2}{c\text{V}-1}$$

and

$$\text{V} = \frac{\text{tr}\{(\mathbf{B}\Sigma)^2\}}{\{\text{tr}(\mathbf{B}\Sigma)\}^2} + \frac{\text{tr}\{(\mathbf{A}\Sigma)^2\}}{\{\text{tr}(\mathbf{A}\Sigma)\}^2}.$$

To use either Box's original method, or its modification, we need to substitute an estimate for Σ in the formulae above. We could use the REML estimate given earlier. Although this goes against the spirit of the approach, which is to base the analysis on OLS estimators, it has the advantage of convenience. An unbiased estimator of the covariance matrix *can* be obtained from the residuals around the OLS estimators, but this requires calculations not implemented in standard software. The steps required are described in the first edition of this book (Jones and Kenward, 1989, pages 287–289), and an estimate of the covariance matrix is given there for the current example.

To examine the performance of these two procedures we return to Table 5.26, where the sizes and powers are presented for the same settings used earlier for the small sample adjusted empirical based approach. Again these results are wholly typical of those obtained across a wider range of settings as presented in Skene and Kenward (2010a). It can be seen that the original Box method is a little conservative in the smaller sample settings, and the modified version improves upon this. The actual test sizes are acceptably close to the nominal, so we are in a position to compare the observed power with that of the empirical based procedure. Here we see a great difference, accentuated, as expected, in the smaller samples. The power of the empirical procedure is markedly inferior, making it unacceptable as a competitor of the Box based procedures. The large variability of the empirical estimator of error is here undermining the performance of the associated test statistic. Our conclusion is that the modified Box procedure should be used if an analysis is required that is robust to the true covariance structure of the data.

We close by applying the various procedures to the overall treatment comparison in Example 5.8, on 3 d.f. We saw earlier, that a conventional fixed subjects effects analysis produced an F-test for this of 6.02 on 3 and 36 d.f., with a resulting P-value of 0.002. The corresponding empirical based test, with the Mancl–DeRouen small sample adjustment, has a P-value of 0.005. Finally, using the modified Box procedure and the REML estimate of the covariance matrix, we get ν_2 and λ estimated as 36.9 and 0.93, respectively. This implies a scaled F-statistic (F/λ) of 5.61, on 3 and 36.9 d.f., giving a P-value of 0.003, in this example close to the result from the fixed subject effects analysis. None of the results from the different approaches differs greatly here.

5.8.3.5 *Permutation test*

A final alternative, and a very simple, robust method that can be used when treatment is not adjusted for carry-over, is a randomization test. Under the null hypothesis of no treatment effects, all subjects have sequences of responses that should not differ systematically. Under the null hypothesis, the empirical distribution of the ANOVA F-test for treatment effects can therefore be approximated by re-calculating the F-statistic following random reallocation of subjects to sequences. The empirical distribution of the F-statistics obtained from 10,000 such re-randomizations is shown in Figure 5.8, and the position of the observed F-statistic (6.08) is marked. This is an extreme value and corresponds to a significance probability of 0.0036, very close to that obtained above from the modified Box procedure and hence not far from the OLS analysis with fixed subject effects.

5.9 Case study: an analysis of a trial with many periods

5.9.1 *Example 5.9: McNulty's experiment*

McNulty (1986) described a series of experiments to show that the perceived velocity of a moving point on a computer screen is affected by relative cues, such as the presence of either vertical or horizontal lines and the amount of

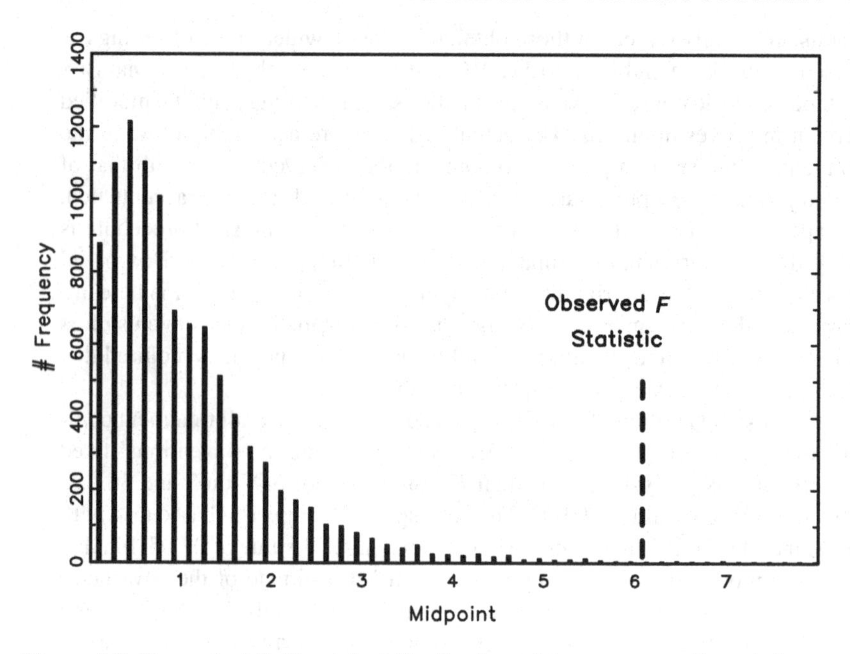

Figure 5.8: Example 5.8: Empirical distribution of the treatment F-statistics.

spacing between them. In her Experiment 1, she asked 16 subjects with good eyesight to determine the perceived velocity of a moving dot on a computer screen under eight different conditions. The relative cues were introduced using one of four possible background displays on the computer screen. The dot moved vertically in an upward direction at a constant velocity, which was set to be either 2.88 cm/sec or 6.42 cm/sec. The perceived visual velocity was measured by the subject equating this perceived velocity with the velocity of a moving belt that the subject was unable to see but was able to touch with one hand and vary its speed with the other. The eight treatments in this experiment consisted of the 2×4 combinations of Speed (S1 = 2.88 cm/sec, S2 = 6.62 cm/sec) and Display (D1, D2, D3 and D4). Display D1 consisted of two horizontal marks 3 cm long, 0.8 mm thick and placed 15 cm apart. The marks were placed centrally on the screen and the dot moved vertically upward between them, traveling a distance of 15 cm. Display D2 consisted of a dark blank field. Display D3 was made up of two vertical marks, each of length 15 cm, thickness 0.8 mm and with a lateral separation between the marks of 1.5 cm. Display D4 was like D3 except the lateral separation between the marks was 3 cm. For displays D1, D3 and D4 the vertical motion of the dot was as for D2.

The design of the experiment was based on the 8×8 Williams square shown in Table 5.27, which gives the order in which the treatments were

Table 5.27: Example 5.9: Williams Latin square used in McNulty's experiment.

Subject	Order of presentation (given twice)							
1 and 9	1	2	8	3	7	4	6	5
2 and 10	2	3	1	4	8	5	7	6
3 and 11	3	4	2	5	1	6	8	7
4 and 12	4	5	3	6	2	7	1	8
5 and 13	5	6	4	7	3	8	2	1
6 and 14	6	7	5	8	4	1	3	2
7 and 15	7	8	6	1	5	2	4	3
8 and 16	8	1	7	2	6	3	5	4

Table 5.28: Example 5.9: Treatment labels in McNulty's experiment.

Treatment	Display	Speed
1	1	1
2	1	2
3	2	1
4	2	2
5	3	1
6	3	2
7	4	1
8	4	2

presented to the subjects in each of two successive replicates. The coding of the eight treatment labels is given in Table 5.28. Each subject was given the presentation order twice in succession, making this a design with 16 periods. The complete plan of the experiment is given in Table 5.29. Note that this design is not balanced for carry-over effects. Additional carry-over effects, over and above those present in each of the four 8×8 Williams squares, are present in Period 9. Subjects 1 and 9 have additional carry-over effects of Treatment 5 in period 9, subjects 2 and 10 have additional carry-over effects of Treatment 6 in period 9, and so on.□□□

The data obtained in the experiment are presented in Table 5.30. The data from Periods 1 to 8 are given as replicate 1 and the data from Periods 9 to 16 as replicate 2.

5.9.2 *McNulty's analysis*

McNulty (1986) ignored the cross-over structure of the design and averaged the data for each treatment combination over the two replicates. She then used these as raw data for an analysis of variance of a factorial design with factors

Table 5.29: Example 5.9: Complete design for Experiment 1.

Subject	Period															
	1	2	3	4	5	6	7	8	9	10	11	12	13	14	15	16
1	1	2	8	3	7	4	6	5	1	2	8	3	7	4	6	5
2	2	3	1	4	8	5	7	6	2	3	1	4	8	5	7	6
3	3	4	2	5	1	6	8	7	3	4	2	5	1	6	8	7
4	4	5	3	6	2	7	1	8	4	5	3	6	2	7	1	8
5	5	6	4	7	3	8	2	1	5	6	4	7	3	8	2	1
6	6	7	5	8	4	1	3	2	6	7	5	8	4	1	3	2
7	7	8	6	1	5	2	4	3	7	8	6	1	5	2	4	3
8	8	1	7	2	6	3	5	4	8	1	7	2	6	3	5	4
9	1	2	8	3	7	4	6	5	1	2	8	3	7	4	6	5
10	2	3	1	4	8	5	7	6	2	3	1	4	8	5	7	6
11	3	4	2	5	1	6	8	7	3	4	2	5	1	6	8	7
12	4	5	3	6	2	7	1	8	4	5	3	6	2	7	1	8
13	5	6	4	7	3	8	2	1	5	6	4	7	3	8	2	1
14	6	7	5	8	4	1	3	2	6	7	5	8	4	1	3	2
15	7	8	6	1	5	2	4	3	7	8	6	1	5	2	4	3
16	8	1	7	2	6	3	5	4	8	1	7	2	6	3	5	4

observers, display and speed. The resulting analysis of variance is given in Table 5.31. To allow for the fact that measurements from the same subject are correlated, she used the Greenhouse–Geisser correction to the degrees of freedom in the F-tests (not reported here), which is not strictly valid in the cross-over context. The means for each combination of display and speed are given in Table 5.32. A plot of the mean perceived speed for each type of display for each speed is given in Figure 5.9. These are the means averaging over subjects, replicates and periods.

5.9.3 Fixed effects analysis

The design in Table 5.29 is a cross-over design with 16 measurements on each subject and should be analyzed as such. We begin by using the basic fixed effects model (5.1) and following that we look at the recovery of between-subject information using random subjects effects (as in Section 5.3). Such analyses are appropriate when the number of periods is not large and some stability of the response can be assumed for the duration of the trial. However, the current design is typical of many in psychology and related disciplines in which there are many periods. Here there are 16; there exist more extreme designs with many times this number. With such long sequences of measurements we need to start considering the repeated measurements structure of the data, as was done earlier in Section 5.7 for repeated measurements *within* periods. We need to consider two main issues. First, the covariance structure implied by the simple model may be too simple for the longer sequences of measurements.

Table 5.30: Example 5.9: Data from McNulty's Experiment 1.

		Period							
		1	2	3	4	5	6	7	8
		9	10	11	12	13	14	15	16
S	R	Perceived speed (cm/sec)							
1	1	2.356	7.056	8.021	2.258	2.869	6.385	7.007	2.954
1	2	4.138	7.581	9.681	1.782	2.710	5.628	5.518	2.429
2	1	1.990	0.463	0.573	8.741	15.712	5.323	3.687	9.840
2	2	6.409	0.537	2.795	3.845	9.535	5.359	4.602	5.774
3	1	0.097	5.200	6.275	4.407	2.405	7.508	2.099	4.187
3	2	1.001	3.003	6.910	6.995	5.909	5.127	4.956	2.490
4	1	1.562	0.769	1.538	7.850	13.136	2.453	2.222	8.668
4	2	2.881	3.259	1.990	7.459	8.143	2.453	5.115	9.498
5	1	1.428	3.442	0.671	0.744	0.219	3.467	3.076	0.952
5	2	0.598	2.112	1.111	0.512	0.695	1.990	4.224	0.976
6	1	3.796	1.208	2.124	4.150	3.601	3.919	2.869	7.557
6	2	7.227	3.711	4.859	6.861	6.360	5.860	3.919	13.417
7	1	2.356	5.115	7.215	2.661	5.323	6.763	3.577	1.184
7	2	5.738	6.604	8.106	5.188	6.763	8.497	7.447	1.941
8	1	3.577	4.315	6.006	12.269	10.670	2.661	5.909	3.857
8	2	13.283	3.674	2.624	8.607	9.168	1.513	4.663	3.821
9	1	2.063	4.456	3.845	1.831	1.306	1.477	3.687	1.501
9	2	2.099	5.384	5.371	1.294	2.246	2.551	5.347	2.234
10	1	4.749	1.416	2.954	2.099	3.149	2.429	1.526	3.418
10	2	3.247	2.014	1.916	2.075	2.576	1.867	1.880	2.966
11	1	0.634	5.786	11.549	4.761	4.431	9.706	7.288	3.540
11	2	0.988	3.284	6.714	4.651	3.845	12.001	6.580	3.967
12	1	3.442	5.493	3.369	7.911	9.425	4.248	4.822	6.983
12	2	3.540	5.005	3.210	8.863	5.225	2.466	4.785	6.031
13	1	1.220	2.209	1.416	1.013	1.269	2.356	5.432	1.660
13	2	1.538	2.283	3.564	1.867	1.892	3.809	4.798	1.953
14	1	1.404	2.637	2.392	2.661	1.367	3.540	2.356	5.640
14	2	5.384	2.466	2.917	5.872	5.213	3.723	2.515	7.007
15	1	0.817	4.053	4.004	2.722	1.452	5.909	3.039	1.550
15	2	2.673	4.212	6.543	2.246	1.867	5.628	4.016	2.368
16	1	3.577	2.527	1.526	6.397	6.397	2.160	1.831	1.867
16	2	3.857	2.038	2.759	7.667	3.284	1.758	2.551	2.844

S: subject, R: replicate. (Reproduced with the permission of Dr. Pauline McNulty.)

We have already touched on this topic in Section 5.8. Second, estimating many separate period parameters can be inefficient if these show some clear pattern or trend that can be modeled. We address these two issues after the simple analyses.

As a first step we ignore the factorial structure of the treatments and fit model (5.1) with first-order carry-over added. The resulting analysis of variance is given in Table 5.33. Note that we are using type 2 sums of squares (each

Table 5.31: Example 5.9: McNulty's analysis of variance (data averaged over replicates).

Source of variation	SS	DF	MS	F-test	P-value
Between Subjects	216.47	15	14.43		
Within Subjects					
Speed (A)	263.41	1	263.41	77.62	< 0.001
Speed×Observers (Error A)	50.90	15	3.39		
Display (B)	104.50	3	34.83	14.09	< 0.001
Display×Observers (Error B)	111.27	45	2.47		
Speed×Display (C)	15.24	3	5.08	4.73	0.006
Speed×Display×Observers (Error C)	43.37	45	1.08		
Total	810.45	127			

Table 5.32: Example 5.9: Treatment combination means (each of 16 observations).

	Display				
Speed	D1	D2	D3	D4	Mean
S1	3.14	1.73	3.34	2.67	2.72
S2	6.91	3.60	6.04	5.79	5.59
Mean	5.02	2.67	4.69	4.23	

term adjusted for other terms to which it is *not* marginal) because the carry-over effects are not orthogonal to subjects, periods or treatments. If carry-over effects are left out of the model, then the type 1, 2 and 3 sums of squares coincide because of the orthogonality of the design.

From Table 5.33 there is no evidence of significant difference between the eight carry-over effects and so these are dropped from the model. The resulting analysis of variance is given in Table 5.34. The differences among the treatments are highly significant, and we need to explore and describe these differences in terms of the 2×4 factorial structure of the treatments.

From Table 5.35 it is clear that there is a real interaction between display and speed. This means that the effect of changing the levels of speed is not the same for each level of display. To determine the nature of these differences we examine the two-way table of speed-by-display means given in Table 5.32. These are the same ones as used in McNulty's analysis; however, their standard errors will be different as we have fitted a (different) model to the raw data. To determine the nature of the interaction we examine the pairwise difference between the eight means using t-tests and adjusting for multiple testing using

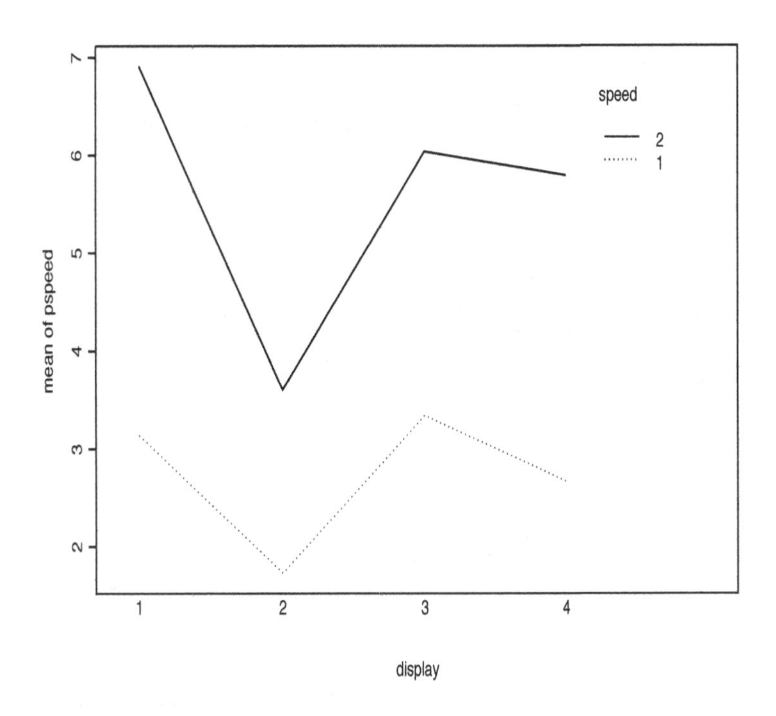

Figure 5.9: Example 5.9: Plot of display means at each speed.

the `simulate` option to the `lsmeans` command in `proc mixed`. None of the resulting P-values was borderline: the largest value below 0.05 was 0.0217 and of those above 0.05 the smallest was 0.1392. The conclusions were different for each speed. For Speed 2 the average perceived speeds obtained when displays

Table 5.33: Example 5.9: Fitting treatment and carry-over effects (type 2 sums of squares).

Source of variation	SS	DF	MS	F-test	P-value
Between Subjects	429.642	15	28.643		
Within Subjects					
Period	115.12	15	7.67	2.80	< 0.001
Treatment	756.09	7	108.01	39.36	< 0.001
Carry-over	29.94	7	4.28	1.56	0.149
Residual	578.97	211	2.74		
Total	1920.56	255			

Table 5.34: Example 5.9: F-tests after dropping carry-over effects.

Source of variation	SS	DF	MS	F-test	P-value
Between Subjects	432.94	15	28.862		
Within Subjects					
Period	112.44	15	7.50	2.68	<0.001
Treatment	766.28	7	109.47	39.19	<0.001
Residual	608.901	218	2.79		
Total	1920.56	250			

Table 5.35: Example 5.9: Factorial effects for treatments.

Source of variation	SS	DF	MS	F-test	P-value
Between Subjects	432.94	15	28.86		
Within Subjects					
Period	112.44	15	7.50	2.68	<0.001
Display	208.99	3	69.67	24.94	<0.001
Speed	526.81	1	526.81	188.61	<0.001
Display$\times$Speed	30.47	3	10.16	3.64	0.104
Residual	608.91	218	2.79		
Total	255	1920.56			

D1, D3 and D4 were used were not significantly different from each other. However, display D2 had a significantly lower average perceived speed than each of D1, D3 and D4. For speed 1 the conclusions were not so clear cut. While D2 still gave the lowest perceived speed, the increases in speed produced when displays D1, D3 and D4 were used formed more of a continuum in the order D2, D4, D1 and D3. In this ordering D1 and D3 gave a significantly higher average perceived speed than D2, with D4 intermediate between D2 and (D1, D3). D4 was not significantly different from either D2 or D1. There was no significant difference between D1 and D3.

In summary, it appears that when using displays D1 and D3 at either speed, the same perceived speed is obtained. At each speed display D2 produces a significantly lower perceived speed than either D1 or D3. The effect of using display D4 depends on which speed is being used. At the lower speed, D4 produces an average perceived speed that is between that of D2 and D1, but not one that is significantly different from either. At the higher speed D4 gives a significantly higher perceived speed than D2, but not one that is significantly different from any of either D1 or D3.

Within the scope of our fixed effects model, we have probably obtained most if not all of the relevant information present in the data from this experiment, and would not continue with further analyses except to check that none of the assumptions made in our model was badly violated. However, for

Table 5.36: Example 5.9: Factorial effects for treatments and carry-overs (type 2 SS).

Source of variation	SS	DF	MS	F-test	P-value
Between Subjects	429.64	15	28.64		
Within Subjects					
Period	115.12	15	7.67	2.80	< 0.001
Treatment					
Display	203.76	3	67.92	24.75	< 0.001
Speed	525.53	1	525.53	191.53	< 0.001
Display×Speed	26.79	3	8.93	3.25	0.023
Carry-over					
Display	27.15	3	9.05	3.30	0.021
Speed	0.10	1	0.10	0.04	0.852
Display×Speed	2.70	3	0.90	0.33	0.805
Residual	578.97	211	2.74		
Total	1920.561	255			

the purposes of illustration and to learn more about the carry-over effects in this trial, we will continue and add effects to our model that account for any carry-over effects of the display and speed factors. To do this we add terms to the model for the carry-over effects of Display and Speed and the interaction of these carry-over effects. It might be, for example, that the effect of using a particular display is still present when the next display is used. If this were the case, there would be a significant carry-over effect of factor Display. Similarly, for speed. A significant interaction of carry-over effects for Display and Speed would mean that the size of the carry-over effects of one factor depended on the size of the carry-over effects of the other. The analysis of variance for this augmented model is given in Table 5.36. We can use type 1 tests here because, in this step, we are principally interested in the carry-over effects.

There is no evidence of any interaction between the factorial carry-over effects, or any significant carry-over of the Speed effect. However, there is a significant carry-over effect of Display. Removing the insignificant carry-over effects from the model gives the analysis of variance in Table 5.37. A comparison of the pair-wise differences between the Display carry-over effects reveals that there is a significant difference between the carry-over effects of Displays D1 and D3 ($\hat{\lambda}_{D1} = 0.452$, $\hat{\lambda}_{D3} = -0.465$, standard error of each = 0.304). The size of this difference is 0.92 and the corresponding P-value for the test of whether this is zero is 0.0167, adjusted for multiplicity using the `adjust` option. The interpretation of this is that the perceived speed of the moving dot in the current period is increased after seeing Display D1 in the previous period and decreased after seeing D3, irrespective of which display is in the current period. The least squares means for the eight factorial combinations,

Table 5.37: Example 5.9: Factorial effects for treatments and carry-over of display (type 2 SS).

Source of variation	SS	DF	MS	F-test	P-value
Between Subjects	430.58	15	28.71		
Within Subjects					
Period	124.29	15	8.29	3.06	0.001
Treatment					
Display	203.76	3	67.92	25.10	<0.001
Speed	526.81	1	526.81	194.69	<0.001
Display$\times$Speed	30.47	3	10.16	3.75	0.012
Carry-over					
Display	27.15	3	9.05	3.34	0.020
Residual	581.76	215	2.71		
Total	1920.56	255			

adjusted for the carry-over effect of Display, are given in Table 5.38. The effect on these means of the adjustment is to change the conclusions for Speed 2. Whereas before D4 was intermediate between D2 and D1, after adjustment D4 was significantly higher than D2 and not different from D3. However, D4 and D1 were significantly different. In other words, (D4, D3 and D1) form a group with D4 = D3 and D3 = D1, but D4 and D1 are unequal.

Before leaving the analysis of these data using a fixed effects model, we note that when the model used to produce Table 5.36 was augmented with terms for the interaction of the direct factorial effects and the carry-over effects of the factorial effect, a significant interaction between the direct effect of speed and its carry-over effects was detected (P-value = 0.014). It appears that the carry-over effects of the two levels of speed are the same when they meet the slower speed, but are significantly different (adjusted P-value < 0.001) when they meet the higher speed. In the absence of any methodological explanation why such an effect might occur, we are inclined at the moment to attribute its significant P-value to chance, rather than as an indication of a real effect, particularly as we did not detect a significant carry-over effect of the Speed main effect in the earlier analysis.

Table 5.38: Example 5.9: Least squares means, adjusted for carry-over effect of display.

	Display			
Speed	D1	D2	D3	D4
S1	3.19	1.73	3.23	2.62
S2	6.97	3.61	5.92	5.75

Table 5.39: Example 5.9: Random subjects effects model.

Source of variation	NDF	DDF	Type 2 F-test	P-value
Period	15	211	2.82	< 0.001
Treatment				
Display	3	211	24.76	< 0.001
Speed	1	211	191.49	< 0.001
Display × Speed	3	211	3.25	0.023
Carry-over				
Display	3	211.2	3.32	0.021
Speed	1	211.2	0.03	0.869
Display × Speed	3	211.2	0.34	0.799

5.9.4 *Random subject effects and covariance structure*

We now take the steps described in Section 5.3.1 and change the subject effects from fixed to random. We first repeat the analysis in terms of the factors distance and speed, including fixed effects for period, distance, speed and the carry-over effects of distance and speed. The analysis of variance for the model, in the style generated by `proc mixed`, is given in Table 5.39. Note that the F-tests and denominator degrees of freedom have been calculated according to the `ddfm=kenwardroger` option. This analysis differs from the earlier one as displayed in Table 5.36 only insofar as there is between-subject information to recover. In the absence of carry-over effects, the period and treatment effects are orthogonal to subjects, there would be no between-subject information to recover, and the two analyses would be identical for inferences about the fixed effects. The inclusion of carry-over effects has introduced a very small degree of nonorthogonality into the analysis, and so the two analyses differ, but only to a very slight extent. This is most apparent from the denominator degrees of freedom of the carry-over effects, which have changed from 211 in the fixed effects analysis to 211.2 for that with random effects.

However, given the long sequences of repeated measurements on each subject, we might question the adequacy of the simple random effects covariance structure, although in the present setting, with only 16 subjects, we should not expect to be able to make very definitive statements about the appropriate covariance structure for these data. In particular, we cannot estimate an unstructured matrix, as there are too few residual degrees of freedom. To give some idea as to the adequacy of the simple random effects structure we can fit a more complex model that extends it, and then assess through the likelihood the contribution of this extension. If the contribution is minimal, we have some support for the existing structure (although other extensions cannot be ruled out). On the other hand, a non-negligible contribution implies both that the original model was inadequate and that the extended model is better, but not that the latter is itself necessarily adequate. The extension must represent a compromise between generality, to explore departures from the simple model, and parsimony, for the sake of efficiency. For this we chose the **first-order antedependence (ante(1))** structure. This introduces both serial dependence (that is, dependence that decreases with increasing time interval) and allows changes in variance over time. For details see Kenward (1987). We can assess through the likelihood the contribution of this additional structure. For this we compare the values of −2logl, where logl is the maximized REML log likelihood under the given covariance structure. For this comparison it is important that the fixed effects structure is the same for both. The random effects model used above was fitted using the following `proc glimmix` commands (we use `glimmix` rather than `mixed` here because we will be making use of some of its specific features below).

```
proc glimmix;
  class subject period display speed discarry spcarry;
  model perspeed = period display speed display*speed discarry
                           spcarry  discarry*spcarry /
                           ddfm=kenwardroger htype=2;
  random subject;
run;
```

This produces $-2\text{logl} = 992.8$. Adding the AD(1) structure, we use:

```
...
  random subject;
  random period / type=ante(1) subject=subject residual;
...
```

and this gives $-2\text{logl} = 930.9$, with a resulting difference of 61.9 on 31 degrees of freedom. Assuming a χ^2_{31} distribution for this likelihood ratio statistic under the null hypothesis produces a P-value of 0.001. Although we should not take the χ^2 approximation too seriously in this small setting, there is clear evidence here that the random effects structure is too simple. It is interesting to compare inferences under the two covariance structures. The F-tests for the fixed effects under the extended structure are given in Table 5.40. In this case, the conclusions are broadly similar between the two analyses, but note how the reduction of degrees of freedom associated with the AD(1) component has caused a decrease in sensitivity of certain comparisons, most notably that for periods. We cannot expect such similarity whenever an inappropriate simpler covariance structure is used, and it is good practice to allow sufficient flexibility in the structure to accommodate the patterns seen in the data.

5.9.5 Modeling the period effects

In analyses of long sequences of repeated measurements where responses over time do not change sharply it is common practice to impose some smooth form

Table 5.40: Example 5.9: Random subjects and AD(1) covariance structure.

Source of variation	NDF	DDF	Type 2 F-test	P-value
Period	15	27.66	2.15	0.043
Treatment				
Display	3	95.12	20.78	<0.001
Speed	1	35.32	128.19	<0.001
Display×Speed	3	105.8	1.50	0.218
Carry-over				
Display	3	96.22	2.77	0.046
Speed	1	52.57	0.27	0.609
Display×Speed	3	89.73	0.14	0.935

on the time profiles. In the current setting this translates into modeling the period effects. While these effects are not of prime interest in a cross-over trial, such modeling can improve efficiency if there is nontrivial nonorthogonality between periods and treatments. The current design is not far from orthogonality, for the models considered, so we would not expect to gain much here by such modeling, but we pursue it for the purposes of illustration. Similarly, with 16 periods, any gain is not expected to be significant, but when there are many tens of periods, or even hundreds, as can happen, then such approaches become much more important.

One obvious model to consider for the period profile is a low-order polynomial, and we begin by replacing the 15 period effects by a quadratic. This allows an underlying trend plus some curvature in the time profile. Having defined the variate px to have the same values as period, but not declared as a class variate, we use the following model statement, with the other parts of the model structure unchanged:

```
...
model perspeed = px px*px display speed display*speed
                      discarry spcarry discarry*spcarry
                      / ddfm=kenwardroger htype=2;
...
```

This produces the F-tests displayed in Table 5.41. The results are very similar to those obtained earlier with period as a categorical variate, except that the evidence for a carry-over effect associated with display is diminished. The estimated period profiles calculated using categorical effects and the quadratic model are plotted in Figure 5.10. Because of the absence of an absolute origin, these profiles have been mean centered. The quadratic is arguably too simple for the observed profile (this could be checked formally with a Wald test for lack of fit and is in this case highly significant) and we anyway need to consider in general whether simple polynomials are likely to be appropriate for

Table 5.41: Example 5.9: Results using a quadratic period profile.

Source of variation	NDF	DDF	Type 2 F-test	P-value
Linear (px)	1	29.5	4.80	0.036
Quadratic (px*px)	1	47.7	2.36	0.131
Treatment				
Display	3	117.0	20.28	<0.001
Speed	1	46.4	156.62	<0.001
Display×Speed	3	128.0	3.48	0.018
Carry-over				
Display	3	123.0	2.19	0.093
Speed	1	71.0	0.27	0.604
Display×Speed	3	119.0	0.82	0.483

long sequences of repeated measurements. Unless the period effect is limited to a simple trend over time, a low-order polynomial is unlikely to be satisfactory: these are *global* models that impose properties that must hold over the full profile. For example, a quadratic polynomial imposes a constant degree of curvature throughout the time period. This is unlikely to be realistic. Because modeling the period profile is of secondary interest, the main aim being to capture the main features in a reasonably parsimonious fashion, this is an ideal setting for *nonparametric* or *semiparametric* smoothing. This can be approached in a variety of ways; for a full development of the subject see Lin and Carroll (2009). We choose to take a convenient route here that is a simple extension of basic polynomial modeling: the use of regression splines.

The essence of the approach is as follows. The overall interval of interest, here the 16 periods, is divided into several sub-intervals. The boundaries between the sub-intervals are called **knots**. Within each interval the response is represented by a polynomial. In practice a cubic is often used for this, hence the term "cubic spline," but this is not essential for the general method. To ensure that the individual polynomials meet smoothly at the knots and so produce an overall smooth curve, the lower-order derivatives (e.g., up to 2nd for a cubic spline) are set to to be equal at the knots. With this basic setup it would be possible, but very tedious, to work out, through appropriate algebraic manipulation, an explicit form for the subsequent model. Most importantly, the representation is still linear in the parameters, and so can be a term in a conventional linear predictor. Given K knots and a polynomial of degree M within the sub-intervals, such a regression spline has $K+M+1$ free parameters. The degree of smoothing is determined by M and the placement and number of the knots. There is a huge literature on knot selection; see, for example, Ruppert et al. (2003). Here we take an ad hoc approach to this, using $M=3$ in keeping with conventional practice and, given that we do not expect very rapid changes in period effects, using just three equally spaced knots ($K=3$). This implies

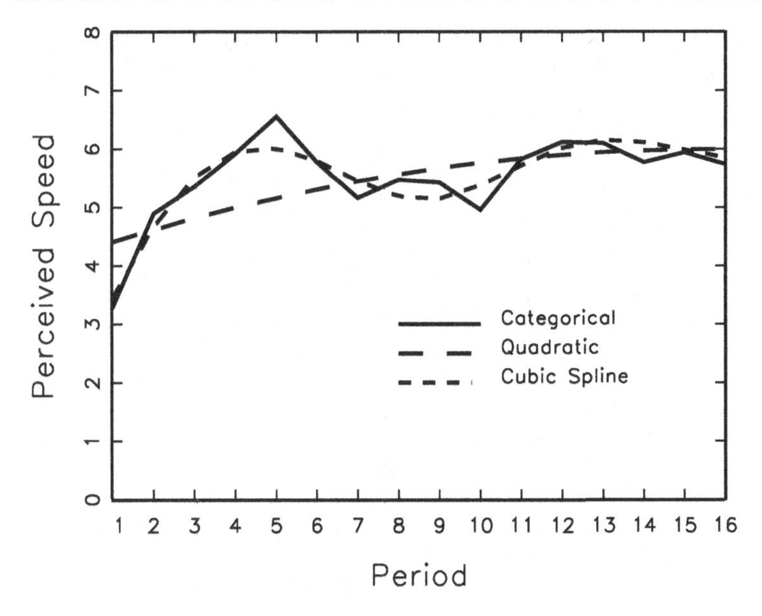

Figure 5.10: Example 5.9: Fitted period profiles from the 15 period cross-over trial.

that there are four sub-intervals and a total of seven parameters. In practice, when we use such a regression spline as part of a linear predictor, one d.f. will be absorbed by the intercept, so in this example we are replacing the 15 categorical period d.f. by 6 regression spline d.f.

To avoid tedious bespoke derivation of the variates associate with the spline model, there are available several forms of **basis functions** which can be used to build up the required model. These can be obtained through straightforward calculations once the knots and limits of the whole interval are given, and various implementations of these calculations exist in statistical packages. For example, in proc glimmix we can use the effect statement for this, which takes the generic form

```
effect [effect-name] = <effect-type> ([var-list]
                       < / effect-options>);
```

where [effect-name] = spline for the calculation of spline terms. Options provide two sorts of spline basis: <basis> = bspline and <basis> = tpf, the former referring to the so-called **B-spline** basis and the latter to the **Truncated Power Function (TPF)**. Appropriate use of these two can lead to exactly the same fitted model the B-spline basis has close connections with so-called **penalized splines**, which we touch on at the end of this section. For our purposes here, we use the TPF basis. This is surprisingly simple. Here are the seven columns of this for the three equally spaced knots applied to the 16 periods:

1	1	1	1	0.00	0.000	0.0000
1	2	4	8	0.00	0.000	0.0000
1	3	9	27	0.00	0.000	0.0000
1	4	16	64	0.00	0.000	0.0000
1	5	25	125	0.02	0.000	0.0000
1	6	36	216	1.95	0.000	0.0000
1	7	49	343	11.39	0.000	0.0000
1	8	64	512	34.33	0.000	0.0000
1	9	81	729	76.77	0.125	0.0000
1	10	100	1000	144.70	3.375	0.0000
1	11	121	1331	244.14	15.625	0.0000
1	12	144	1728	381.08	42.875	0.0000
1	13	169	2197	561.52	91.125	0.4219
1	14	196	2744	791.45	166.375	5.3594
1	15	225	3375	1076.89	274.625	20.7969
1	16	256	4096	1423.83	421.875	52.7344

The first four columns correspond to an overall cubic; the final three are additional shifted power functions that are truncated to zero on the left of the three knots. To incorporate this spline regression term for the periods we can use the following `proc glimmix` code, noting how the `period` term is replaced by the `perspl` term generated by the `effect` statement:

```
proc glimmix;
  class sub period dis spe disc spec;
  effect perspl = spline( px / basis = tpf degree=3 knotmethod =
  equal(3)); model resp = perspl dis spe dis*spe discarry spcarry
                          discarry*spcarry / ddfm=kenwardroger
                           htype=2;
  random sub;
  random period / type=ante(1) subject=sub residual;
run;
```

The fitted cubic spline is plotted in Figure 5.10 along with the categorical period effects and the fitted quadratic polynomial, and the resulting Wald tests are given in Table 5.42. The results are very similar to those from the previous analyses; in particular, there is no suggestion at all of a carry-over effect associated with display. The use of modeling the period profile has added little to the present analysis, but is more relevant in the analysis of longer cross-over designs and of small (in terms of numbers of subjects) unbalanced designs with more than a few periods.

To finish this section, we note that there is a second rather different ap-

Table 5.42: Example 5.9: Results with a cubic regression spline for the period profile.

Source of variation	NDF	DDF	Type 2 F-test	P-value
Period Spline	6	25.56	4.14	0.005
Treatment				
Display	3	98.83	20.90	< 0.001
Speed	1	37.12	131.46	< 0.001
Display×Speed	3	114.6	1.56	0.204
Carry-over				
Display	3	101.1	2.72	0.048
Speed	1	59.91	0.14	0.712
Display×Speed	3	96.98	0.24	0.865

proach to fitting splines in the linear mixed model framework. This uses an algebraic equivalence between a so-called **smoothing (or penalized) spline** and a best linear unbiased predictor (BLUP) from a very particular linear mixed model. Such models can be fitted in `glimmix` using particular options on the `random` statement; indeed, such an approach was used for this example in the previous edition of this book. Such a formulation has the advantage of allowing the data a more direct role in determining the degree of smoothing, but has the interpretational disadvantage of splitting the model for the outcome between the fixed effects and the random effects components. A further issue lies in the appropriate inference for such models – even though the linear mixed model can be used in a numerical sense to fit the model, it does not follow automatically that this model provides the appropriate inferential framework. For a thorough exposition of smoothing splines and the linear mixed model, see Welham (2009).

Chapter 6

Analysis of discrete data

6.1 Introduction

6.1.1 Modeling dependent categorical data

At the time of the first edition of this book, Jones and Kenward (1989), the methodology available for binary and categorical cross-over data was rather limited and amounted largely to a somewhat ad hoc collection of tests based on simple contingency tables. An exception to this was the Mainland–Gart test for direct treatment effect from a two-period two-treatment trial with binary data described in Section 2.13. Although introduced there in the context of a contingency table, Gart (1969) gave a derivation for this in terms of a logistic regression model and Altham (1971) considered the same model from a Bayesian viewpoint. Since the time of the first edition, interest in the analysis of repeated and correlated categorical data has grown enormously and since the early 1990s there has been available a much wider range of methodology; see, for example, Chapters 7–11 of Diggle et al. (2002) and Molenberghs and Verbeke (2000). These changes were reflected in the second edition of this book, and only minor developments of an evolutionary nature have occurred since, mainly computational. These have been incorporated in this chapter.

The starting point for analyzing dependent categorical data is the construction of an explicit model; although early techniques usually involved some form of model, this was often defined only implicitly. The choice of model and interpretation of the parameters is central to an informed comparison of the different approaches and highlights a key feature of analysis in these settings: there is no single "natural" choice of model such as, for example, the multivariate normal linear model used extensively in the previous chapter. The parameters of different models may have quite different interpretations and ideally the first step in an analysis is to identify the appropriate model. In practice, the situation is a little less clear cut; there are relationships between different models that allow some linking of functions of parameters, and different models can often lead to similar substantive conclusions.

In this chapter we review and consider the application to cross-over data of the current main approaches to the analysis of correlated discrete data. Particular attention will be paid to comparisons of types of model and the interpretation of the parameters of these and also to the consequences of small sample size, a common issue in typical cross-over trials. We consider first binary data.

Table 6.1: Example 6.1: Binary data from a four-period cross-over trial.

Joint	Sequence			
Outcome	ABCD	BDAC	CADB	DCBA
(0,0,0,0)	1	0	1	1
(0,0,0,1)	0	1	1	0
(0,0,1,0)	1	1	0	1
(0,0,1,1)	1	0	0	0
(0,1,0,0)	1	1	1	0
(0,1,0,1)	1	1	1	2
(0,1,1,0)	1	1	1	2
(0,1,1,1)	0	1	1	0
(1,0,0,0)	1	0	1	0
(1,0,0,1)	1	1	0	0
(1,0,1,0)	1	0	1	0
(1,0,1,1)	2	0	0	1
(1,1,0,0)	1	1	1	0
(1,1,0,1)	0	2	2	4
(1,1,1,0)	2	3	3	0
(1,1,1,1)	4	9	5	10
Total	18	22	19	21

Techniques have been more thoroughly explored for this setting and the exposition is somewhat simpler. We examine how the techniques for binary data can be generalized to the categorical setting, particularly for the important special case of an ordinal response. We complete the chapter by looking briefly at some other types of responses, namely, counts and survival times.

6.1.2 Types of model

6.1.2.1 Example 6.1

Consider as an example a four-period four-treatment trial (Kenward and Jones (1992)) the results of which are summarized in Table 6.1. Eighty subjects were allocated at random to four sequence groups, with treatments labeled A, B, C and D. For each subject, at the end of each period, an efficacy measurement was recorded as failure (0) or success (1), so at the end of the trial each subject had one of 16 possible outcomes: (0,0,0,0), (0,0,0,1), ..., (1,1,1,1). The numbers of subjects who responded with each of these outcomes are presented in Table 6.1 in the form of a contingency table with columns corresponding to sequence groups and rows to joint outcomes.□□□

6.1.2.2 *Marginal models*

As with continuous data from a cross-over trial, the aim of the analysis is to explain the variation in the observed responses in terms of period, treatment and possible other effects, such as carry-over. Following conventional approaches to the analysis of binary data, we relate a linear model involving these effects to a function of the success probability. As before, let Y_{ijk} be the response observed on subject k in group i in period j, in this case, binary. We can write for a model with period and direct treatment effects

$$g\{\mathrm{E}(Y_{ijk})\} = g\{P(Y_{ijk} = 1)\} = \mu + \pi_j + \tau_{d[i,j]}. \tag{6.1}$$

The construction on the right hand side of (6.1) is just the same as used earlier in Equation (5.1) and the effects carry over their associations, although not their strict meanings.

The function relating the success probability to this linear component or *linear predictor* is represented by $g(\cdot)$. We term $g(\cdot)$ the link function, noting that some authors use this for its inverse. The use of the identity function would imply that the probabilities are modeled directly on a linear scale. This is usually avoided in practice because it is typically not sensible to expect treatment or other effects to act additively across the whole range of possible probabilities. Common choices of the function such as the logit and probit have a form for which the inverse is sigmoid in shape. These have the added advantage of mapping values of the linear predictor to the appropriate (0,1) interval for probabilities. In other words, any calculable linear predictor will correspond to a genuine probability. This is not true when the probabilities are modeled on the linear scale. We note in passing that these sigmoid functions are fairly linear for probabilities between about 0.2 and 0.8, and if, for a particular example, the observed probabilities lie in this range, then there is often little to choose between an analysis on the linear and transformed scales. Given the typical small size of cross-over trials, there is also usually little practical difference among the functions mentioned above, and we will use the logit function almost exclusively in the following, pointing out where necessary if there is any restriction on the choice of link function for a particular analysis. Thus the logit version of (6.1) can be written

$$\mathrm{logit}\{P(Y_{ijk} = 1)\} = \ln\left\{\frac{P(Y_{ijk} = 1)}{1 - P(Y_{ijk} = 1)}\right\} = \mu + \pi_j + \tau_{d[i,j]}$$

or equivalently,

$$\mathrm{E}[Y_{ijk}] = P(Y_{ijk} = 1) = \frac{e^{\mu + \pi_j + \tau_{d[i,j]}}}{1 + e^{\mu + \pi_j + \tau_{d[i,j]}}}.$$

Effects in this model are **log odds-ratios**. To see this, let $\pi_{d,j}$ be the probability that a randomly chosen subject responds with a 1 in period j under treatment

d. The the treatment effect $\tau_a - \tau_b$ can expressed as the log odds-ratio

$$\tau_a - \tau_b = \ln\left\{\frac{\pi_{a,j}/(1-\pi_{a,j})}{\pi_{b,j}/(1-\pi_{b,j})}\right\}. \tag{6.2}$$

This type of model has been termed *marginal* or *population averaged* (Zeger et al. (1988)). The model determines the average success probability over all individuals from the population under consideration for the given covariate values (treatment, period and so on). It is marginal with respect to the observations in other periods. That is, the same model for the marginal probabilities would be used if different subjects were used in different periods (albeit without the need to allow for within-subject dependence as well). Such a model might be regarded as appropriate if, for example, we wished to summarize results in the form of success probabilities under different treatments averaging over period effects. Such statements are population averaged in nature. One objection to the use of such models in a *trial setting* is that the subjects rarely represent a random sample from any well-defined population and so the idea of averaging over this population, or making random draws from it, lacks credibility.

6.1.2.3 Subject-specific models

The marginal model presented above is not a complete one for the observations: it does not define the form of within-subject dependence. Hence the marginal model cannot tell us the whole story about the comparative behavior of one individual on different treatments, and this is particularly relevant if subgroups of individuals have quite different patterns of behavior across the treatments in the trial. The marginal model would simply average over this behavior and, when the link function is not the identity, the resulting marginal model can misrepresent the average behavior in each subgroup. The likelihood of this actually occurring in practice depends on the particular setting, but does require rather large differences in behavior among the subgroups to have substantial impact. Models that directly address individual patterns of behavior are termed *subject-specific*. A very simple subject-specific model that is often used in practice parallels the subject effects model met in Chapter 5, (5.1):

$$\text{logit}\{P(Y_{ijk}=1 \mid s_{ik})\} = \mu + \pi_j + \tau_{d[i,j]} + s_{ik}, \tag{6.3}$$

for s_{ik} an effect associated with the (ik)th subject. It is assumed that the observations from a subject are conditionally independent given the subject effect. In the various linear models used in Chapter 5 for which the expectation and linear predictor are on the same scale, the parameters in both the marginal and subject-specific models have the same interpretation. The extra terms have implications for the error structure. With a nonidentity link function this is no longer necessarily true and the corresponding parameters in (6.1) and (6.3) do not in general represent equivalent quantities. This also underlies the problem of averaging over disparate sub-groups mentioned above in the context of marginal models. The parameters in the subject-specific model modify a particular subject's underlying probability, determined by s_{ik}. This does not mean, however, that functions of these subject-specific parameters cannot have an interpretation that applies globally. For example, within-subject odds-ratios will be the same for all subjects with common covariates. Extending the earlier notation, let $\pi_{a,j,s}$ be the probability that a subject with effect s under treatment a in period j responds with a 1. Then from (6.3)

$$\tau_a - \tau_b = \ln\left\{\frac{\pi_{a,j,s}/(1-\pi_{a,j,s})}{\pi_{b,j,s}/(1-\pi_{b,j,s})}\right\}, \tag{6.4}$$

which is the same for all s. But we do emphasize that this is not the same quantity as the marginal log odds-ratio in (6.2).

Marginal probabilities can be obtained from subject-specific ones by taking expectations over the distribution of the subject effects. In general, however, the model structure (linear additive model on a logit scale, for example) on which the subject specific probabilities are based will not carry over to the resulting marginal probabilities. There are exceptions to this, and if normally distributed subject effects are used, then, to a close approximation for the logit link, and exactly for the probit link, the marginal model will have the same structure with the parameters scaled downwards in absolute size (Zeger et al., 1988). Newhaus et al. (1991) show more generally that for any distribution of the subject effects there is a sense in which parameters are attenuated in the marginal model. Good discussions of the distinction between population averaged and subject-specific models can be found in Zeger et al. (1988), Zeger (1988), Newhaus et al. (1991), and Diggle et al. (2002).

In this chapter we concentrate on marginal and simple subject-specific models for categorical cross-over data. The most important analyses can be formulated in terms of one or other of these two classes of model. Two alternative forms of model for dependent categorical data are the *transition* and *multivariate log-linear*; see Diggle et al. (2002), Chapter 7, for example. The former are of more relevance for modeling the probabilities of transition from one category to another in longer sets of repeated measurements and the latter are more suitable for analyses in which the association structure of the data is of prime interest, rather than a nuisance to be accommodated, as in the present context.

6.2 Binary data: subject effect models

6.2.1 Dealing with the subject effects

Recall from (6.3) the logistic representation of the simple subject-specific model:

$$\text{logit}\{P(Y_{ijk}=1 \mid s_{ik})\} = \mu + \pi_j + \tau_{d[i,j]} + s_{ik},$$

where s_{ik} is an effect associated with the (ik)th subject, sometimes called in this context a *latent variable*. Conditional on this effect, the repeated measurements from this subject are assumed to be independent. It is tempting to use conventional logistic regression to fit such a model and obtain inferences. However, an important feature of such latent variable models in the non-normal setting is the inconsistency of the maximum likelihood estimates, a result that is well-known in the analysis of matched pair case-control studies (Breslow and Day, 1980, Chapter 7), a setting that is closely related to the current setup. The inconsistency arises because the number of parameters increases at the same rate as the number of subjects and this means that the usual asymptotic results do not apply. Two possible routes are used in practice to avoid this difficulty. First, a conditional likelihood analysis can used in which the subject effects are eliminated. Second, the subject effects can be assumed to follow some distribution; the resulting model is a special case of the generalized linear *mixed* model (Diggle et al., 2002, Chapter 9). We now look in turn at these two routes, comparing and contrasting them as we proceed. We begin with the conditional likelihood approach.

6.2.2 *Conditional likelihood*

6.2.2.1 *Mainland–Gart test*

We consider first the conditional likelihood approach because this leads, in the 2×2 setting, to the commonly used **Mainland–Gart** test (Section 2.13). In general, a conditional likelihood analysis can be constructed whenever there exist sufficient statistics for the nuisance parameters, in this case the subject effects. Such statistics exist only for particular combinations of distribution and link: the binomial/logit combination is one such example. The general approach is to use in place of the full likelihood for the data the likelihood derived from the distribution of the data *conditional on the observed values of these sufficient statistics*. By definition, this conditional likelihood is free of the nuisance parameters, and conventional methods are then applied to this to make inferences about the remaining parameters of interest. The approach is analogous to an analysis with fixed subject effects in the normal linear model, and all information contained in the sufficient statistics is lost in the process. In the present two-period binary setting the sufficient statistics for the subject effects are simply the subject totals. Omitting details of the derivation, the test for treatment effect in the absence of carry-over effect is the test for no association in the 2×2 contingency table of *preference data*:

Group	(0,1)	(1,0)
1 (AB)	n_{12}	n_{13}
2 (BA)	n_{22}	n_{23}

obtained by discarding the nonpreference columns from the full 4×2 table, presented in Table 2.35. This is the Mainland–Gart test (Mainland, 1963; Gart,

1969) for treatment effect described in Section 2.13. Note that the related test introduced by Prescott, also described in Section 2.13, is not an example of a conditional likelihood analysis because it uses the nonpreference outcomes.

Tests for the *period* effect (adjusted for treatment) can be constructed in exactly the same way as for the Mainland–Gart and Prescott tests, by interchanging n_{22} and n_{23}. If a test is to be made for *carry over*, then this cannot be done using conditional likelihood: all the direct information is contained in the subject sums and this is discarded through the conditioning process. We return to this test when we consider the random subject effects model below.

6.2.2.2 Mainland–Gart test in a logistic regression framework

The emphasis in Section 2.13 was on the calculation of simple tests for direct treatment effect. To establish the framework for estimation and the analysis for other, less simple designs, we now introduce more formally the underlying subject-specific logistic regression model. First we see how the odds-ratio measuring association in the Mainland–Gart test is related to the treatment effect in this underlying model.

For the 2×2 design we can express the linear predictor in a simple way if we set $\pi_1 = 0, \pi_2 = \pi, \tau_A = 0$ and $\tau_B = \tau$. For one individual (with subject effect s, say), the linear predictor corresponding to each period in each sequence can be expressed:

	Period	
Sequence	1	2
AB	$\mu + s$	$\mu + \pi + \tau + s$
BA	$\mu + \tau + s$	$\mu + \pi + s$

Conditionally on s, the two observations from this individual are assumed to be independent. So the conditional probabilities of the *joint* outcomes, (0,0), (0,1) and so on, are simply obtained from the products of the individual probabilities. For example, the probability of an (0,1) outcome in sequence AB is

$$P_{01}(AB \mid s) = \frac{1}{1+e^{\mu+s}} \times \frac{e^{\mu+\pi+\tau+s}}{1+e^{\mu+\pi+\tau+s}}.$$

The conditional probabilities in the 2×2 table for the Mainland–Gart test are then:

Group	(0,1)	(1,0)
1 (AB)	$\frac{1}{1+e^{\mu+s}} \frac{e^{\mu+\pi+\tau+s}}{1+e^{\mu+\pi+\tau+s}}$	$\frac{e^{\mu+s}}{1+e^{\mu+s}} \frac{1}{1+e^{\mu+\pi+\tau+s}}$
2 (BA)	$\frac{1}{1+e^{\mu+\tau+s}} \frac{e^{\mu+\pi+s}}{1+e^{\mu+\pi+s}}$	$\frac{e^{\mu+\tau+s}}{1+e^{\mu+\tau+s}} \frac{1}{1+e^{\mu+\pi+s}}$

Now the odds-ratio in this table is

$$\phi = \frac{P_{01}(AB \mid s)P_{10}(BA \mid s)}{P_{01}(BA \mid s)P_{10}(AB \mid s)},$$

which, after some simplification, reduces to

$$\phi = e^{2\tau}.$$

Thus the odds-ratio in this table is the square of the odds-ratio in the original logistic regression model. Using standard asymptotic results for *log* odds-ratio estimators (Cox and Snell, 1989) we have that

$$\mathrm{V}(\ln\hat{\phi}) \simeq \frac{1}{n_{12}} + \frac{1}{n_{13}} + \frac{1}{n_{22}} + \frac{1}{n_{23}} = v \text{ say.} \tag{6.5}$$

Hence an asymptotic 95% confidence interval for $\hat{\tau}$ is given by

$$\exp\{\ln(\hat{\phi}/2) \pm 1.96\sqrt{\hat{v}}/2\}.$$

6.2.2.3 *Small sample issues*

These results are asymptotic and will not work sufficiently well in small problems, such as the one described in Example 2.5 in Chapter 2. In this example, it will be recalled, there were two centers. The problems of small data sets are highlighted by the presence of the zero cell in Center 2 of Example 2.5, for which the crude log-odds ratio is not even defined. This does not affect the calculation of the score test used in Section 2.13 (the conventional chi-squared test) provided there are no zero margins, but raises strong doubts about its behavior in this setting. Alternatively, modifications can be made to the odds-ratio estimator and its associated measure of precision, to improve the small-sample behavior and to ensure its existence when there are zero cells. Cox and Snell (1989) (p.32) suggest adding one half to each cell and modifying the variance estimator accordingly:

$$V_A = \frac{(n_{12}+n_{13}+1)(n_{12}+n_{13}+2)}{(n_{12}+n_{13})(n_{12}+1)(n_{13}+1)} + \frac{(n_{22}+n_{23}+1)(n_{22}+n_{23}+2)}{(n_{22}+n_{23})(n_{22}+1)(n_{23}+1)}.$$

A simpler method is to replace the zero cell only by one half and use this figure in the original variance formula (6.5).

At the end of Section 5.7 the point was made that, in the absence of carry-over or treatment-by-period interaction in the model, small sample tests can the obtained by a re-randomization (or permutation) procedure. It is interesting to use this here, to compare how the various procedures for testing the Mainland–Gart odds-ratios actually perform in the current setting. In fact, there are only a finite number of configurations for the re-randomized data. Using a large number of re-randomizations (of subjects to groups) we estimate implicitly, with a high degree of accuracy, the probabilities associated with these configurations. Fisher's exact test does this using the analytical probabilities for each configuration (under the null hypothesis), but is different in one other respect from the current re-randomization based method. Fisher's exact test conditions on the nonpreference totals and so the only re-allocation occurs within the preference cells. In the re-randomization approach, all subjects are re-randomized. We should therefore expect small differences from Fisher's test, and these differences give an indication of the impact of the conditioning in this setting.

We apply the re-randomization procedures to the Mainland–Gart test calculated for the results in Center 2 of Example 2.5. In Table 6.2 we give the probabilities calculated using the asymptotic χ_1^2 approximation for four tests: (1) conventional chi-squared (as in Section 2.13), (2) conventional chi-squared with Yates' correction, (3) the Wald test using the estimate and variance obtained after adding one half to all preference cells and (4) the Wald test using the estimate and variance obtained after adding one half to zero cells only. For comparison, Table 6.2 also contains the significance probabilities obtained from 1 million re-randomizations for these same four test statistics. The simplicity of the tests themselves means that the computation involved in this takes only few minutes. It is not even necessary to use conventional test statistics for this approach. We could use instead any measure of departure from the null hypothesis, such the odds-ratios from (3) and (4), or even the count in one of the cells of the Mainland–Gart table. These would all give the same significance probabilities under re-randomization as the conventional chi-squared statistic. For comparative purposes, we also show the probabilities that each test generates when we restrict the re-randomizations to those subjects who show a preference. This generates numerically the same hypergeometric probabilities that underly Fisher's exact test.

The re-randomization based, or conditional exact, sampling distributions of the test statistics are discrete, and in small samples, may have only few support points. This means that nominal test sizes cannot be achieved exactly and some have argued that this implies that such procedures are conservative. This view is open to debate, but a good compromise is to use so-called mid-P procedures in discrete problems. These attempt to accommodate the strongly discrete sampling distribution of the exact test statistic by combining probabilities of more extreme configurations with one half the probability of the observed configuration. It has been argued that such tests have more useful long-run behavior; see, for example, Lancaster (1961) and Agresti et al. (1993). The current re-randomization tests give us a good opportunity to illustrate this modification, so Table 6.2 contains *P*-values calculated both in the conventional way and using mid-*P* procedures.

There are several points to note from these results. First, Yates' adjusted test and the restricted re-randomization tests are close (as expected) to Fisher's exact test ($P = 0.061$). Second, all the tests give identical re-randomization based results apart from (3), which is not greatly dissimilar. Finally, apart from Yates' corrected procedure, the asymptotic procedures are, in this example, more conservative than the small-sample procedures based on

Table 6.2: Example 2.5: Center 2: Significance probabilities from asymptotic and re-randomization versions of the Mainland–Gart test.

	Asymptotic	R-randomization based		
Statistic	χ_1^2	Conventional	mid-P	Restricted
(1)	0.014	0.021	0.014	0.061
(2)	0.066	0.021	0.014	0.061
(3)	0.063	0.036	0.029	0.061
(4)	0.024	0.021	0.014	0.061

(1) and (2) conventional chi-squared tests, without and with Yates' correction; (3) and (4) Wald tests based on tables with one half added to (3) all cells and (4) only zero cells.

re-randomization. The comparison of the results from the full and restricted re-randomizations suggest that some information has been lost in the latter approach, but we must be careful not overgeneralize the results from this single example.

6.2.2.4 Conditional logistic regression

The re-randomization procedure provides some insights into the various approaches to inference that we might make using the Mainland–Gart test in small samples, but is unfortunately rather limited. It can only be used for models restricted to period and direct treatment effects. More importantly, it is limited to overall treatment tests. We therefore return now to the conditional likelihood procedures based on the subject effects logistic regression model. In this model there are two levels, or degrees, of conditioning that can be used.

First, we can just condition on the sufficient statistics for the subject effects and apply asymptotic results to the resulting conditional likelihood. This is usually what is implied by the term *conditional logistic regression*. It can be done directly in a number of computer packages, for example, Stata (procedure `clogit`). In SAS the `logistic` procedure can be used in which the `strata` statement identifies the class variable on which conditioning is to be done; in the cross-over setting this will be the subject identifier.

Second, and importantly in small problems, the conditioning process can be continued further to eliminate from the likelihood all the parameters except those about which inferences are being made. This produces *conditional exact inferences* that generalize Fisher's exact procedure for the 2×2 table. Further, it is possible to produce conditional exact confidence intervals and tests for specific comparisons. This is computationally infeasible except in small samples, but this is not a real issue, as it is in just such settings that such an approach is of value. This is conveniently done using the `exact` facility of the SAS `genmod` procedure, from release 12.1.

As an illustration of the use of conditional exact procedures for estimation we consider again Center 2 from Example 2.5. Suppose we wish to estimate a 95% confidence interval for the treatment log odds-ratio from Center 2 (B versus A). The following genmod code sets up the exact analysis, with the variables taking obvious names:

```
proc genmod data=ex25;
 class sub cen per trt / param=ref;
 where cen=2;
 model y = sub per trt / dist=binomial;
 exact 'exact treatment effect' trt / estimate=both cltype=exact;
run;
```

This generates the results for the exact treatment effect:

```
                    The GENMOD Procedure

                 Exact Conditional Analysis

      Conditional Exact Tests for 'exact treatment effect'

                                            --- p-Value ---
       Effect   Test             Statistic    Exact      Mid

       trt      Score               5.5000   0.0606   0.0455
                Probability         0.0303   0.0606   0.0455


     Exact Parameter Estimates for 'exact treatment effect'

                         Standard     95% Confidence    Two-sided
Parameter   Estimate      Error          Limits          p-Value  Type

trt    1   -1.1331*          .     -Infinity  -0.1315   0.0606  Exact

          NOTE: * indicates a median unbiased estimate.

                   Exact Odds Ratios for 'exact treatment effect'

                               95% Confidence      Two-sided
Parameter      Estimate            Limits            p-Value   Type

trt         1     0.322*         0      0.877        0.0606   Exact

          NOTE: * indicates a median unbiased estimate.
```

There are some points to note here. First, as is not unusual in such problems, the zero in the table has meant that one end of the exact confidence interval is at $-\infty$ or ∞. Second, the exact 2-sided P-value is precisely the value obtained from the Fisher's exact version of the Mainland–Gart test in

Table 6.2; in this very simple setting these two do indeed coincide. Third, an alternative P-value is displayed, the so-called mid-P value, which we have met earlier. For comparison with the exact confidence interval, the two modified log odds-ratio estimates introduced above (one half added to all and zero cells, respectively) produce the following asymptotic 95% confidence intervals: $(-6.53, 0.17)$ and $(-5.89, -0.41)$. Again these reflect the (asymptotic) significance of the associated Wald tests.

To illustrate the role of conventional conditional logistic modeling (not exact) we now take the analysis of Example 2.5 further. Suppose that the results from the two centers are to be combined in one analysis, and we make the assumption that the period and treatment effects are the same in both centers. The model based approach allows us to make the necessary extension in a natural way. We could, for example, simply introduce center as an additional effect, to give the linear predictor:

$$\text{logit}\{P(Y_{cijk} = 1 \mid s_{cik})\} = \mu + \pi_j + \gamma_c + \tau_{d[i,j]} + s_{cik}, \tag{6.6}$$

for γ_c an effect associated with center c, $c = 1, 2$. This model can then be treated as any other logistic regression model in a conditional likelihood or conditional exact analysis. Note, however, that because center is a between-subject term it is eliminated along with the subject effects in the conditional analysis, and the use of this model in this setting is equivalent to a simple pooling of the data from the two centers. To confirm this, we can calculate the "Mainland–Gart" odds-ratio from the pooled table:

Group	(0,1)	(1,0)	Total
1 (AB)	2	7	9
2 (BA)	6	5	11
Total	8	12	20

For the B versus A comparison we need, the log odds-ratio from this table is -1.44, with an estimated asymptotic SE equal to 1.01. The Wald statistic is then -1.43. Suppose we now fit the logistic regression model (6.3) using conditional likelihood to the combined data:

```
proc logistic data=ex25;
  class sub cen per trt / param=ref;
  strata sub;
  model y = cen per trt;
run;
```

giving:

Analysis of Maximum Likelihood Estimates

Parameter		DF	Estimate	Standard Error	Wald Chi-Square	Pr > ChiSq
cen	1	0	0	.	.	.
per	1	1	-0.5352	0.5024	1.1350	0.2867
trt	1	1	-0.7175	0.5024	2.0400	0.1532

Apart from the factor of 2 expected from the earlier results, and very small rounding differences in the SEs, it can be seen that these are equivalent to those obtained from the Mainland–Gart table above.

Additional within-subject effects such as period-by-center or treatment-by-center interaction could be estimated simply using a suitably extended version of this model, but we would need good substantive reasons for examining such terms and sufficient power to make the process worthwhile.

To summarize, we can use a conditional likelihood analysis to draw inferences from a subject effects logistic regression model for cross-over data. The advantage of this approach is that we need make no assumptions about the distribution of the subject effects, although it is assumed that other effects (like treatment and period) are consistent across subjects. In very small samples or, more accurately, samples with few preference responses, for which asymptotic results are not reliable, we can, with appropriate software, construct conditional exact analyzes which provide both tests and confidence intervals for direct treatment (and other) effects. One disadvantage of the conditional approach is that all between-subject information is lost. This implies that relevant information on direct treatment effects may be lost from inefficient designs, inferences cannot be made about between-subject terms like center effects, and population-averaged summaries cannot be constructed from the analysis. In a typical trial setting we would not regard any of these as serious drawbacks.

6.2.2.5 Random subject effects

To recover the between-subject information from a subject effects based analysis, a random-effects model may be used. A natural choice of distribution for the subject effects is the normal, given that the transformed scale of the linear predictor is the scale upon which we expect effects to be approximately additive. The resulting model is an example of a **generalized linear mixed model.** The associated likelihood is obtained by integrating over the distribution of the subject effects. As an illustration, consider again the 2×2 cross-over design. We saw earlier that, conditional on the subject effect for one subject, s_{ik} say, the probability for the joint outcome for that subject (y_{i1k}, y_{i2k}) can be written as the product of the two separate probabilities:

$$\begin{aligned}
\mathrm{P}(Y_{i1k} = y_{i1k}, Y_{i2k} = y_{i2k} \mid s_{ik}) &= \frac{e^{y_{i1k}(\mu+\pi_1+\tau_{d[i,1]}+s_{ik})}}{1+e^{\mu+\pi_1+\tau_{d[i,1]}+s_{ik}}} \\
&\times \frac{e^{y_{i2k}(\mu+\pi_2+\tau_{d[i,2]}+s_{ik})}}{1+e^{\mu+\pi_2+\tau_{d[i,2]}+s_{ik}}}.
\end{aligned}$$

For the likelihood we need the expectation of this joint probability with respect to the distribution of s_{ik}, $f(s)$, say:

$$\mathrm{P}(Y_{i1k} = y_{i1k}, Y_{i2k} = y_{i2k}) = \int \mathrm{P}(Y_{i1k} = y_{i1k}, Y_{i2k} = y_{i2k} \mid s) f(s) ds.$$

This integral can be solved analytically only for special combinations of link and subject effects distribution, such as the probit combined with the normal distribution. More generally, numerical techniques can be employed provided the random effects structure is relatively simple. Analyses based on such integrated likelihoods can be done in a relatively straightforward way using Guassian quadrature (and other types of numerical integration) in SAS `proc glimmix` and `proc nlmixed`. Other statistical packages, such as Stata and MLwiN, have facilities for random subject effects analyses in a logistic regression context, and full Bayesian versions can be implemented using Markov chain Monte Carlo methods in WinBUGS and SAS `proc mcmc` (Spiegelhalter et al., 2000).

We now show how model (6.3) together with the assumption of normally distributed subject effects,

$$s_{ik} \sim \mathrm{N}(0, \sigma_s^2),$$

can be fitted using SAS `proc glimmix`; for such standard problems this is typically much more straightforward than `proc nlmixed`, which gains great flexbility at the expense of such simplicity. As an illustration, we again turn to the the data from Center 2 of Example 2.5, the trial on cerebrovascular deficiency.

```
proc glimmix data=ex25 method=quad(qcheck);
  where cen=2;
  class sub per trt;
  model y = per trt / dist=binary;
  random intercept / subject=sub;
  estimate "treatment B vs A" trt -1 1;
run;
```

The `method=quad` option of the `proc glimmix` statement requests adaptive Gasussian quadrature for the numerical integration to calculate the full marginal likelihood. If this is omitted, the default method (i.e., omitting method=) is an approximate one, an example of so-called pseudo-likelihood. This typically has poor behavior with binary data with random Gausssian effects and so should not be used in settings like this. However, the adaptive Gaussian quadrature is not itself guaranteed to provide a sufficiently precise estimate of the maximum likelihood estimator and it is important to confirm with a fair degree of certainty that the solution is indeed the one required. To help with this, proc glimmix includes several tools, one of which is the qcheck option included in the code above. This performs an adaptive recalculation of the objective function (2 log likelihood) at the solution, using increasing numbers of quadrature points, starting from the number used in the optimization. It is also possible to over-ride the adaptive selection of quadrature points and impose a fixed number, using qpoints=. Up to a limit, an increased number of points typically implies increased precision for the calculation of the likelihood, the main disadvantage being increased computation time. With small to moderately sized cross-over trials, this is less of an issue and below the results from the adaptive quadrature will be compared with those of a fixed, but large, number of points.

From the above code we obtained the key parameter estimates:

```
                    Covariance Parameter Estimates

                                                        Standard
          Cov Parm       Subject     Estimate              Error

          Intercept      sub           19.2756           11.5125


                   Type III Tests of Fixed Effects

                             Num         Den
        Effect                DF          DF      F Value       Pr > F

        per                    1          65         1.60       0.2103
        trt                    1          65         4.43       0.0391


                                  Estimates

                                  Standard
Label                 Estimate       Error      DF    t Value    Pr > |t|

treatment B vs A      -1.7065     0.8106      65     -2.11     0.0391
```

The results from the qcheck option are below, and these do suggest that this analysis is not sufficiently close to the optimum.

Adaptiveness of Quadrature at Solution

Quadrature Points	Objective Function	---Relative Difference to--- Converged	Previous
9	136.61945388		
11	136.36540174	-0.001859561	-0.001859561
21	136.35181693	-0.001958996	-0.000099621
31	136.36096489	-0.001892037	0.0000670909

The analysis is therefore repeated with a large fixed number, 31, of quadrature points, i.e., using `proc glimmix ... method=quad(qpoints=31)`. Increasing this to 51 points had minimal effect on the results. For 31, these were as follows:

Covariance Parameter Estimates

Cov Parm	Subject	Estimate	Standard Error
Intercept	sub	24.3118	18.6818

Type III Tests of Fixed Effects

Effect	Num DF	Den DF	F Value	Pr > F
per	1	65	1.61	0.2094
trt	1	65	4.04	0.0486

Estimates

Label	Estimate	Standard Error	DF	t Value	Pr > |t|
treatment B vs A	-1.8602	0.9256	65	-2.01	0.0486

The differences from the earlier analysis under adaptive quadrature are small in a substantive sense, but not wholly negligible. The greatest difference is in the estimates of the between-subject variance. This is both very large ($\hat{\sigma}_s^2 = 24.4$) but also very poorly estimated. This large between-subject variability is a consequence of the small proportion of preference outcomes. The dominance of (0,0) and (1,1) outcomes implies very high within-subject dependence. The large estimated value for σ_s^2 in turn has a major impact on the absolute size of the treatment effect estimate. This subject-specific estimate increases in absolute size relative to its marginal counterpart as σ_s^2 increases. By comparison with these results, the modified estimates obtained from the conditional likelihood Mainland–Gart odds-ratios earlier are -1.59 (0.85) and -1.57 (0.70) for halves added to zero cells and all cells, respectively. These are fairly consistent with the random effects estimate, although a little smaller both in size and SE. The Wald test calculated from the random effects estimate of treatment effect is 4.04, with associated $P = 0.04$. We can also calculate a likelihood ratio test for the treatment effect. Under the current model $-2\text{logl} = 136.3$. Dropping treatment and refitting produces $-2\text{logl} = 142.7$, giving a difference of 6.4 on 1 d.f. The associated tail probability from the χ_1^2 distribution is 0.01, a rather more extreme result, and one that is more consistent with the small sample tests based on re-randomization. The discrepancy between the Wald and LR procedures suggests that the asymptotic properties of these tests are not holding particularly well in this setting.

The high degree of within-subject dependence has important implications for the interpretation of the treatment effect in this model. This can be seen very clearly in the original 2×4 table. Even though there is some evidence that abnormal readings are more likely to be seen under treatment B, this effect is confined to a small minority of the subjects observed. When averaged over the subjects in the trial (a population averaged view) the odds-ratio, or difference in probabilities, is comparatively small.

We now extend this analysis to include both centers, paralleling that done earlier using conditional logistic regression. We return to the combined model (6.6) with a simple center effect and no interactions (6.6):

$$\text{logit}\{P(Y_{cijk} = 1 \mid s_{cik})\} = \mu + \pi_j + \gamma_c + \tau_{d[i,j]} + s_{cik}.$$

The `proc glimmix` code for the single center is extended in an obvious way, again using 31 fixed quadrature points:

```
proc glimmix data=ex25 method=quad(qpoints=31);
  class sub cen per trt;
  model y = cen per trt / dist=binary;
  random intercept / subject=sub;
  estimate "treatment B vs A" trt -1 1;
run;
```

producing the following estimates:

```
                  Covariance Parameter Estimates

                                                         Standard
          Cov Parm      Subject     Estimate              Error

          Intercept     sub            11.6863            6.0406


                   Type III Tests of Fixed Effects

                          Num        Den
        Effect             DF         DF     F Value      Pr > F

        cen                 1         98        1.49      0.2246
        per                 1         98        0.91      0.3431
        trt                 1         98        1.85      0.1769


                               Estimates

                                     Standard
Label                   Estimate        Error       DF    t Value    Pr > |t|

treatment B vs A       -0.6509       0.4785       98      -1.36      0.1769
```

The treatment estimates and SEs from both the conditional and random effects analyses are very similar, with a slightly smaller absolute value using the random subject effects model. Note that we also now have an estimate of the center effect, albeit a rather imprecise one. The Wald test for a zero treatment effect is produced automatically. We could, if we wish, use the likelihood ratio test as an alternative. The value of $-2\log l$ from the above fit is 222.9 and from the fit with treatment omitted, $-2\log l = 224.8$, a difference of 1.9. The associated tail probability from the χ_1^2 distribution is $P = 0.17$, a very similar result to the Wald test. We do see from the combined data that there is no real evidence of a treatment effect, unlike the analysis of Center 2 alone. The difference in treatment effect between the centers could be investigated formally using the center-by-treatment interaction. Such terms can be added to the model in an obvious way. We do not expect sufficient power in the present setting to justify such a test so we do not pursue it here.

We can summarize the differences between the three approaches to the subject specific model, (1) conditional, (2) conditional exact and (3) random subject effects, through the inferences they produce for the treatment effect from the analysis of both centers. By combining the centers we reduce the influence of small sample issues in the comparison, particularly those associated with the zero cell in Center 2. We have discussed these issues in some detail

Table 6.3: Example 6.2: Inferences for the B-A treatment difference, both centers.

Analysis	Estimate	SE	P	95% CI
1. Conditional	−0.718	0.502	0.153	(−1.702, 0.267)
2. Conditional Exact (mid-P)	−0.680	0.488	0.131	(−2.010, 0.412)
3. Random Effects	−0.651	0.478	0.177	(−1.598, 0.298)

earlier. In very small samples, to ensure validity, we would recommend either the use of the conditional exact procedures or, where applicable, rerandomization tests.

The three sets of results are presented in Table 6.3. The results from the tests are very consistent. Given this, it is surprising that the conditional exact confidence intervals are so much more conservative than the other two. This is due to the use of the mid-P conditional scores test. The exact confidence interval presented is directly associated with the more conservative exact test obtained by doubling the one sided-probability, for which $P = 0.31$.

Before moving on to higher-order designs, we note that similar procedures can be used to test for carry-over in the 2×2 setting, not forgetting the issues that this raises, as discussed in Section 2.7. For this we just need to include a period-by-treatment interaction in the model:

```
proc glimmix data=ex25 method=quad(qpoints=31);
  class sub cen per trt;
  model y = cen per trt per*trt / dist=binary;
  random intercept / subject=sub;
run;
```

There is no conditional or conditional exact analog of this analysis because the carry-over effect is part of the between-subject stratum, all the information in which is removed when conditioning on the subject effects. The resulting estimate of carry-over is, in terms of the interaction, −0.88 with an SE of 1.77. Predictably, the corresponding Wald statistic is far from significant.

An alternative and very simple test for carry-over, introduced by Altham (1971), is the test for association in the 2×2 contingency table of *non-preference* responses:

Group	(0,0)	(1,1)
1 (AB)	n_{11}	n_{14}
2 (BA)	n_{21}	n_{24}

Combining the two centers, we get the following table:

12	29
13	26

The conventional chi-squared statistic for testing association in this table is equal to 0.15, and comparing this with the χ_1^2 distribution we get $P = 0.69$, a result that is wholly consistent with the previous analysis.

6.2.2.6 *Higher-order designs*

The subject-specific logistic regression model (6.3) provides us with an immediate extension of the previous analyses to higher-order designs. Consider the four-period four-treatment design, Example 6.1. First these data are arranged by observation:

subject	period	treatment	response
1	1	1	0
1	2	2	0
1	3	3	0
1	4	4	0
2	1	3	0
...			
79	4	1	1
80	1	4	1
80	2	3	1
80	3	2	1
80	4	1	1

Procedures based on the conditional likelihood can be obtained in exactly the same way as described above for the extended 2×2 design. In principle, conditional exact procedures could be used, but given the number of subjects and number of observations per subject, the necessary calculations become somewhat more burdensome and, arguably, are less important in this setting.

The random subject effects model can also be fitted using SAS `proc glimmix` in just the same way as earlier for Example 2.1. Again we start with adaptive Gaussian quadrature and examine the convergence through `qcheck`. Here the results seem very stable, and using 31 fixed quadrature points gives essentially the same results.

```
proc glimmix data=ex61 method=quad(qcheck);
  class sub per trt;
  model y = per trt / dist=binary;
  random intercept / subject=sub;
  estimate "B vs A" trt -1 1 0 0;
  estimate "C vs A" trt -1 0 1 0;
  estimate "D vs A" trt -1 0 0 1;
run;
```

Table 6.4: Example 6.1: Results from the subject specific analyses; estimates are log odds-ratios.

	Conditional		Random subjects	
Effect	Estimate	SE	Estimate	SE
B-A	−0.683	0.393	−0.679	0.392
C-A	−0.015	0.404	−0.071	0.404
D-A	−0.371	0.399	−0.405	0.398
Overall tests				
Wald	4.08	($P = 0.25$)	4.85	($P = 0.18$)
LR	4.16	($P = 0.25$)	3.90	($P = 0.27$)
Estimate of σ_s^2			1.56	(SE 0.68)

The main results from the conditional and random effects analyses are summarized in Table 6.4. The overall test for treatment effect is on 3 degrees of freedom and, as before, can either be obtained using likelihood ratio or Wald procedures. Both are presented. One point to note from these two analyses is the high degree of consistency between them. In the absence of carry-over in the model, this design is completely balanced: subjects, periods and treatments are all orthogonal. Hence there is effectively no between-subject information to recover, and both analyses are essentially using the same information. The small differences between the two sets of results, which would not be seen with a conventional linear regression model, are due to the nonlinearity of the link function and nonconstant variance of the binary responses. It follows that unless we want to calculate marginal effects from this analysis we have nothing to lose by using the conditional likelihood approach, and this relies on fewer assumptions than the random subject analysis. To obtain marginal effects with the latter model we could integrate using the observed estimate of σ_s^2 (equal to 1.56 in this example). Recall, however, that in theory a logistic regression model cannot simultaneously hold exactly in both the subject-specific and marginal settings, so care must be taken in mapping corresponding parameters from one model to the other. However, as mentioned earlier, an approximate mapping does hold when normal subject effects are used in the logistic model and this improves as σ_s^2 decreases. It is therefore not without meaning in this setting to consider obtaining such marginal effects through integration. Alternatively, if the effects in a marginal model are of direct interest, we can start with such a model. We consider this next.

Table 6.5: Example 6.1: Raw marginal probabilities.

Group	A	B	C	D
ABCD	0.67	0.56	0.67	0.50
BDAC	0.68	0.73	0.68	0.86
CADB	0.79	0.58	0.68	0.58
DCBA	0.81	0.67	0.86	0.71

6.3 Binary data: marginal models

6.3.1 Marginal model

The logistic form of the simple marginal model introduced at the start of this chapter (6.1) can be written

$$\text{logit}\{\text{E}(Y_{ijk})\} = \text{logit}\{P(Y_{ijk} = 1)\} = \mu + \pi_j + \tau_{d[i,j]}. \qquad (6.7)$$

In such a model we are concerned with modeling the marginal probabilities of success or failure in each period. Consider Example 6.1, the four-period four-treatment trial. The raw estimates of these marginal probabilities from each sequence group are the simple proportions given in Table 6.5. The aim of the analysis is to fit model (6.7) to these probabilities. Although this introduces the parameters of interest, it does not provide a complete description of the distribution of the data because it does not refer in any way to the statistical dependence among the repeated measurements. The underlying distribution is product-multinomial: the counts in each row of Table 6.1 follow a multinomial distribution and those in different rows are assumed to be independent. The multinomial probabilities correspond to each *joint* outcome and the marginal model does not define these. To complete the definition of the joint probabilities, additional structure must be imposed and this determines, in some form, the dependence among the repeated measurements. Typically the expression of the joint probabilities in terms of the marginal parameters will be complicated; indeed, with more than two times of measurement there will usually be no explicit expression for these; they will exist only as solutions of sets of equations. This implies that an analysis that requires a fully parameterized representation of the joint probabilities, that is, a likelihood based analysis, will be comparatively convoluted. For a good discussion of this point see Liang et al. (1992), Section 2, or Diggle et al. (2002), Section 8.2. Although likelihood analyses have been developed for these settings, they are not as yet available for routine use. We concentrate here on more accessible nonlikelihood methods. Some example of full likelihood marginal analyses in the two-period two-treatment setting can be found in Kenward and Jones (1994).

Koch et al. (1977) extended the weighted least squares approach of Grizzle (1965) for modeling categorical data to the multivariate and repeated measurement setting. A model such as (6.7) is specified for the expected values of the observations in each period, but the variances and covariances are not modeled, but estimated using the marginal one-way and two-way tables of counts from each sequence group. Using these, empirical generalized least squares (EGLS) is used to fit the model and as a basis for inference. This avoids the need to model explicitly the dependence structure of the repeated measurements. The method is implemented in the SAS `catmod` procedure and so has the advantage of ready access. However, the method requires very large sample sizes for acceptable behavior; indeed, with moderate to small sample sizes the required statistics may not even exist due to singularities in the estimated variance-covariance matrix. The SAS `proc catmod` manual recommends on average 25 subjects for each combination of period and group, which implies a total of about $25 \times p \times s$ subjects for a cross-over trial with p periods and s sequences. For example, this amounts to 400 subjects for the four-period four-treatment sequence trial used here as an example. Some simulation results for a parallel group trial are given by Kenward and Jones (1992) and these tend to confirm these sample size recommendations. Useful discussions of this approach are given by Zeger (1988) and Agresti (1989). Lipsitz and Fitzmaurice (1994) use the method as a basis for power calculations for repeated measurements trials with binary outcomes. While the approach has some advantages in terms of flexibility, the restriction in sample size means that it is rarely applicable in the cross-over setting.

An alternative to the EGLS approach that suffers far less from problems with sample size and is comparatively simple to use in practice is based on the use of generalized estimating equations (GEE). The literature on this has grown rapidly following the introduction of the method to a biometric audience. Principal early references are White (1982), Liang and Zeger (1986), Zeger and Liang (1986). A current overview is given in Chapter 8 of Diggle et al. (2002), with a very thorough account in Molenberghs and Verbeke (2000). We consider the estimating approach in its simplest form (sometimes called GEE1) in which only the marginal probabilities are modeled. Additional sets of equations can be added for estimating measures of dependence (correlations, odds-ratios, risk-ratios) to produce so-called GEE2, and other approaches can be developed from this starting point, but the gain in possible efficiency from this is matched by some loss of simplicity. See, for example, Diggle et al. (2002), Section 8.2.

In the GEE1 approach a generalized linear model is used to represent the marginal observations at each time of measurement and in the process of estimation the variances are calculated from the current marginal model parameters. No attempt is made to model the correlations between the repeated measurements. Instead a fixed "working" correlation matrix is used and this leads, with some minor provisos, to consistent estimates of the model parameters whatever the true correlation structure (Liang and Zeger, 1986; Zeger and Liang, 1986). Subsequently, inferences about the model parameters are based on estimates of error that are robust to misspecification of the correlations, the so-called **sandwich** or **empirical** estimator.

The whole approach is particularly simple when the identity matrix is used for the working correlation matrix and this would appear to be the most widely used implementation. We term this the independence estimating equation (IEE) implementation of GEE1. There are some advantages to the use of IEE. Pepe and Anderson (1994) show how a nonidentity working correlation matrix *may* lead to inconsistency when there are time-dependent covariates, although this does not apply to the cross-over setting where the sequences of time-dependent covariates (treatments) are randomized at the start of the trial. In general, provided the marginal model is correct, the IEE approach will produce consistent estimators. One objection to the use of IEE is possible inefficiency. In the cross-over setting this will be an issue only for inefficient designs, that is, when a nontrivial amount of information is contained in the between-subject stratum. In such settings it is probably better anyway to consider the random effects subject-specific models.

In some applications of GEE1 the working correlation matrix is re-estimated at each cycle of the estimation procedure, as described in Liang and Zeger (1986). To avoid issues with structural inconsistency (McCullagh and Nelder, 1989, Section 9.3) and possible inconsistency of estimators (Crowder, 1995) such an approach is probably best avoided with cross-over trials.

In summary, we consider only the IEE version of GEE1 for cross-over trials. Two main questions arise about the performance of this approach with categorical data from cross-over trials. First, is there likely to be much loss of efficiency in using the independence assumption for estimation? Second, is the empirical estimator sufficiently reliable in small samples? Arguably the latter represents the weakest component of the simple independence implementation of the estimating equation method to be used here. We have already indicated that the loss of efficiency is likely to be negligible in efficient designs. Sharples and Breslow (1992) describe a simulation study of the GEE method for logistic regression with a very simple covariate structure. They suggest that little is lost in terms of bias and efficiency using the independence assumption, and the empirical estimator of error performed acceptably well in terms of bias down to sample sizes of 50 units. Kenward and Jones (1994) augment these results with some simulations addressed specifically to the cross-over setting. Binary data were simulated from the four-period four-treatment design of Example 6.1. The loss in efficiency through the use of the IEE estimators was negligible, and the estimated SEs performed well for sample sizes of 40 and above. Somewhat surprisingly, the actual 5% and 1% test sizes based on Wald statistics were acceptable even with a trial size of only 20. More recently, there have been several proposals for improving the small sample behavior of the sandwich estimator, and subsequent inferences; see, for example, Fay and Graubard (2001), Kauermann and Carroll (2001), Mancl and DeRouen (2001), Pan and Wall (2002). The IEE procedure can be used in the current setting in a straightforward way with SAS `proc genmod` and `proc glimmix`, with the latter incorporating some of the small sample adjustment. Facilities for GEEs are also available in several other packages, for example, Stata, Splus and R. We will use `proc glimmix`, as it allows us to see the impact of applying the small sample adjustments. As we have seen before, it is precisely in the cross-over setting that small sample issues are likely to arise. We apply it first to Example 2.1, the pair of cross-over trials from the trial on cerebrovascular deficiency. Following the subject-specific analysis we fit a model with a center effect but no interactions:

$$\text{logit}\{P(Y_{cijk}=1)\} = \mu^M + \pi_j^M + \gamma_c^M + \tau_{d[i,j]}^M.$$

The superscript M has been added to the parameters in this model to emphasize their distinction from the parameters in the subject effects model. The following `proc glimmix` commands will fit this model using IEE and will produce sandwich estimates of precision. Note that the effects estimates are identical to those that would be obtained using ordinary logistic regression in which all observations are assumed independent.

```
proc glimmix data=bk25 empirical;
  class sub cen per trt;
  model y  = cen per trt / dist=binary s;
  random _residual_ / subject=sub type=vc;
  estimate 'Centre (2-1)'  cen -1 1;
  estimate 'Period (2-1)'  per -1 1;
  estimate 'Direct Treatment Effect (B-A)'  trt -1 1;
run;
```

The parameter estimates and empirical SEs produced by this fit are presented in Table 6.6 alongside the corresponding estimates and SEs from the random subject effects analysis, together with the Wald statistics. It can be seen how the effects estimates have been attenuated in the marginal analysis by a very consistent amount; the ratios of the corresponding estimates are around 2.4. The SEs are attenuated to a similar degree, however, and the resulting inferences based on the Wald tests are almost identical in the two analyses. This is typically the case with these types of model in a cross-over setting that is largely confined to within-subject information. The degree of attenuation is directly related to the size of the within-subject dependence.

We can also use small sample procedures to adjust the calculation of the standard errors. These are selected as qualifiers to the `empirical` option. Two are considered here: (1) `empirical=root`, which uses the residual approximation in Kauermann and Carroll (2001), and (2) `empirical=firores`, the proposed adjustment in Mancl and DeRouen (2001). In this example these produce standard errors for the treatment effect of 0.199 and 0.201, respectively. Both are very close indeed to the simple unadjusted estimator, 0.197.

Table 6.6: Example 2.5: Both centers: estimated log odds-ratios from the subject-specific and marginal analyses.

	Subject-Specific		Marginal	
Effect	Estimate (SE)	Wald	Estimate (SE)	Wald
Center (2-1)	1.174 (0.960)	1.22	0.482 (0.387)	1.24
Period (2-1)	−0.449 (0.471)	−0.95	−0.179 (0.198)	−0.91
Treatment (B-A)	−0.650 (0.478)	−1.36	−0.268 (0.197)	−1.36

Table 6.7: Example 6.1: Estimated treatment effects, log odds-ratios, from the subject specific and marginal analyses.

	Subject-Specific		Marginal	
Effect	Estimate (SE)	Wald	Estimate (SE)	Wald
B-A	−0.679 (0.392)	1.73	−0.537 (0.325)	1.24
C-A	−0.071 (0.404)	0.18	−0.081 (0.323)	0.25
D-A	−0.405 (0.398)	1.02	−0.341 (0.276)	1.24
Overall (type 3) tests				
Wald	4.85	$(P = 0.18)$	3.70	$(P = 0.31)$

The between-subject variance is considerably smaller in Example 6.1, the four-treatment trial (6.4). Here we should expect less attenuation. The basic model (6.7) can be fitted using the following `glimmix` instructions. The overall treatment test is on three degrees of freedom and requires calculation of a Wald statistic; the type 3 tests are produced by default and here, in the absence of interactions, these are equivalent to type 2 tests.

```
proc glimmix data=ex61 empirical;
  class sub per trt;
  model y = per trt / dist=binary;
  random _residual_ / subject=sub type=vc;
  estimate "B vs A" trt -1 1 0 0;
  estimate "C vs A" trt -1 0 1 0;
  estimate "D vs A" trt -1 0 0 1;
run;
```

The two sets of analyses, subject-specific and marginal, are summarized in Table 6.7. The attenuation affect can again be seen, but is less marked here because of the smaller within-subject dependence. Again the inferences from the two analyses are very similar.

As in Section 6.2, we could also approach small sample tests using randomization procedures, at least with simple model structures. Recall that these procedures need not be applied to conventionally justified test statistics, because the validity of the procedure is based on the empirical calculation of the sampling distribution under re-randomization. For example, a logistic regression based statistic could be calculated under the assumption that all observations are independent. One could even use an ANOVA treatment sum of squares. The choice of statistic *will* affect the power of the resulting procedure, but not its validity.

6.4 Categorical data

6.4.1 *Example 6.2: Trial on patients with primary dysmenorrhea*

As an example of a cross-over trial with an ordinal response, we consider the data from a trial to investigate the effects of placebo (A) and low (B) and high (C) dose analgesics on the relief of pain in subjects with primary dysmenorrhea (Kenward and Jones, 1992). A three-period design was used with all six sequences. Eighty-six subjects were randomized to the sequences, achieving approximate balance, with group sizes ranging from 12 to 16. At the end of each treatment period each subject rated the amount of relief obtained as none, moderate or complete, and we label these 1, 2 and 3, respectively. Over the period of the trial each subject produced 1 of 27 possible joint outcomes: (1,1,1), (1,1,2), ... (3,3,3). The resulting data are summarized in Table 6.8.□□□

6.4.2 *Types of model for categorical outcomes*

There is range of ways in which we can approach a categorical response, irrespective of the complications introduced by having repeated measurements. With a binary outcome we have used linear models for functions, principally the logit, of the success probability. With categorical data we can associate *several* probabilities with each observation, or more precisely, $C-1$ independent probabilities for a C category response. We can then consider several alternative sets of functions that might be considered appropriate for equating to a linear predictor. Denote by $\pi_i \dots \pi_C$ the probabilities associated with a C category response Y. Some possible functions, based on the logit link, are

- Generalized (or adjacent category) logits:

$$\ln\left(\frac{\pi_c}{\pi_1}\right) \quad \left[\ln\left(\frac{\pi_c}{\pi_{c-1}}\right)\right] \quad c = 2,\dots,C.$$

- Cumulative logits:

$$\ln\left(\frac{\sum_{i=c}^{k} \pi_i}{\sum_{i=1}^{c-1} \pi_i}\right) = \ln\left\{\frac{\mathrm{P}(Y \geq c)}{\mathrm{P}(Y < c)}\right\} \quad c = 2,\dots,C.$$

Table 6.8: Example 6.2: Data from the trial on pain relief.

	Sequence Group						
Outcome	ABC	ACB	BAC	BCA	CAB	CBA	Total
(1,1,1)	0	2	0	0	3	1	6
(1,1,2)	1	0	0	1	0	0	2
(1,1,3)	1	0	1	0	0	0	2
(1,2,1)	2	0	0	0	0	0	2
(1,2,2)	3	0	1	0	0	0	4
(1,2,3)	4	3	1	0	2	0	10
(1,3,1)	0	0	1	1	0	0	2
(1,3,2)	0	2	0	0	0	0	2
(1,3,3)	2	4	1	0	0	1	8
(2,1,1)	0	1	1	0	0	3	5
(2,1,2)	0	0	2	0	1	1	4
(2,1,3)	0	0	1	0	0	0	1
(2,2,1)	1	0	0	6	1	1	9
(2,2,2)	0	2	1	0	0	0	3
(2,2,3)	1	0	0	0	0	0	1
(2,3,1)	0	0	0	1	0	2	3
(2,3,2)	0	0	0	0	0	0	0
(2,3,3)	0	2	0	0	1	0	3
(3,1,1)	0	0	0	1	0	2	3
(3,1,2)	0	0	2	0	2	1	5
(3,1,3)	0	0	3	0	4	1	8
(3,2,1)	0	0	0	1	0	0	1
(3,2,2)	0	0	0	1	0	0	1
(3,2,3)	0	0	0	0	0	0	0
(3,3,1)	0	0	0	0	0	1	1
(3,3,2)	0	0	0	0	0	0	0
(3,3,3)	0	0	0	0	0	0	0
Total	15	16	15	12	14	14	86

- Continuation-ratio logits:

$$\ln\left(\frac{\pi_c}{\sum_{i=1}^{c-1}\pi_i}\right) = \ln\left\{\frac{\mathrm{P}(Y=c)}{\mathrm{P}(Y<c)}\right\} \quad c=2,\ldots,C.$$

The generalized logits are most commonly used when the categories have no ordering, as models based on these have an invariance to re-ordering of the categories. The other two are clearly based on a particular ordering, and so are arguably more appropriate in an ordinal setting, such as the pain relief trial. The continuation-ratio model is not invariant to reversal of the scale and so tends to be used more where the direction (e.g., low to high) has a specific substantive meaning which does not operate in reverse simply by relabeling. Finally, the cumulative logits are very commonly used as the basis for analyses of ordinal data, particularly when constrained to have a *proportional* structure. That is, if a linear predictor (less intercept) η, corresponds to a particular observations then this is held constant for each cumulative logit, allowing only the intercept (or so-called *cut-point* parameter) to differ among these:

$$\ln\left\{\frac{\mathrm{P}(Y \geq c)}{\mathrm{P}(Y < c)}\right\} = \mu_j + \eta, \;\; c = 2,\ldots,C.$$

This is called a **proportional odds model** (McCullagh, 1980) and can be derived in terms of an underlying latent distribution for the outcome, which is assumed to be categorized to produce the ordinal observation. Another view of the proportional odds model is that it represents a set of logistic regression models. The cth cumulative logit can be regarded as a simple logit for a new binary variable obtained by combining categories c and above to define a success. There are $C-1$ such binary variables and it is assumed that, apart from the intercepts, the same logistic regression model (with linear predictor η) fits each. This generates a parsimonious, powerful, and easily interpretable way of modeling ordinal data because there is only a single odds-ratio for each effect, but the proportionality assumption need not always hold. Global tests exist for proportionality in such models, and typically these compare the fitted model with one based on generalized logits (which saturate the probabilities). Alternatively, one can examine proportionality term by term in the linear predictor using so-called **partial proportional odds** models (Peterson and Harrell, 1990; Lall et al., 2002). In the following we principally use the proportional odds model and its extensions, but will make some references to the generalized logit approach, which has one advantage in terms of conditional exact testing.

6.4.3 Subject effects models

6.4.3.1 Proportional odds model

Example 6.2 has an ordinal response and so we begin by considering a proportional odds model for this. We can extend the subject effects logistic regression model to this setting in a very natural way by adding the subject effect to the common linear predictor:

$$\mathrm{logit}\{P(Y_{ijk} \geq c \mid s_{ik})\} = \mu_c + \pi_j + \tau_{d[i,j]} + s_{ik}, \;\; c = 2,\ldots,C. \tag{6.8}$$

Of the two approaches to the subject effects model used earlier in a binary setting, only the random one can now be applied. The necessary sufficient statistics for the subject effects do not exist in the proportional odds model, and so a conditional likelihood cannot be constructed. However, the random subject effects analysis proceeds very much as before. SAS `proc glimmix` can be used to fit the model. The structure is very much as before, with the choice of a multinomial response distribution (`dist=multinomial`) defaulting to a proportional odds structure:

```
proc glimmix data=ex62 method=quad(qcheck);
  class sub per trt;
  model y (descending) = per trt / dist=mult;
  random intercept / subject=sub;
  estimate "treatment B vs placebo" trt -1 1 0;
  estimate "treatment C vs placebo" trt -1 0 1;
  estimate "treatment C vs B" trt 0 -1 1;
run;
```

The estimates are very stable with respect to the number of qpoints, and in all fits the estimate of the subject variance tends to zero. There is no evidence at all of any within-subject dependence. So the resulting estimates and standard errors are the same as would be obtained from a conventional proportional-odds regression in which all the data were assumed to be independent. The estimated log odds-ratios for the treatment effects are as follows.

Label	Estimate	Standard Error	DF	t Value	Pr > |t|
treatment B vs placebo	2.0413	0.3274	167	6.23	<.0001
treatment C vs placebo	2.4156	0.3327	167	7.26	<.0001
treatment C vs B	0.3743	0.2841	167	1.32	0.1895

The differences from placebo are highly significant, but the low and high doses exhibit very similar behavior.

6.4.3.2 *Generalized logit model*

Before turning to marginal models for this problem we briefly consider a conditional likelihood analysis. As mentioned above, the required sufficient statistics do not exist for the subject effects proportional odds model (6.8), so a conditional likelihood cannot be constructed using this approach. The required sufficient statistics do exist, however, for the generalized logit model with subject effects. For a generic cross-over design this model can be written

$$\ln\left(\frac{\pi_c}{\pi_1}\right) = \mu_c + \pi_{cj} + \tau_{cd[i,j]} + s_{cik}, \quad c = 2,\ldots,C.$$

This is an extension of the Rasch model, commonly used in the social sciences (Ansersen, 1977). An important feature of this model is that all parameters, including the subject effects, are allowed to take different values for the different logits, i.e., it does not display the parsimony of the proportional odds model.

To some extent this reflects the lack of natural ordering in the categories, and such a model would be appropriate for an unordered categorical response. It is less well suited to an ordinal outcome, although some aspect of the ordered nature can be introduced by regressing on the category scores. The unstructured treatment effects $\tau_{2a},\ldots,\tau_{Ca}$ are replaced by

$$\tau_{ca} = c\tau_a, \quad c = 2,\ldots,C.$$

Tests for treatment effects based on this model are generalizations of the Cochran–Armitage trend test (Armitage, 1955). Somewhat surprisingly perhaps, analyses based on this regression based generalized logit model and the proportional odds model can be similar in overall conclusions. This follows from the approximate linearity in the central range of the logistic transformation. For probabilities between about 0.2 and 0.8, the logit relationship is approximately linear and in this range it can be shown that the two types of logit (cumulative and generalized) actually lead to similar models. In analyses where fitted probabilities are more extreme, differences between the approaches are likely to be more marked.

For the conditional likelihood analysis we need to condition on the sufficient statistics for the subject effects. These are the joint outcomes *ignoring order* and conditioning on these produces a likelihood with a conventional log-linear form (Conaway, 1989). Kenward and Jones (1991) show how such log-linear analyses can be constructed in a compact way for general cross-over designs. Agresti and Lang (1993) explore equivalences between such a conditional analysis and that produced by a nonparametric approach with random effects and the use of quasi-symmetric log-linear models. For details of the analysis of Example 6.2 under this model we refer the reader to Kenward and Jones (1991).

A further simplification takes place when there are only two periods, for then the sufficient statistic for subject (i,k) who responds with x in Period 1 and y in Period 2 is the pair of outcomes $R = \{(x,y),(y,x)\}$. Conditioning on the outcome being a member of this set, we get

$$\begin{aligned} & \operatorname{logit}[P\{Y_{i1k} = x, Y_{i2k} = y \mid (x,y) \in R\}] \\ = \;& \pi_{x1} + \tau_{xd[i,1]} + \pi_{y2} + \tau_{yd[i,2]} - \pi_{y1} - \tau_{yd[i,1]} - \pi_{x2} - \tau_{xd[i,2]}. \end{aligned}$$

This is a standard logistic regression model, but one without an intercept, and conditional exact procedures for logistic regression can be applied to this for very small sample sizes.

6.4.4 *Marginal models*

6.4.4.1 *Proportional odds model*

We now consider fitting a marginal proportional odds model to the data from Example 6.2. Given the very small size of the between-subject variance

Table 6.9: Example 6.2: Estimated log odds-ratios for the treatment effects from the random subject effects and marginal analyses.

	Random subjects		Marginal (IEE)	
Effect	Estimate	SE	Estimate	SE
B-placebo	2.041	0.327	2.041	0.367
C-placebo	2.416	0.333	2.416	0.371
C-B	0.374	0.284	0.374	0.252
Overall tests				
Wald	57.3		43.2	

estimated from the random subject effects analysis, we should expect very similar results from a marginal model. For this problem we need to use the `genmod` procedure not `glimmix` used earlier for binary outcomes because, at present, the latter does not incorporate the empirical estimate of error with the proportional odds model.

```
proc genmod data=ex62 descending;
  class sub per trt;
  model y = per trt / dist=mult;
  repeated subject = sub / type=ind;
  estimate "treatment B vs A" trt -1 1 0;
  estimate "treatment C vs A" trt -1 0 1;
  estimate "C vs B" trt 0 -1 1;
run;
```

The results from this fit, and that of the earlier random subjects analysis for comparison, are presented in Table 6.9. With σ_s^2 effectively estimated as zero, the random effects analysis produces the likelihood estimates and SEs under the assumption of independence. The IEE analysis therefore provides exactly the same estimates, with SEs slightly changed by the sandwich modification. Essentially the analyses give the same results.

6.4.4.2 Partial proportional odds model

The proportional odds analyses rest on the assumption that the effects in the linear predictor (period, treatment) are consistent among the $C-1$ cumulative logits, that is, the proportional odds assumption holds. Departures from this assumption imply that there are effects that are not consistent between the $C-1$ logistic regressions of the binary variables defined by the $C-1$ cut-points. This assumption can be examined term by term by looking at the cut-point-by-period and cut-point-by-treatment interactions. A *partial proportional odds* model is one in which some of these interactions are present, but not all (Peterson and Harrell, 1990; Lall et al., 2002). Now, because of the way in which the proportional odds model is formulated in standard software, these interactions cannot simply be added to the linear predictor. Instead we can reformulate the analysis in terms of dependent binary outcomes and let the empirical variance estimator accommodate the dependencies among these.

In a general setting, a C category ordinal random variable Y_{ijk} can be re-expressed as $C-1$ binary **correlated** responses Z_{ijkc}:

$$Z_{ijkc} = \begin{cases} 1 & Y_{ijk} \geq c \\ 0 & Y_{ijk} < c \end{cases} \qquad c = 2, \ldots C.$$

The proportional odds model for Y_{ijk}

$$\text{logit}\{\text{P}(Y_{itj} \geq c)\} = \mu_c + \pi_j + \tau_{d[i,j]}, \;\; c = 2, \ldots, C$$

implies a logistic regression model for each binary response:

$$\text{logit}\{\text{P}(Z_{ijkc} = 1)\} = \mu_c + \pi_j + \tau_{d[i,j]}, \;\; c = 2, \ldots, C.$$

We can add to this model interactions between the existing terms and each level of the cut-point, c:

$$\text{logit}\{\text{P}(Z_{ijkc} = 1)\} = \mu_c + \pi_j + \tau_{d[i,j]} + (\mu\pi)_{c,j} + (\mu\tau)_{c,d[i,j]}, \;\; c = 2, \ldots, C.$$

The terms $\{(\mu\pi)_{c,j}\}$ and $\{(\mu\tau)_{c,d[i,j]}\}$ represent departures from the assumption of proportionality and can be examined to assess this assumption. If all the binary observations were independent, this model could be fitted using conventional logistic regression. However, the analysis needs to accommodate both dependence among observations from the same subject and among observations derived from the same ordinal response. A simple, but rather crude, method that can use existing GEE software is to restructure the data in terms of these binary variables, fit a logistic model and let the empirical variance estimator take care of the correlations among these binary responses.

We now illustrate this with the data from Example 6.2. First, every ordinal response Y is replaced by two new binary responses Z_1 and Z_2:

$$Z_{c-1} = \begin{cases} 1 & Y \geq c \\ 0 & Y < c \end{cases} \qquad c = 2, 3.$$

The two sets of binary variables are then combined in one data set, thus doubling the number of observations. A factor (or class variate) is introduced to distinguish between the two new binary outcomes (called `cut`, say), and all other variates (subject, period and treatment) are duplicated exactly. Thus the new data set takes the form shown in Table 6.10.

The full marginal model, with both interactions, can then be fitted as follows:

Table 6.10: Example 6.2: Data set restructured for fitting a partial proportional odds model.

sub	per	trt	cut	y	z
1	1	1	1	1	0
1	2	3	1	1	0
1	3	2	1	1	0
1	1	1	2	1	0
1	2	3	2	1	0
1	3	2	2	1	0
...					
21	1	1	1	1	0
21	2	3	1	2	1
21	3	2	1	3	1
21	1	1	2	1	0
21	2	3	2	2	0
21	3	2	2	3	1
...					
86	1	3	1	3	1
86	2	2	1	3	1
86	3	1	1	1	0
86	1	3	2	3	1
86	2	2	2	3	1
86	3	1	2	1	0

```
proc genmod data=ex62_restructured descending;
  class cut period treatment sub;
  model resp = cut period treatment cut*period
                   cut*treatment / dist = b wald type3;
  repeated subject=sub / type=ind;
run;
```

We are interested in the overall contribution of the interactions, so we first examine the Wald tests:

```
Wald Statistics For Type 3 GEE Analysis

                              Chi-
Source              DF      Square    Pr > ChiSq

period               2        5.28        0.0715
treatment            2       39.37        <.0001
cut                  1       66.51        <.0001
cut*period           2        3.77        0.1515
cut*treatment        2        0.49        0.7814
```

The interactions are both small and so the proportional odds assumption would appear to be acceptable in this example. If this were not the case for the treatment effects, then different treatment odds-ratios would need to be presented for each cut-point, and the overall treatment test would be on $(c-1)(t-1)$ degrees of freedom rather than $(t-1)$.

6.5 Further topics

6.5.1 *Count data*

There are many different ways in which counts may arise in a cross-over trial. The Poisson distribution is a natural *starting point* for modeling these. The Poisson log-linear analog of the logistic subject effects model (6.3) can be written:

$$Y_{ijk} \mid s_{ik} \sim \text{Po}(\eta_{ijk})$$

for

$$\ln(\eta_{ijk}) = \mu + \pi_j + \tau_{d[i,j]} + s_{ik}.$$

To avoid distributional assumptions for s_{ik} we might consider a conditional likelihood analysis, again using the analogy with the logistic model. The Poisson log-linear model has a very special property with respect to such an analysis: identical results are obtained whether we simply estimate the subject effects as fixed parameters or construct the conditional likelihood formally and use this. The simplest approach therefore is to fit a Poisson log-linear model with fixed subject effects. In `proc genmod` we could use the following generic form:

```
proc genmod;
  class sub per treat;
  model resp =  sub per treat / dist = poisson;
run;
```

This will of course remove all between-subject information from the analysis. If we wish to recover this, a (normal based) random subjects analysis is simply constructed in `proc glimmix`; this would follow the same structure seen previously, with the `poisson` option for the distribution.

However, when comparing subject-specific and marginal analyses, there is an important difference between analyses that use a log link and those that use a logistic link. We have seen in the latter case that effects in the model are attenuated when we move from subject-specific to analogous marginal models, with the degree of attenuation depending on the size of the subject effects variance. The same is *not* seen with a log link. In this situation only the intercept differs between the two types of model. The reason is as follows. Let η be the linear predictor without the subject effect; then

$$\begin{aligned}\text{Marginal mean} &= \mathrm{E}_S[e^{\eta+s}] \\ &= \mathrm{E}_S[e^{\eta}] \times \mathrm{E}_S[e^{s}] \\ &= e^{\eta} \times e^{\kappa} \\ &= e^{\eta+\kappa}\end{aligned}$$

where, because $s \sim \mathrm{N}(0, \sigma_s^2)$,

$$e^{\kappa} = e^{\sigma_s^2/2}, \text{ i.e., } \kappa = \sigma_s^2/2.$$

Hence the intercept has a quantity $\sigma_s^2/2$ added to it in the marginal model.

We have seen that the modeling of count data from cross-over trials is relatively straightforward *provided* the Poisson distribution provides a reasonable approximation. However, in many settings the Poisson distribution is in fact a rather poor model for count data. For example, events, or episodes, from one subject in one treatment period may well be mutually correlated, or the underlying rate may change with time during the period. Typically, the consequence of such departures is that the observed variability of the observations is greater than that predicted by the Poisson model. This is called **over-dispersion** (McCullagh and Nelder, 1989, Section 6.3.2). When using a Poisson model for count data, the possibility of overdispersion needs to be considered. There are several ways in which this could be done. The underlying Poisson assumption could be changed, with the negative binomial a popular choice, or additional random effects can be added to the Poisson model. The interplay between random effects and components for overdispersion is a subtle one, however. For recent developments, see Molenberghs et al. (2010). Further discussion of the analysis of count data in the context of the 2×2 design can be found in Longford (1998).

6.5.2 *Time to event data*

Although not an example of categorical data, analyses for event, or failure, time data have much in common with those met already. Time to event data is often met in the survival context, one that is self-evidently incompatible with cross-over designs. However, other forms of repeatable events may be used as an outcome. France et al. (1991) give an example in the context of a trial on treatment for angina in which time to stopping an exercise was the outcome of interest. One could approach such data using parametric models for the event times; the log normal distribution is one obvious candidate. A full model based analysis would require incorporation of within-subject dependence. If the only interest were in constructing a valid test for treatment effect in the absence of carry-over, then the randomization based tests introduced in Section 5.5 could be used to provide robust analyses, following estimation methods that ignore the dependence. The presence of censoring raises further complications, however. One possible approach uses the Cox proportional hazards model (Cox, 1972). Kalbfleish and Prentice (1980) develop the use of this model to paired event time data, and France et al. (1991) extend this to the 2×2 cross-over design, producing a procedure closely related to the Mainland–Gart test. Alternatively, other multivariate generalizations of the Cox model might be considered, for example, Oakes (1986).

6.5.3 *Issues associated with scale*

One common feature of nearly all the models used in this chapter is the use of a nonlinear scale linking the effects of interest, typically direct treatment, to the mean outcome of the response. We have already touched on the relevance of scale in Section 6.1 when contrasting marginal and subject-specific models. We emphasized that, in general, the parameters in these classes of model have different interpretations. More strictly, except in very special cases, a nonlinear model cannot hold simultaneously both at the marginal and subject-specific levels. The impact in terms of model specification of adding terms such as covariates or subject effects to nonlinear models has been explored in detail by a number of authors; see, for example, Gail et al. (1984), Struthers and Kalbfleisch (1986) and Cramer (1991), pp. 36–39. It is important that this is borne in mind when results from cross-over trials are compared with, or as in done in meta-analysis, combined with, "equivalent" treatment comparisons from parallel group and other designs. It may well be that different basic quantities are being estimated. Curtin et al. (1995) discuss this in the context of meta-analysis for binary data that may include cross-over trials, and Ford et al. (1995) give a good example of the problems that this may cause for proportional hazards models, with explicit reference to the 2×2 cross-over trial.

Chapter 7

Bioequivalence trials

7.1 What is bioequivalence?

The early phase of drug development is concerned with determining the safe and effective dose to give patients in future clinical trials. In this carefully planned phase very low doses of an active drug are given to a small number of healthy human volunteers to determine the pharmacokinetics (PK) of the drug. Assuming an orally administered drug is being studied, PK is concerned with obtaining information on the absorbtion, distribution, metabolism and elimination of the drug. Quite often PK is referred to as what the body does to the drug. An important outcome of a PK study is an assessment of how much of the active constituents of the drug reaches its site of action. As this cannot be easily measured directly, the concentration of drug that reaches the circulating bloodstream is taken as a surrogate. The concentration of drug that is in the blood is referred to as its bioavailability. It is assumed that a drug with a larger bioavailability than another will also be such that a greater amount of its active ingredients reaches the intended site of action. Two drugs which have the same bioavailability are termed bioequivalent. See FDA Guidance (FDA, 1992, 1997, 1999b, 2000, 2002). Statistical approaches to determining bioequivalence are described in FDA Guidances (FDA, 1992, 1997, 1999a, 2001). There are a number of reasons why trials are undertaken to show two drugs are bioequivalent. Among them are (i) when different formulations of the same drug are to be marketed, for instance, in solid tablet or liquid capsule form; (ii) when a generic version of an innovator drug is to be marketed; (iii) when production of a drug is scaled up and the new production process needs to be shown to produce drugs of equivalent strength and effectiveness to the original process. In all of these situations there is a regulatory requirement to show that the new or alternative version of the drug is bioequivalent to what is considered to be its original version.

In the following we will refer to the original or innovator version of the drug under consideration as the Reference or R. The new or alternative version of the drug will be referred to as the Test or T. Test and Reference are compared in cross-over trials that use healthy volunteers as the subjects. In a 2×2 trial, for example, each subject is given a single dose of T and R and blood samples are taken at a series of time points subsequent to dosing. Each blood sample is then assayed to determine the concentration of drug in the blood plasma. Often the blood sampling is taken more frequently during what is expected to be the

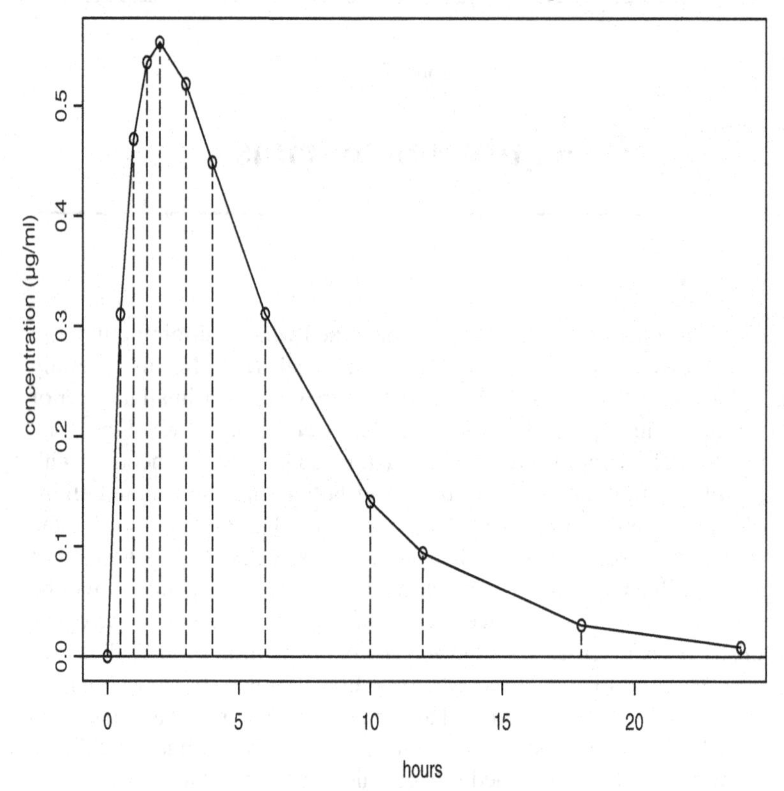

Figure 7.1: Observed concentration-time profile for a single subject in a given period.

absorption phase of the drug and then less frequently during the elimination phase. For each subject and period the concentrations of drug in the blood are plotted against the corresponding sampling times to give a concentration-time profile for that subject and period. A typical profile is given in Figure 7.1.

Once the drug gets past the stomach and into the small intestine, it begins to be absorbed into the blood, eventually reaching a peak concentration. From then on, the concentration diminishes as the drug is eliminated from the body. The area under the profile is referred to as the Area Under the Curve or AUC. The AUC is taken as a measure of exposure of the drug to the subject. The peak or maximum concentration is referred to as Cmax and is an important safety measure. For regulatory approval of bioequivalence it is necessary to show from the trial results that the mean values of AUC and Cmax for T and R are not significantly different. The AUC is calculated by adding up the areas of the regions identified by the vertical lines under the plot in Figure 7.1 using an arithmetic technique such as the trapezoidal rule (see, for example, Welling (1986), 145–149, Rowland and Tozer (1995), 469–471). Experience (e.g., Guidance (FDA, 1992, 1997, 1999b, 2001)) has dictated that AUC and

Cmax need to be transformed to the natural logarithmic scale prior to analysis if the usual assumptions of normally distributed errors are to be made. Each of AUC and Cmax is analyzed separately and there is no adjustment to significance levels to allow for multiple testing (Hauck et al. (1995)). We will refer to the derived variates as log(AUC) and log(Cmax), respectively.

In bioequivalence trials there should be a wash-out period of at least five half-lives of the drugs between the active treatment periods. If this is the case, and there are no detectable pre-dose drug concentrations, there is no need to assume that carry-over effects are present and so it is not necessary to test for a differential carry-over effect (FDA Guidance, FDA (2001)). The model that is fitted to the data will be the one used in Section 5.3 of Chapter 5, which contains terms for subjects, periods and treatments. An example of fitting this model will be given in the next section. To simplify the following discussion we will refer only to log(AUC); the discussion for log(Cmax) is identical.

For a thorough review of bioequivalence we refer the reader to Patterson and Jones (2006).

All the analyses considered in the following are based on summary measures (AUC and Cmax) obtained from the concentration-time profiles. If testing for bioequivalence is all that is of interest, then these measures are adequate and have been extensively used in practice. However, there is often a need to obtain an understanding of the absorption and elimination processes to which the drug is exposed once it has entered the body, e.g., when bioequivalence is not demonstrated. This can be done by fitting compartmental models to the drug concentrations obtained from each volunteer. These models not only provide insight into the mechanisms of action of the drugs, but can also be used to calculate the AUC and Cmax values. See, for example, Lindsey et al. (2000).

The history of bioequivalence testing dates back to the late 1960s and early 1970s (see, for example, Patterson and Jones (2006)). The regulatory implications of bioequivalence testing are also described in Patterson and Jones (2006) and so we do not repeat these here.

At the present time, average bioequivalence (see Section 7.2) serves as the current international standard for bioequivalence testing using a 2×2 cross-over design. Alternative designs (e.g., replicate cross-over designs) may be also utilized for drug products to improve power (see Patterson and Jones (2006)).

7.2 Testing for average bioequivalence

The now generally accepted method of testing for average bioequivalence (ABE) is the two-one-sided-tests procedure (TOST) proposed by Schuirmann (1987). It is conveniently done using a confidence interval calculation. Let μ_T and μ_R be the (true) mean values of log(AUC) (or log(Cmax)) when subjects are treated with T and R, respectively.

ABE is demonstrated if the 90% two-sided confidence interval for $\mu_T - \mu_R$ falls within the acceptance limits of $-\ln 1.25 = -0.2231$ and $+\ln 1.25 = 0.2231$. These limits are set by the regulator (FDA Guidance (FDA, 1992, 2001, 2002)) and when exponentiated give limits of 0.80 and 1.25. That is, on the natural scale, ABE is demonstrated if there is good evidence that

$$0.80 \leq \exp(\mu_T - \mu_R) \leq 1.25.$$

We note that symmetry of the confidence interval is on the logarithmic scale, not on the natural scale.

The method gets its name (TOST) because the process of deciding if the 90% confidence interval lies within the acceptance limits is equivalent to rejecting both of the following one-sided hypotheses at the 5% significance level:

$$H_{01}: \mu_T - \mu_R \leq -\ln 1.25$$
$$H_{02}: \mu_T - \mu_R \geq \ln 1.25.$$

Example

The derived data given in Tables 7.1 and 7.2 are from a pharmacokinetic study that compared a test drug (T) with a known reference drug (R). The design used was a 2×2 cross-over with 24 healthy volunteers in the RT sequence group and 25 in the TR sequence group. Each volunteer should have provided both an AUC and a Cmax value. However, as can be seen, not all volunteers had sufficient data to make this possible and there are several missing values.

The subject-profile plots (see Chapter 2) for those subjects that had values in both periods for log(AUC) and for log(Cmax) are given in Figure 7.2. It is clear that for Subject 4 in the TR sequence both log(AUC) and log(Cmax) are unusually low in the second period. These plots have been drawn using a modified version of the Splus-code given in Millard and Krause (2001), Chapter 7.

The SAS code to calculate the confidence intervals for log(AUC) and log(Cmax) as needed for the TOST analysis is given below, where we fit a mixed model using SAS `proc mixed`. This model fits a random term for subjects within sequences. Using a mixed model we can produce an analysis that includes the data from all subjects, including those with only one value for AUC or Cmax. However, including the subjects with only one response does not change the results in any significant way and so we will report the results obtained using the subsets of data that have values in both periods for AUC (45 subjects) and Cmax (47 subjects). These results are the same as would be obtained by fitting a model with fixed subject effects.

Table 7.1: Bioequivalence trial: RT sequence.

Subject	AUC Test	AUC Ref	Cmax Test	Cmax Ref
1	79.34	58.16	2.827	2.589
3	85.59	69.68	4.407	2.480
5	.	121.84	.	5.319
8	377.15	208.33	11.808	9.634
10	14.23	17.22	1.121	1.855
11	750.79	1407.9	6.877	13.615
13	21.27	20.81	1.055	1.210
15	8.67	.	1.084	0.995
18	269.40	203.22	9.618	7.496
20	412.42	386.93	12.536	16.106
21	33.89	47.96	2.129	2.679
24	32.59	22.70	1.853	1.727
26	72.36	44.02	4.546	3.156
27	423.05	285.78	11.167	8.422
31	20.33	40.60	1.247	1.900
32	17.75	19.43	0.910	1.185
36	1160.53	1048.60	17.374	18.976
37	82.70	107.66	6.024	5.031
39	928.05	469.73	14.829	6.962
43	20.09	14.95	2.278	0.987
44	28.47	28.57	1.773	1.105
45	411.72	379.90	13.810	12.615
47	46.88	126.09	2.339	6.977
50	106.43	75.43	4.771	4.925

Note: Reproduced with permission from Patterson (2001a).

```
data bio2x2;
input subject sequence $ period form $ AUC CMAX ;
logauc=log(AUC);
logcmax=log(CMAX);
datalines;
1   RT   2 T   79.34  2.827
1   RT   1 R   58.16  2.589
3   RT   2 T   85.59  4.407
3   RT   1 R   69.68  2.480
5   RT   2 T     .      .
5   RT   1 R  121.84  5.319
.    .   . .     .      .
.    .   . .     .      .
.    .   . .     .      .
```

(Continued)

(Continued)

```
40  TR   1 T   62.23  3.025
40  TR   2 R   64.92  3.041
41  TR   1 T   48.99  2.706
41  TR   2 R   61.74  2.808
42  TR   1 T   53.18  3.240
42  TR   2 R   17.51  1.702
46  TR   1 T     .    1.680
46  TR   2 R     .      .
48  TR   1 T   98.03  3.434
48  TR   2 R  236.17  7.378
49  TR   1 T 1070.98 21.517
49  TR   2 R 1016.52 20.116;
run;
proc mixed data=bio2x2;
class sequence subject period form;
model logauc=sequence period form/ ddfm=kenwardroger;
random subject(sequence);
lsmeans form/pdiff cl alpha=0.1;
estimate 'ABE for logAUC' form -1 1; run;

proc mixed data=bio2x2;
class sequence subject period form;
model logcmax=sequence period form/ ddfm=kenwardroger;
random subject(sequence);
lsmeans form/pdiff cl alpha=0.1;
estimate 'ABE for logCmax' form -1 1;
run;

AUC - Analysis
Covariance Parameter Estimates
Cov Parm                   Estimate
SUBJECT(SEQUENCE)            1.5465
Residual                     0.1987
Type 3 Tests of Fixed Effects
                 Num       Den
  Effect         DF        DF      F Value     Pr > F
  SEQUENCE        1        43         0.33     0.5672
  PERIOD          1        43         0.29     0.5947
  FORM            1        43         1.06     0.3080
Estimates
                                 Standard
```

(Continued)

(Continued)

```
 Label                  Estimate        Error
 ABE for logAUC          0.09699      0.09401
 DF        t Value       Pr > |t|
 43         1.03         0.3080
 Least Squares Means
                                      Standard
 Effect  FORM           Estimate       Error
 FORM    R                4.4143      0.1970
 FORM    T                4.5113      0.1970

Differences of Least Squares Means
 Effect     FORM          _FORM          Estimate
 FORM       R               T            -0.09699
  DF        t Value     Pr > |t|         Alpha
  43        -1.03       0.3080          0.1
 Standard
  Error
 0.09401

 Differences of Least Squares Means
 Effect     FORM          _FORM    Lower          Upper
 FORM       R               T     -0.2550       0.06104
```

The 90% confidence interval for $\mu_T - \mu_R$ is $(-0.0610,\ 0.2550)$ for log(AUC) and $(-0.0871,\ 0.1887)$ for log(Cmax), where it will be noted that the signs have been reversed compared to those in the SAS output. Exponentiating the limits to obtain confidence limits for $\exp(\mu_T - \mu_R)$ gives (0.9408, 1.2905) for AUC and (0.9166, 1.2077) for Cmax. A graphical summary of these results is given in Figure 7.3. Here, to show the overall pattern and the essential details, we have plotted all the T/R ratios in the left plot and only those ratios which are less than 2.5 in the right plot. Also given in the plots are the confidence intervals as vertical bars and the null hypothesis value of 1 and the acceptance limits as dotted horizontal lines. These plots have been drawn using a modified version of the Splus-code given in Millard and Krause (2001), Chapter 7.

```
Cmax - Analysis
Covariance Parameter Estimates
Cov Parm                  Estimate
SUBJECT(SEQUENCE)          0.7294
Residual                   0.1584
Type 3 Tests of Fixed Effects
                Num       Den
 Effect          DF        DF     F Value     Pr > F
 SEQUENCE         1        45        0.18     0.6730
 PERIOD           1        45        0.11     0.7456
 FORM             1        45        0.38     0.5390
Estimates
                                          Standard
 Label                Estimate             Error          DF
 ABE for logCmax       0.05083            0.08211         45
t Value     Pr > |t|
 0.62       0.5390
Least Squares Means                 Standard
 Effect  FORM       Estimate          Error
    FORM     R       1.2619       0.1375
    FORM     T       1.3128       0.1375

Differences of Least Squares Means
 Effect     FORM          _FORM          Estimate
 FORM       R               T            -0.05083
 DF        t Value      Pr > |t|       Alpha
 45        -0.62         0.5390          0.1
 Standard
  Error
 0.08211

 Differences of Least Squares Means
 Effect     FORM          _FORM     Lower          Upper
 FORM       R              T       -0.1887       0.08707
```

The interval for AUC is not contained within the limits of 0.8 to 1.25, but the one for Cmax is. Therefore, T cannot be considered bioequivalent to R, as it fails to satisfy the criterion for AUC.

If we had fitted the mixed model to the full set of data, the confidence intervals for $\mu_T - \mu_R$ would have been $(-0.0678, 0.2482)$ for log(AUC) and $(-0.0907,\ 0.1843)$ for log(Cmax).

No analysis is complete until the assumptions that have been made in the modeling have been checked. As in Chapter 2, we can check the normality of

Table 7.2: Bioequivalence trial: TR sequence.

Subject	AUC Test	AUC Ref	Cmax Test	Cmax Ref
2	150.12	142.29	5.145	3.216
4	36.95	5.00	2.442	0.498
6	24.53	26.05	1.442	2.728
7	22.11	34.64	2.007	3.309
9	703.83	476.56	15.133	11.155
12	217.06	176.02	9.433	8.446
14	40.75	152.40	1.787	6.231
16	52.76	51.57	3.570	2.445
17	101.52	23.49	4.476	1.255
19	37.14	30.54	2.169	2.613
22	143.45	42.69	5.182	3.031
23	29.80	29.55	1.714	1.804
25	63.03	92.94	3.201	5.645
28	.	.	0.891	0.531
29	56.70	21.03	2.203	1.514
30	61.18	66.41	3.617	2.130
33	1376.02	1200.28	27.312	22.068
34	115.33	135.55	4.688	7.358
38	17.34	40.35	1.072	2.150
40	62.23	64.92	3.025	3.041
41	48.99	61.74	2.706	2.808
42	53.18	17.51	3.240	1.702
46	.	.	1.680	.
48	98.03	236.17	3.434	7.378
49	1070.98	1016.52	21.517	20.116

Note: Reproduced with permission from Patterson (2001a).

the studentized residuals by plotting histograms and normal probability plots. The histograms of the studentized residuals and normal probability plots for log(AUC) and log(Cmax) are given in Figure 7.4. We note that in a two-period cross-over trial the two residuals for each subject are equal in magnitude and of opposite signs. Hence the plots in Figure 7.4 are only for the residuals from the first period (we could, of course, have chosen the second period). There is clear evidence that the residuals for log(AUC) are not normally distributed and some evidence that the residuals from log(Cmax) are not normally distributed. We will not look further here for reasons to explain the lack of normality.

An alternative analysis might be to use nonparametric methods to overcome the lack of normality (see Section 2.12 in Chapter 2). However, such an approach may not receive regulatory approval.

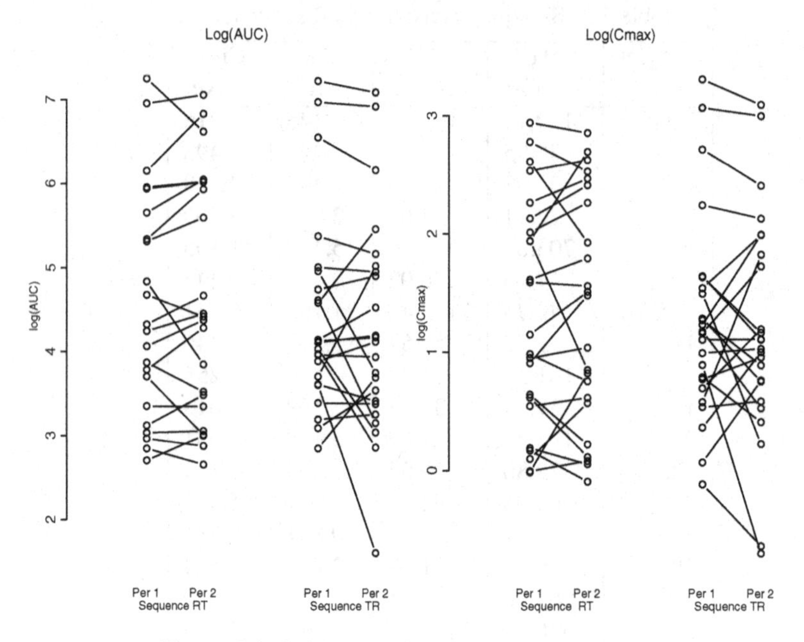

Figure 7.2: Subject profile plots for 2×2 trial.

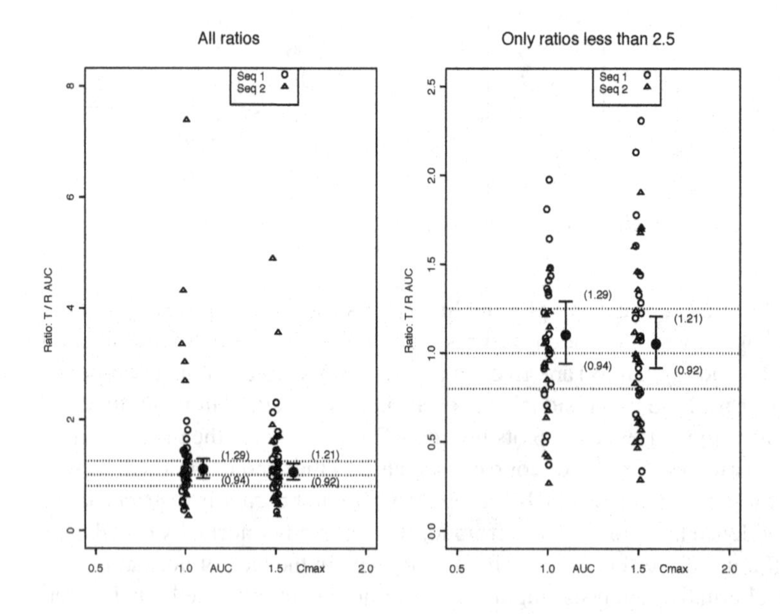

Figure 7.3: Ratios (T/R) for AUC and Cmax for 2×2 trial.

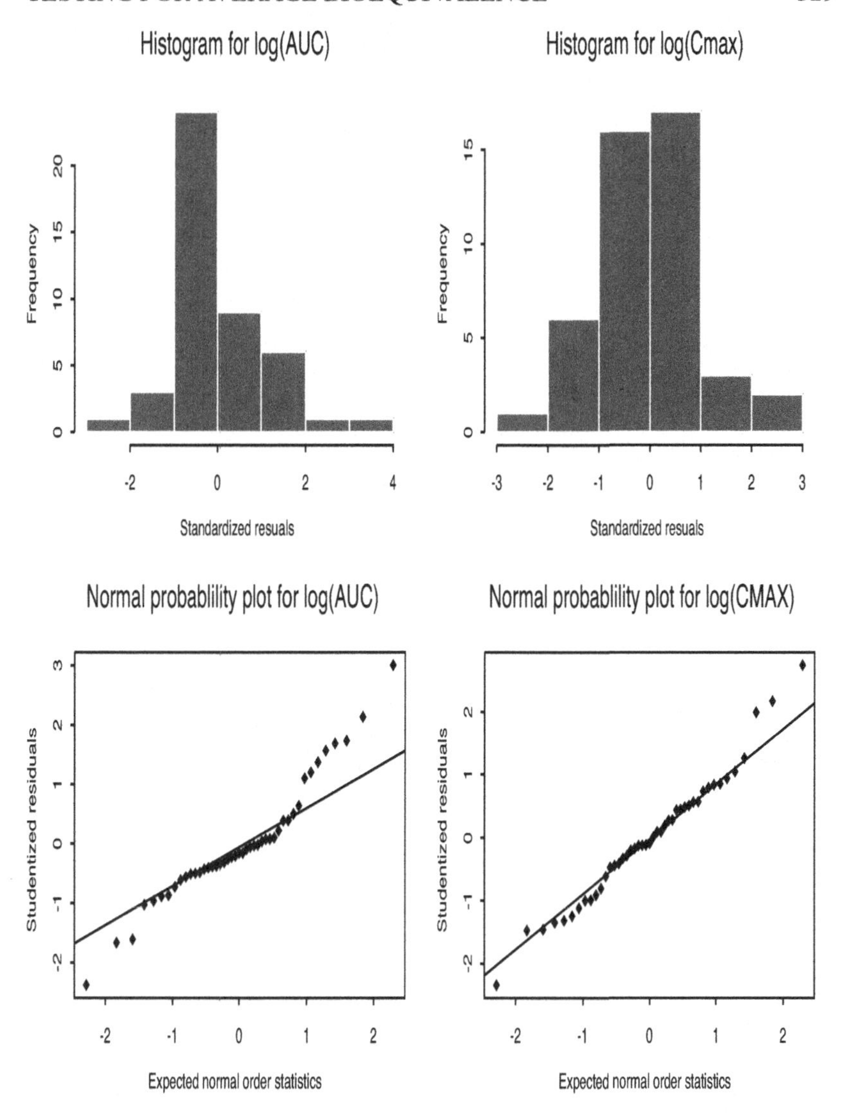

Figure 7.4: Histograms and normal probability plots for 2×2 trial.

The power and sample size for a bioequivalence trial can conveniently be calculated using the R package PowerTOST (Labes (2013).

We do not say more on bioequivalence studies and refer the reader to Patterson and Jones (2006).

In Chapters 11, 12 and 13, we consider sample size re-estimation in a bioequivalence trial.

Chapter 8

Case study: Phase I dose–response noninferiority trial

8.1 Introduction

This case study is based on a Phase I double-blind trial to estimate the dose response of an active drug (D) using a surrogate endpoint, sGaw (specific conductance), in healthy volunteers using whole body plethysmography. sGaw represents airway conductance in the larger conducting airways and is considered to be a a useful surrogate for forced expiratory volume in one second (FEV_1). It is hoped that if taken into further development the active drug will provide an effective treatment for patients suffering from chronic obstructive pulmonary disease (COPD) .

A secondary objective of this trial was to show that at least one dose of D was noninferior to a control treatment (A).

An interesting feature of this trial was that, although it was to use five periods, an interim analysis was planned after four periods had been completed. The aim of the interim was to determine the optimal allocation of doses in the fifth period.

The sequences used in the four-period design are given in Table 8.1. Here A is thc control, B is Placebo and C, D and E are doses of the active drug measured in units of fine particle dose (fpd): C = 5, D = 17 and E = 51. The fpd for the doses chosen in the fifth period could be as high as 155.

In the absence of carry-over effects in the linear model for the responses, this design has high efficiency for each pair-wise comparison with A (94.89) and relatively high efficiency of the remaining pair-wise comparisons (B vs C, 87.50; B vs D, 89.53; B vs E, 89.53; C vs D, 89.53; C vs E, 89.53; D vs E, 87.50). If carry-over effects are included in the linear model, the average efficiency drops to 66.23. As carry-over effects are not expected, this design is suitable for its intended purpose.

Table 8.1: Incomplete block design for six treatments.

Sequence	Periods			
1	A	C	D	E
2	A	C	D	B
3	B	D	E	A
4	C	E	A	D
5	C	E	A	B
6	D	A	B	E
7	D	A	B	C
8	E	B	C	A

8.2 Model for dose response

The relationship between sGaw and the fine particle dose was expected to be well approximated by a three-parameter Emax model. The equation of the Emax curve is

$$E[Y|fpd] = e0 + \frac{emax \times fpd}{fpd + ed50}. \tag{8.1}$$

An example of such a model is plotted in Figure 8.1. Here $e0$ is the response of Placebo, $e0 + emax$ defines the maximum response and $ed50$ is the

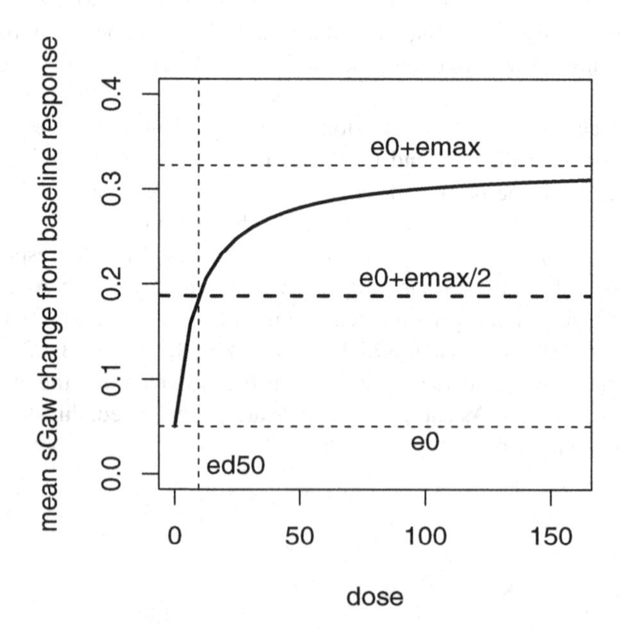

Figure 8.1: Emax model for sGaw change from baseline response.

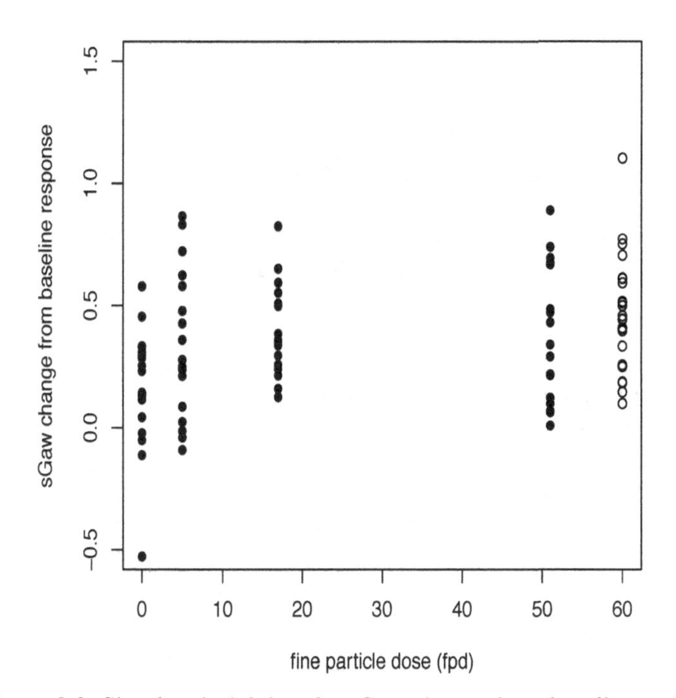

Figure 8.2: Simulated trial data for sGaw change from baseline response.

fpd that gives a response of $e0 + emax/2$, i.e., an fpd that gives 50% of the effect compared to Placebo. The horizontal lines in Figure 8.1 indicate the levels of these three responses and the vertical line identifies the $ed50$.

Due to reasons of confidentiality, the actual data from this trial cannot be reproduced here. Instead we use data simulated from the illustrative model plotted in Figure 8.1, augmented with simulated data for the control treatment A. Also, period effects were added to the simulated data.

The simulated trial data are plotted in Figure 8.2, where the closed symbols are for the doses of D and the open symbols are for A, the control. The plotted points for A have been placed at the extreme right of the plot for convenience and do not represent a sample of responses at fpd = 60.

Some typical SAS code to fit this model using `proc nlmixed` is given below, where the $ed50$ parameter has been fitted as the exponential of $\log(ed50)$:

```
proc nlmixed data=emaxdata cov ecov corr alpha=0.1
parms  led50=2.5
e0=0.17
emax=0.25
control=0.36
wssigma2=0.02
        bs2=0.02
        p2=-0.004 p3=0.052 p4=-0.052;
if fpd ne 18 then
       Funct= u + e0 + (per2*p2)+(per3*p3)+(per4*p4) +
      ( (emax*(fpd)) / ( exp(led50) + (fpd) ) );
else
   Funct= u + e0 + (per2*p2)+(per3*p3)+(per4*p4)+ control;
    bounds wssigma2>0, bs2>0, vmax>0.1;
model     cfb24~normal(Funct,wssigma2);
random    u~normal(0,bs2) subject=patnum;
predict   funct out=nlmixedb;
estimate 'Effect at fpd  5 -PBO' (vmax*5 /(exp(led50) + 5));
estimate 'Effect at fpd 17 -PBO' (vmax*17/(exp(led50) + 17));
estimate 'Effect at fpd 51 -PBO' (vmax*51/(exp(led50) + 51));
    estimate 'Effect at Control-PBO' control;
 run;
```

The estimated values of the parameters and their standard errors are given in Table 8.2. A notable feature is the presence of significant period effects. The number of degrees of freedom for the t-tests is 23.

The least squares means of each dose group and the pairwise comparisons of these means with Placebo are given in Table 8.3.

The fitted Emax curve is plotted in Figure 8.3.The large open circle symbols on the plot indicate the values of the fitted dose and control group means.

Table 8.2: Parameter estimates for sGaw trial.

Parameter	Estimate	Std Err	t-value	Pr $> \|t\|$
ed50	1.276	1.064	1.20	0.2425
e0	0.307	0.057	5.40	$<.0001$
emax	0.212	0.050	4.25	0.0003
control vs Placebo	0.261	0.042	6.24	$<.0001$
σ_W^2	0.017	0.003	6.00	$<.0001$
σ_B^2	0.035	0.011	3.09	0.0052
period 2 vs 1	−0.155	0.038	−4.12	0.0004
period 3 vs 1	−0.076	0.038	−2.00	0.0571
period 4 vs 1	−0.215	0.038	−5.61	$<.0001$

Table 8.3: Least squares means and contrast estimates for sGaw trial.

Contrast	LS mean	Std Err	t-value	Pr > $\|t\|$
fpd 5	0.430	0.054	7.99	$< .0001$
fpd 17	0.482	0.048	9.99	$< .0001$
fpd 51	0.504	0.054	9.25	$< .0001$
control	0.568	0.052	10.89	$< .0001$
fpd 5 vs Placebo	0.124	0.049	2.53	0.0189
fpd 17 vs Placebo	0.175	0.039	4.48	0.0002
fpd 51 vs Placebo	0.198	0.042	4.70	$< .0001$
control vs Placebo	0.261	0.042	6.24	$< .0001$

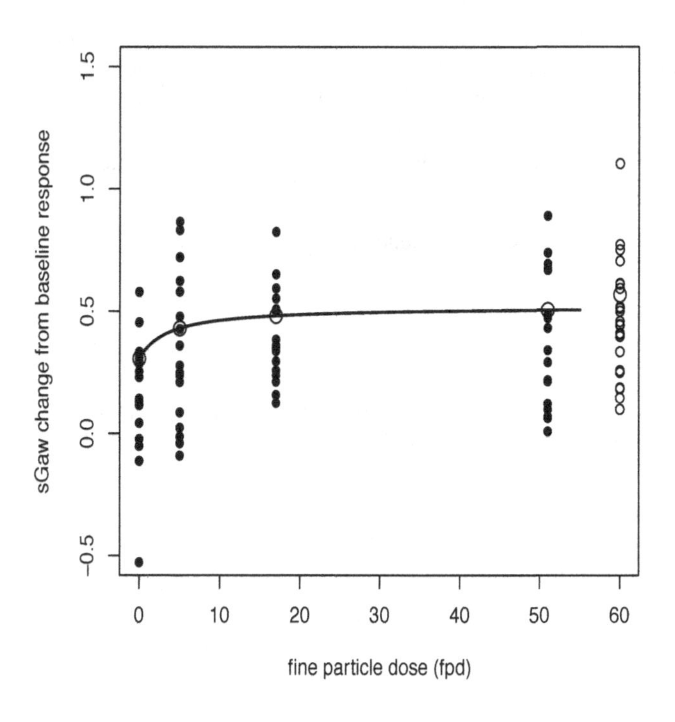

Figure 8.3: Fitted means for Emax model and control treatment.

From Tables 8.2 and 8.3 we can see that all the doses and control give significantly higher mean responses than Placebo. In addition, the mean response increases monotonically with increasing dose. Therefore, the first of the trial's objectives, that of showing a significant dose response, has been achieved.

8.3 Testing for noninferiority

The second objective of the trial was to show that there was a dose that was not inferior to control. The criterion for noninferiority was that the lower bound of a one-sided 90% confidence interval, for the ratio of the contrast for a dose compared to the contrast for control, was greater than 0.6.

Let μ_d denote the true mean for dose d, $d > 0$, μ_B, the true mean for Placebo and μ_A the true mean for the control. The ratio of interest is

$$R = \frac{\mu_d - \mu_B}{\mu_A - \mu_B} \,. \tag{8.2}$$

The estimated value of R for dose fpd = 51, given the values in Tables 8.2 and 8.3, is $\hat{R} = \frac{0.198}{0.261} = 0.76$.

To obtain the lower limit of a one-sided 90% confidence interval for R, we use Fieller's theorem (Fieller (1940)).

Let a denote the estimate of the difference in means of fpd 51 and Placebo and let b denote the estimate of the difference in means of the control and Placebo. Further, let v_{11}, v_{22} and v_{12} denote the variances of a and b, respectively, and their covariance.

Let $g = t^2 s^2 v_{22}/b^2$, where t is the upper 0.95 percentile of the central t-distribution on 23 degrees of freedom and $s = \sqrt{\sigma_W^2}$.

The lower limit of the 90% confidence interval is then given by

$$\frac{1}{1-g}\left[R - g\frac{v_{12}}{v_{22}} - \frac{t\,s}{b}\sqrt{v_{11} - 2\,R\,v_{12} + R^2\,v_{22} - g\left(v_{11} - \frac{v_{12}^2}{v_{22}}\right)}\,\right] . \tag{8.3}$$

For our dataset, $R = 0.7583301$, $s = 0.1297690$, $t = 1.319460$, $v_{11} = 0.001774$, $v_{22} = 0.001752$ and $v_{12} = 0.000987$. The lower limit is then 0.582, which, being lower than 0.6, means that fpd 51 cannot be claimed to be non-inferior to the control treatment.

As a result of the interim analysis, the decision is to use the fifth period of the design with one or more doses at fpd > 51.

8.4 Choosing doses for the fifth period

As the results of the interim indicated that none of the doses used in the first four periods of the design were noninferior to the control treatment, it was decided that the trial would be extended to include a fifth period. The doses available for this period were fpd = 102 and fpd = 155.5. It was also decided that Placebo would also be used in the fifth period, to assess safety and to avoid aliasing the two new doses with the effect of the fifth period. However, due to the requirement of obtaining as much information as possible about the two new doses, it was decided that the control treatment would not be used in the fifth period.

To increase the chance of concluding one of the new doses is noninferior to the control, it is desirable to minimize the width of the lower confidence interval on the estimated ratio $\hat{R}$, as defined in the previous section. Therefore, the criterion chosen to determine the doses and their replication in the fifth period was the minimization of the variance of $\hat{R}$.

If $R = a/b$ and the standard error of the estimate of b is relatively small compared to b, then an approximation to the variance of $\hat{R} = \hat{a}/\hat{b}$ is

$$V\left(\frac{\hat{a}}{\hat{b}}\right) = \left[\frac{\hat{a}}{\hat{b}}\right]^2 \left[\frac{V(\hat{a})}{\hat{a}^2} + \frac{V(\hat{b})}{\hat{b}^2}\right]. \tag{8.4}$$

Therefore, as a surrogate for the minimization of $V(\hat{a}/\hat{b})$, we chose the allocation of doses in the fifth period to minimize $V(\hat{a}) + V(\hat{b})$, where $a = V(Control - Placebo)$, $b = V(Dose - Placebo)$ and $Dose = 102$ or 155.5.

Two types of design were searched for. The first only allowed 155.5 and Placebo in the fifth period, to optimize the information gained on the highest dose. The second type allowed both 120 and 155.5 in the fifth period, in the hope that both 120 and 155.5 would be shown to be noninferior.

Some restrictions were also placed on the doses and their replications in the fifth period. Placebo could be allocated to one or two sequences only (i.e., to no more than six subjects) and could not be allocated to a sequence that already contained Placebo.

For the second type of design, dose 155.5 could be allocated to between two and five sequences (i.e., to $6 \leq 15$ subjects) and dose 102 could be allocated to between one and two sequences (i.e., to $3 \leq 6$ subjects). Clearly, the emphasis in this type of design is still on dose 155.5, with some information gained on dose 102.

We look first at the choices for a design of the first type. Table 8.4 gives the 21 possible designs that satisfy our restrictions.

To compare the choices we assume a simple additive model that contains fixed effects for subjects, periods and treatments. We use this model to obtain estimates and their variances of the pair-wise comparisons of the fitted means of each treatment group versus Placebo. For these calculations we have set the within-subject variance equal to 1, as the size of this variance will not affect the choice of design. For simplicity, we have not made use of the fact that some of the treatments are ordered doses. That is, we have not fitted the Emax model to get the contrast variances. We assume that fitting the Emax model may lower the variances of the estimated contrasts, but will not change their rank order in terms of size. The estimated variances of the contrasts are given in Table 8.5, where $V_{CP} = Var(Control - Placebo)$, and $V_{155.5P} = Var(155.5 - Placebo)$.

Table 8.4: Possible treatment allocations for Period 5 (2 = Placebo, 6 = 155.5).

Period 5	Sequence							
choice	1	2	3	4	5	6	7	8
1	6	6	6	6	6	6	2	2
2	6	6	6	6	6	2	6	2
3	6	6	6	2	6	6	6	2
4	6	2	6	6	6	6	6	2
5	2	6	6	6	6	6	6	2
6	6	6	6	6	6	6	6	2
7	6	6	6	6	6	2	2	6
8	6	6	6	2	6	6	2	6
9	6	2	6	6	6	6	2	6
10	2	6	6	6	6	6	2	6
11	6	6	6	6	6	6	2	6
12	6	6	6	2	6	2	6	6
13	6	2	6	6	6	2	6	6
14	2	6	6	6	6	2	6	6
15	6	6	6	6	6	2	6	6
16	6	2	6	2	6	6	6	6
17	2	6	6	2	6	6	6	6
18	6	6	6	2	6	6	6	6
19	2	2	6	6	6	6	6	6
20	6	2	6	6	6	6	6	6
21	2	6	6	6	6	6	6	6

Table 8.5: Period 5 choices ordered by variance.

Period 5	Variance		
choice	V_{CP}	$V_{155.5P}$	$V_{CP}+V_{155.5P}$
1,2,3,4,5,7,8,10,12,13,14,16,19	0.102	0.279	0.381
9,17	0.102	0.283	0.385
6,11,15,18,20,21	0.102	0.480	0.582

The last column gives the sum of the variances of V_{CP} and $V_{155.5P}$, the criterion we will use to compare the choices. The rows of this table are ordered in terms of $V_{CP}+V_{155.5P}$ (all figures are rounded to three decimal places). Clearly the best design is any one of those in the first row of Table 8.4 in which two sequence groups get Placebo.

In the second type of design, we include doses 120 and 155.5. There are 441 designs that satisfy the restrictions and of these the three given in Table 8.6 were chosen as optimal choices under different criteria. The variances obtained

Table 8.6: Possible treatment allocations for Period 5 (2 = Placebo, 6 = 155.5, 7 = 120).

Period 5 choice	Sequence 1	2	3	4	5	6	7	8
1(opt for 155.5)	2	6	6	6	7	2	6	6
2(opt for 120)	6	7	6	6	7	6	2	2
3(opt for sum)	7	6	6	6	7	6	2	2

Table 8.7: Period 5 choices ordered by variance.

Period 5 choice	Variance $V_{CP}+V_{155.5P}$	$V_{CP}+V_{120P}$	$V_{CP}+V_{155.5P}+V_{CP}+V_{120P}$
1	0.395	0.732	1.127
2	0.418	0.519	0.937
3	0.417	0.520	0.937

from these designs are given in Table 8.7, where $V_{120P} = Var(120 - Placebo)$. The first design (choice 1) in Table 8.6 is one of the designs that minimizes the variance of $Var(155.5 - Placebo)$, the second design (choice 2) is one of the designs that minimizes the variance of $Var(120 - Placebo)$ and the third row is one of the designs that minimizes the sum of these two variances. If the comparison of dose 155.5 and Placebo is of primary importance, then the first design in Table 8.6 is optimal. We note that the inclusion of dose 120 in the design has increased the variance of this comparison from 0.279 to 0.293. If both comparisons of doses 155.5 and 120 are of interest, which they probably are, we could choose either of the designs in the second and third rows of Table 8.6. For the purposes of illustration we will choose the design in the third row.

8.5 Analysis of the design post-interim

In the previous section, two possible candidate designs were identified as the ones to take forward into the fifth period. One had Placebo and fpd 155.5 in the fifth period and the other had these two treatments and fpd 120 in the fifth period. Here we will take the design that has both fpd 120 and fpd 155.5 in the fifth period. In particular, we will take the design that has its first four periods as those given in Table 8.1 and whose fifth period has, respectively, the following treatments: F,G,G,G,F,G,B,B, where B = Placebo, F = fpd 120 and G = fpd 155.5.

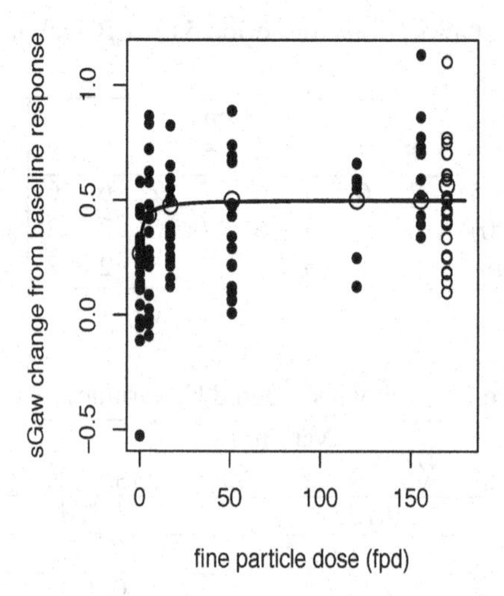

Figure 8.4: Fitted means for Emax model and control treatment for five-period design.

The estimated values of the parameters and their standard errors are given in Table 8.8.The number of degrees of freedom for the t-tests is again 23.

The fitted Emax curve is plotted in Figure 8.4. The large open circle symbols on the plot indicate the values of the fitted dose and control group means. The data and mean for the control treatment have been plotted at fpd = 170, for convenience only.

The estimated means of each dose group and the pairwise comparisons of these means with Placebo are given in Table 8.9.

Table 8.8: Parameter estimates from five-period design.

Parameter	Estimate	Std Err	t-value	Pr $> \|t\|$
led50	1.069	1.063	1.01	0.3247
e0	0.316	0.054	5.88	$<$ .0001
emax	0.189	0.038	4.91	$<$ .0001
control vs Placebo	0.252	0.037	6.75	$<$ .0001
σ_W^2	0.015	0.002	6.93	$<$ .0001
σ_B^2	0.036	0.011	3.20	0.0040
Period 2 vs 1	−0.154	0.035	−4.41	0.0002
Period 3 vs 1	−0.077	0.035	−2.17	0.0410
Period 4 vs 1	−0.215	0.036	−6.03	$<$ .0001
Period 5 vs 1	0.062	0.042	1.45	0.1606

Table 8.9: Mean and contrast estimates for five-period design.

Contrast	Estimate	Std Err	t-value	Pr $>|t|$
fpd 5	0.435	0.052	8.40	$<.0001$
fpd 17	0.477	0.047	10.08	$<.0001$
fpd 51	0.494	0.051	9.61	$<.0001$
fpd 120	0.500	0.054	9.23	$<.0001$
fpd 155.5	0.501	0.055	9.15	$<.0001$
control	0.567	0.051	11.14	$<.0001$
fpd 5 vs Placebo	0.119	0.043	2.78	0.0107
fpd 17 vs Placebo	0.161	0.032	5.01	$<.0001$
fpd 51 vs Placebo	0.179	0.033	5.32	$<.0001$
fpd 120 vs Placebo	0.184	0.036	5.13	$<.0001$
fpd 155.5 vs Placebo	0.185	0.036	5.09	$<.0001$
control vs Placebo	0.252	0.037	6.75	$<.0001$

We will now repeat the test for noninferiority by calculating the lower bound of the 90% one-sided confidence interval for the ratio of the effects of the fpd 155.5 dose and the control (compared to Placebo).

The estimated ratio is $R = 0.185/0.252 = 0.734$. Using Fieller's theorem again, the lower limit is 0.563, which is less than the 0.6 noninferiority boundary. Therefore, the active drug was not taken forward for further development.

Chapter 9

Case study: Choosing a dose–response model

9.1 Introduction

This case study illustrates how a model may be chosen for a dose response relationship when there is uncertainty in the shape of the dose–response curve. The example is based on a real trial where dose-finding was used, but for confidentiality reasons we have changed some aspects and will use simulated data. However, the main features of the design and the analysis have been retained. The drug under study was for the treatment of COPD (chronic obstructive pulmonary disease) and the primary endpoint in the trial was trough forced expiratory volume over 1 second ($TFEV_1$) following seven days of treatment. The endpoint was recorded in liters just prior to 24 hours post-dose. We will refer to the investigational drug as A. Also included in the trial was an active comparator, which we will refer to as B. The main purpose of the study was to evaluate the efficacy of five doses of A (0, 12.5, 25, 50 and 100 μg once a day) and open-label B (18 μg), so that an optimal dose of A could be chosen for future Phase III studies.

The basic design of the trial was of the incomplete block type consisting of 12 sequences in four periods, with three subjects allocated at random to each sequence. The design is given in Table 9.1, where the doses of A (0, 12.5, 25, 50 and 100) are labeled as 1, 2, 3, 4 and 5, respectively, and B is labeled as 6. For a model with carry-over effects, the average efficiency of the pair-wise comparisons is 80.81%. In the absence of carry-over effects, the average efficiency is 88.57%. It was assumed that carry-over effects were unlikely and so the primary analysis assumed a model without carry-over effects. A sample size of three subjects per sequence group, i.e., 36 subjects in total, was sufficient to ensure a power of about 90% for the pairwise comparisons of the four nonzero doses of A versus the zero dose. This assumed a two-sided significance level of 0.05/4 = 0.0125, to allow for multiple testing. The assumed within-subject standard deviation was 0.105 liters and the size of difference to detect between the highest dose and placebo was 0.12 liters.

Table 9.1: Partially balanced design for $t = 6$.

Subject	Period			
	1	2	3	4
1	1	4	2	5
2	4	5	1	2
3	2	1	5	4
4	5	2	4	1
5	2	5	3	6
6	5	6	2	3
7	3	2	6	5
8	6	3	5	2
9	3	6	1	4
10	6	4	3	1
11	1	3	4	6
12	4	1	6	3

9.2 Analysis of variance

The data set for our illustrative analyses contains 36 subjects and is plotted in the left panel of Figure 9.1, with the addition of the sample means for each dose group. Here we have plotted all the data and have not identified the four repeated measurements on each subject. In the right panel of Figure 9.1 is a plot of the sample means, where a dose–response relationship is clearly evident.

In Table 9.2 we show the analysis of variance for the fitted model that includes fixed effects for subjects, periods and treatments. We can see there is strong evidence of a difference between the treatment groups but little evidence of a difference between the periods. The least squares means from this model are given in Table 9.3 and plotted in Figure 9.2, where we have also plotted a horizontal line at 0.12 liters above the placebo (A, dose 0 μg) least squares mean. The dose taken forward into Phase III must achieve this level of improvement over placebo.

If we fit a model with random subject effects, the estimates of the between- and within-subject variances are 0.1269 and 0.0090, respectively. This indicates that the correlation within subjects is very high: $(0.1269/(0.1269+0.0090) = 0.93)$. The tests of the fixed effects (including the Kenward–Roger adjustment) are given in Table 9.4. The least squares means from this model are given in Table 9.5.

These are similar to the results obtained from the fixed-effects model. This is to be expected given the large between-subject variability. Therefore, in the following we will report only the results from the fixed-effects model.

The differences between the least squares means of all the pairwise comparisons are given in Table 9.6. We can see that all doses of A of 25 or higher are significantly better than the placebo dose (using a multiplicity adjusted two-sided significance level of 0.0125).

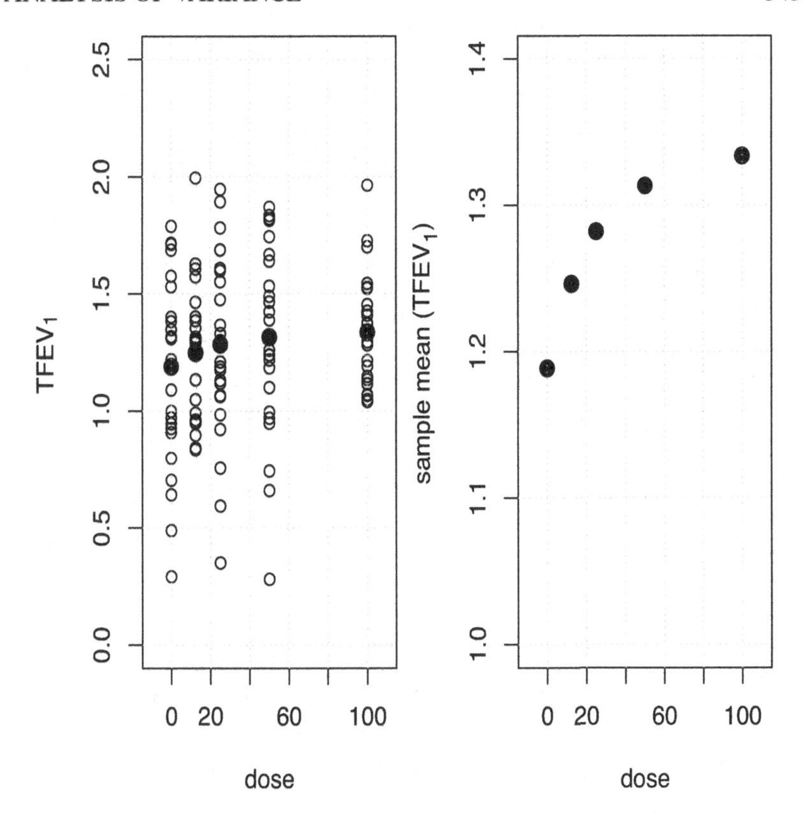

Figure 9.1: Plot of raw data and sample means (left panel) and sample means (right panel) excluding active control.

Table 9.2: Analysis of variance for model with fixed subject effects.

Source	d.f.	SS	MS	F	*P*-value
Subjects	35	18.093	0.5169	57.21	< 0.0001
Periods	3	0.072	0.0239	2.65	0.0531
Treatments	5	0.295	0.0590	6.53	< 0.0001
W-S Residual	100	0.904	0.0090		

Table 9.3: Least squares means from the model with fixed subject effects.

Dose of A	Estimate	Standard Error
0	1.200	0.0204
12.5	1.230	0.0204
25	1.287	0.0204
50	1.325	0.0204
100	1.317	0.0204
B	1.297	0.0204

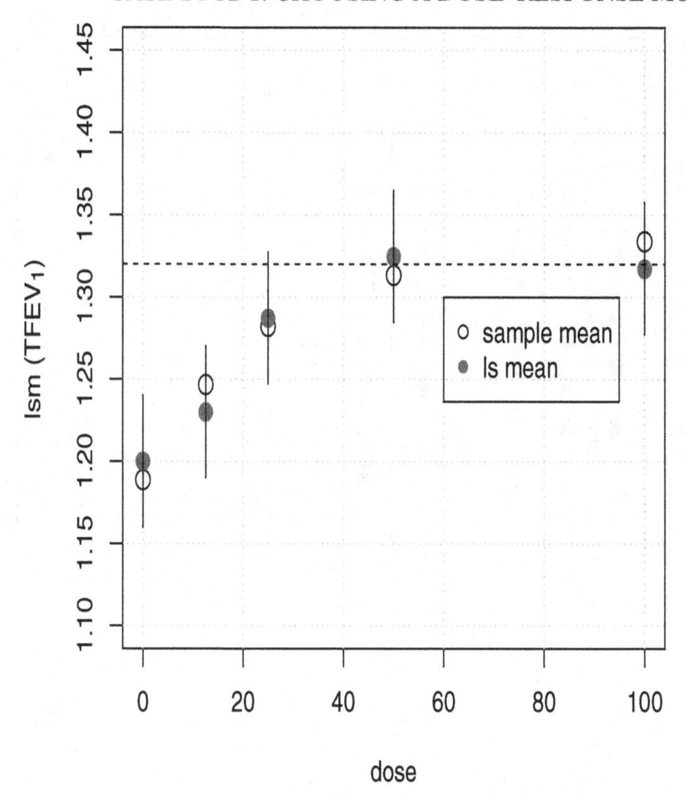

Figure 9.2: LS means (excluding active control).

Table 9.4: Test for fixed effects from model with random subject effects.

Effect	Num d.f.	Den d.f.	F Value	Pr > F
per	3	100	2.65	0.0531
trt	5	100	6.54	< .0001

9.3 Dose–response modeling

We will now consider fitting a dose–response relationship to the data from this trial with the objective of deciding on a model to use for predicting the dose or doses to take forward into Phase III confirmatory trials. Recall that the dose to take forward must achieve an improvement over the placebo dose of 0.12 liters. However, prior to the running of this trial, there was some uncertainty in the shape of the dose–relationship. The functions for some possible shapes are given in Table 9.7. After discussions with the clinical team, four candidate models were selected to represent a range of plausible dose–response shapes for TFEV1. The selection of possible shapes took account of the results of previous studies on the same compound and other drugs for the same indication.

Table 9.5: Least squares means from the model with random subject effects.

Dose of A	Estimate	Standard Error
0	1.200	0.0628
12.5	1.230	0.0628
25	1.287	0.0628
50	1.324	0.0628
100	1.318	0.0628
B	1.297	0.0628

Table 9.6: Differences between the dose least squares means from the model with fixed subject effects.

Parameter	Estimate	Standard Error	*P*-value
12.5 vs 0	0.0307	0.0296	0.3129
25 vs 0	0.0873	0.0296	0.0040
50 vs 0	0.1247	0.0296	<0.0001
100 vs 0	0.1174	0.0296	0.0001
25 vs 12.5	0.0572	0.0296	0.0564
50 vs 12.5	0.0946	0.0296	0.0019
100 vs 12.5	0.0873	0.0296	0.0020
50 vs 25	0.0374	0.0296	0.2101
100 vs 25	0.0301	0.0296	0.3126
100 vs 50	−0.0073	0.0296	0.8057
B vs 0	0.0968	0.0296	0.0015
12.5 vs B	−0.0667	0.0296	0.0266
25 vs B	−0.0095	0.0296	0.7302
50 vs B	0.0279	0.0296	0.3488
100 vs B	0.0206	0.0296	0.4889

Table 9.7: Selection of functions for dose–response relationship.

Name	Function
Sigmoid Emax	$E(y) = E_0 + Emax\frac{dose^{\lambda}}{ED_{50}{}^{\lambda}+dose^{\lambda}}$
Emax	$E(y) = E_0 + Emax\frac{dose}{ED_{50}+dose}$
Logistic	$E(y) = E_0 + \frac{Emax}{1+\exp[(ED_{50}-dose)/\delta]}$
Exponential	$E(y) = E_0 + E_1(\exp(\frac{dose}{\delta}) - 1)$
Quadratic	$E(y) = E_0 + \beta_1 dose + \beta_2 dose^2$
Linear	$E(y) = E_0 + \beta_1 dose$

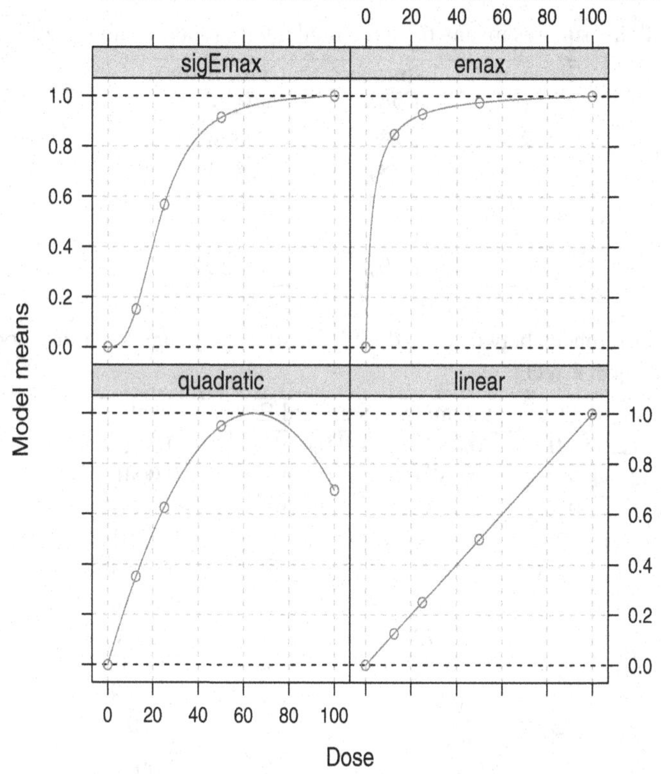

Figure 9.3: Candidate dose–response shapes.

The five shapes were (1) a four-parameter (sigmoid) Emax model, (2) a three-parameter Emax model, (3) a quadratic model and (4) a linear model. These are plotted in Figure 9.3, where the response is scaled to lie in the range 0 to 1.

To fit the models, test hypotheses and make predictions, we will follow the statistical methodology that has been qualified by the European Medicines Agency (see EMA (2014), Bretz et al. (2005), Bornkamp et al. (2009) and Pinheiro et al. (2014)). The steps in this methodology are given in Table 9.8.

Assuming that there are m candidate models, we test the following hypotheses: $H_0^m : \mathbf{c}_m^T \mu = 0$, where $\mu = (\mu_1, \mu_2, \ldots, \mu_k)$ is the vector containing the mean responses at doses $i = 1, 2, \ldots, k$, and $\mathbf{c}_m^T = (c_{m1}, c_{m2}, \ldots, c_{mk})$ is the optimal contrast vector representing model m, subject to $\sum_{i=1}^k c_{mi} = 0$. The coefficients of $\mathbf{c}_m$ are chosen to maximize the power of the test to detect model m, using the test statistics T_m defined below.

Each of the models in the set of candidates is tested using the single contrast test

$$T_m = \frac{\sum_{i=1}^k c_{mi}\hat{\mu}_i}{\sqrt{\widehat{Var}(\sum_{i=1}^k c_{mi}\hat{\mu}_i)}}.$$

Table 9.8: Steps in the MCP-Mod methodology.

	Design
Step 1	Choose set of candidate models
Step 2	Calculate corresponding optimal contrast coefficients
	Analysis
Step 3	Establish if there is a dose–response signal (trend) while controlling the Type I error rate
Step 4	Selection of a single model using appropriate test statistics or other metrics, possibly combined with external data (or model averaging)
Step 5	Dose estimation and selection (e.g., of minimum effective dose or dose that gives x% improvement over placebo)

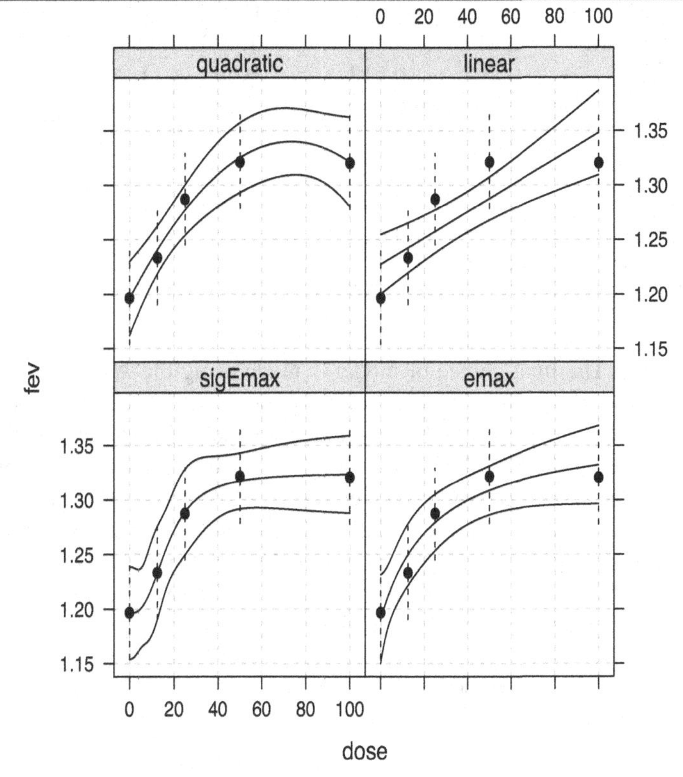

Figure 9.4: Fitted models (with fixed subject effects).

The construction of the optimal contrasts and the remaining steps of the methodology can be conveniently completed using the *DoseFinding* R package (Bornkamp et al. (2014)).

This package calculates the optimal contrast coefficients ($\mathbf{c}_m$, Step 2) and uses these to test for a dose–response trend for each model in the candidate

Table 9.9: Contrast tests.

Multiple Contrast Test — Contrasts				
	sigEmax	emax	quadratic	linear
0	−0.570	−0.866	−0.710	−0.437
12.5	−0.443	0.042	−0.246	−0.409
25	0.037	0.192	0.117	−0.139
50	0.462	0.394	0.607	0.229
100	0.514	0.238	0.231	0.755
Contrast Correlation				
	sigEmax	emax	quadratic	linear
sigEmax	1.000	0.773	0.916	0.908
emax	0.773	1.000	0.898	0.612
quadratic	0.916	0.898	1.000	0.693
linear	0.908	0.612	0.693	1.000
Multiple Contrast Test				
	t-stat	adj-p	AIC	
sigEmax	5.404	< 0.001	−183.9239	
quadratic	5.281	< 0.001	−185.4390	
emax	4.688	< 0.001	−184.1905	
linear	4.626	< 0.001	−175.2283	

set (T_m, Step 3). The final choice of model is made using the AIC value for each model (Step 4). All four fitted models are shown in Figure 9.4, where the observed means and pointwise 95% confidence bands are also plotted. The results of applying the MCP-Mod methodology to our data are given in Table 9.9. It is clear that all models give strong evidence of a significant trend in the mean response as the dose increases. The selected model, using the minimum AIC value (Step 4), is the quadratic model. Finally, the R package estimates the dose that gives an improvement over placebo of 0.12 liters (Step 5) and for each model these are 47.27 (sigEmax), 52.47 (emax), 43.49 (quadratic) and 99.47 (linear).

Based on these results, the recommended dose to take forward into Phase III would be 43.5 μg.

Chapter 10

Case study: Conditional power

10.1 Introduction

To illustrate the use of conditional power we will use the data from a 2×2 Phase III cross-over trial in patients that had difficulty sleeping due to a painful condition. The trial compared an active drug (B) to a placebo (A) on sleep maintenance as measured by the WASO time. WASO (Wake After Sleep Onset) time is a measure of the total time awake during a sleep session after first falling asleep. Decreasing WASO time is beneficial. There was a two-week wash-out period between the two treatment periods. The WASO times were obtained in a sleep laboratory using polysomnography and were assumed to be normally distributed. As with the other case studies, we have changed some of the details of the trial and used simulated data to illustrate its analysis.

At the planning stage of this trial there was some uncertainty regarding the amount by which B would reduce the mean WASO time compared to A. While it was expected that the reduction would be 20 minutes, it could be as low as 15 minutes, which was still considered as clinically meaningful. To allow for this uncertainty, an un-blinded interim analysis was planned when 50% of the subjects in each sequence group had completed both periods. To simplify the description of the analysis, we will assume that there is an equal number of subjects in each sequence group at the interim analysis. The within-subject variance of the WASO times was assumed to be 1200. The trial was planned to have a power of 0.9 to detect a reduction of 20 minutes, assuming a one-sided test with a significance level of 0.025. The planned sample size for the trial was therefore 64 subjects, 32 in each sequence group.

There was no intention to stop the trial at the interim. The aim of the interim was to ensure that the final sample size was sufficient to satisfy a conditional power of 0.9, based on the interim results. We note there was no plan to change the sample size based on an estimate of the within-subject variance (which was assumed to be well estimated at the planning stage) but only to allow for an overestimation of the true reduction in mean WASO time.

10.2 Variance spending approach

At the interim analysis, the number of additional subjects (if any) needed to achieve a conditional power at 0.9 was calculated using the "variance spending approach" described by Fisher (1998). This is a special case of the method described by Cui et al. (1999). See also Jennison and Turnbull (2003).

To describe the variance spending approach, we will follow the exposition given by Jennison and Turnbull (2003), but modified for the 2×2 cross-over trial.

We assume that the cross-over trial is planned to recruit n subjects to each sequence group and an interim analysis is planned when rn subjects in each group have completed the trial, with $0 < r < 1$. After the interim, we assume that the sample size per group for the second stage is changed from $(1-r)n$ to $\gamma(1-r)n$, so that the new total sample size per group is $n^* = rn + \gamma(1-r)n$.

Let y_{ijk} be the WASO time for subject k in period j in sequence group i and define $X_{1k} = (y_{11k} - y_{12k})/2$, $X_{2k} = (y_{21k} - y_{22k})/2$. If $S_1 = \sum_{k=1}^{rn}(X_{1k} - X_{2k})$ and $S_2 = \sum_{k=rn+1}^{n^*}(X_{1k} - X_{2k})$, then $S_1 \sim N(rn\theta, rn\sigma^2)$ and $S_2 \sim N(\gamma(1-r)n\theta, \gamma(1-r)n\sigma^2)$, where θ is the mean reduction in WASO time and σ is the within-subject standard deviation.

Further,

$$W_1 = \frac{S_1}{\sqrt{n}\sigma} \sim N(r\sqrt{n}\frac{\theta}{\sigma}, r)$$

and, conditional on the data at the interim,

$$W_2 = \frac{\gamma^{-\frac{1}{2}} S_2}{\sqrt{n}\sigma} \sim N(\sqrt{\gamma}(1-r)\sqrt{n}\frac{\theta}{\sigma}, (1-r)).$$

Under the null hypothesis that $\theta = 0$, $W_2 \sim N(0, (1-r))$ whatever the data-dependent choice of γ. W_2 is independent of W_1.

The variance-spending test statistic is

$$Z = W_1 + W_2 = \frac{S_1 + \gamma^{-\frac{1}{2}} S_2}{\sqrt{n}\sigma}. \tag{10.1}$$

At the end of the first stage, i.e., at the interim analysis, the conditional power, given that $\theta = \hat{\theta}_1$, is

$$\Phi\left[\frac{\{r + \sqrt{\gamma}(1-r)\}\sqrt{n}\frac{\hat{\theta}_1}{\sigma} - z_{1-\alpha/2}}{\sqrt{(1-r)}}\right],$$

where z_p is the $100p$th percentile of the standard normal distribution.

If we wish to choose γ to give a power of $1-\beta$, then

$$\gamma = \frac{\left[\sqrt{1-r}z_{1-\beta} + z_{1-\alpha/2} - r\sqrt{n}\frac{\hat{\theta}_1}{\sigma}\right]^2}{(1-r)^2 n \frac{\hat{\theta}_1^2}{\sigma^2}}.$$

Table 10.1: WASO times (minutes).

Group AB			Group BA		
	Period			Period	
Subject	1	2	Subject	1	2
1	26.8	96.4	17	71.4	124.6
2	93.6	44.2	18	63.0	48.1
3	80.1	67.1	19	69.4	113.3
4	86.6	66.9	20	23.5	18.8
5	92.9	52.7	21	69.3	71.2
6	19.1	78.8	22	73.3	8.8
7	82.1	108.4	23	145.6	9.2
8	120.2	99.8	24	124.6	130.7
9	18.1	130.6	25	87.4	69.5
10	80.5	91.9	26	67.6	15.8
11	89.4	119.1	27	71.8	46.2
12	77.7	114.4	28	64.0	58.4
13	75.5	5.8	29	118.9	82.2
14	57.6	58.1	30	41.9	52.2
15	59.0	23.1	31	85.3	32.8
16	19.8	102.3	32	49.2	64.3

A confidence interval for θ, as derived by Jennison and Turnbull (2003), is

$$\frac{S_1 + \gamma^{-\frac{1}{2}} S_2}{(r + \sqrt{\gamma}(1-r))n} \pm \frac{z_{1-\alpha/2}\,\sigma}{(r + \sqrt{\gamma}(1-r))\sqrt{n}}. \tag{10.2}$$

10.3 Interim analysis of sleep trial

The simulated data from the 32 subjects (16 per group) at the interim stage are given in Table 10.1. Fitting a model with fixed effects for subjects, periods and treatments gives the results displayed in Table 10.2. We can see that the interim estimates of $\hat{\theta}$ and $\hat{\sigma}$ are 14.397 and 34.422, respectively, indicating that the assumed value (20) for θ, used at the planning stage, was indeed optimistic. Allowing for a mid-course sample size modification was therefore

Table 10.2: Estimates obtained from the interim analysis.

Parameter	Estimate	Std Err	1-sided P-value
θ	14.397	8.605	0.052
σ	34.422	-	-
γ	2.024	-	-

Table 10.3: Second stage WASO times (minutes).

Group AB			Group BA		
	Period			Period	
Subject	1	2	Subject	1	2
33	126.1	108.2	66	83.4	43.1
34	120.1	75.2	67	115.7	98.5
35	151.4	85.6	68	191.2	42.9
36	78.3	14.8	69	52.0	122.2
37	106.6	115.3	70	108.1	34.5
38	74.4	47.9	71	91.1	47.4
39	75.9	81.5	72	40.6	54.6
40	75.3	71.8	73	50.7	50.6
41	104.2	68.5	74	96.3	90.5
42	9.3	132.6	75	64.5	103.7
43	85.4	85.0	76	72.0	38.5
44	70.7	93.6	77	85.9	63.0
45	41.5	70.2	78	124.4	63.6
46	35.9	31.5	79	127.2	64.1
47	56.5	120.9	80	87.5	72.6
48	109.8	64.6	81	59.0	59.2
49	56.3	45.4	82	114.9	94.6
50	60.0	51.0	83	113.4	88.5
51	95.8	63.7	84	58.9	65.3
52	99.8	161.7	85	117.1	44.5
53	32.0	91.8	86	59.9	22.7
54	97.0	85.6	87	90.8	35.0
55	35.4	135.2	88	44.7	56.2
56	16.0	72.0	89	47.4	138.1
57	49.9	133.2	90	70.9	9.7
58	69.7	113.7	91	105.0	93.0
59	76.4	145.4	92	106.8	41.4
60	80.4	113.7	93	76.4	76.1
61	78.1	34.6	94	70.5	24.4
62	36.5	107.6	95	33.3	125.1
63	62.1	89.0	96	54.0	96.2
64	92.9	109.5	97	115.0	134.1
65	87.6	27.7	98	101.3	42.2

prudent planning. The estimated value of γ is 2.0244, leading to a revised total sample size of 32 + 2.0244*32 = 96.78. Rounding this up to the next even number gives the revised total as 98 and a revised value for γ of 2.0625.

To complete the illustrative analysis, we simulated data for a further 33 subjects per group. These data are given in Table 10.3. The value of S_2 from these data, the value of S_1 from the interim data and the estimate of σ from the analysis of data from all 98 subjects are given in Table 10.4. The value of the test statistic given by Equation (10.1) is 2.943, the 95% confidence interval, given by Equation (10.2), but using the t-distribution, is (4.82, 24.77), and the point estimate of θ, taken as the mid-point of this interval, is 14.80. The one-sided P-value, obtained from the standard normal distribution, is 0.002. The conclusion is that the active drug significantly lowers WASO time by about 15 minutes. We note that the usual confidence interval, obtained from fitting the linear model with fixed effects for subjects, periods and treatments, is (5.03, 24.67) and slightly narrower.

Table 10.4: Results from analysis of both stages.

Statistic	Value
$S1$	230.35
$S2$	497.25
σ	34.63

Chapter 11

Case study: Proof of concept trial with sample size re-estimation

11.1 Introduction

This example is based on a Phase II Proof of Concept (PoC), placebo-controlled, study that examined the pain relief of a novel drug in subjects with flare enriched osteoarthritis of the knee. The two treatments in the trial were a novel drug (A) and a placebo (P). The design was a 2×2 cross-over trial, as shown in Table 11.1. The primary endpoint was the Western Ontario and McMaster (WOMAC) Osteoarthritis Index pain subscale score measured at the end of each treatment period. The subscale is the sum of the answers to five questions, where the answer to each question was coded as 0 to 4, giving a maximum total of 20. Each active period lasted two weeks and there was a two-week wash-out period between them. The recorded pain score was subsequently rescaled to lie in the range 0–10, to give the primary endpoint for analysis. Higher scores indicate greater pain.

The aim of the trial was to determine if PoC could be declared and the drug taken forward for further development. Let μ_A and μ_P denote the true means for A and P, respectively, and let σ^2 denote the within-subject variance for the WOMAC score. Given that we expect the active drug to lower the pain score, we define the difference, $\delta = \mu_P - \mu_A$, to give a positive value if A is truly better than P. Three decisions were to be made at the final analysis:

- **Clear PoC Go Forward for A.**
  Clear evidence of efficacy of A. That is, to be 80% sure that A has a greater than 0.9 reduction in the WOMAC pain score compared to P. A meta-analysis of previous studies had determined that the standard treatment, compared to P, had a reduction of this size. The objective, therefore, was not to show just that A is significantly better than P, but to show that it was significantly better by at least 0.9. The PoC Go Forward decision was deemed to have been achieved if the lower limit of a one-sided 80% confidence interval for δ exceeded 0.9.
- **Clear PoC Stop for A.**
  Clear lack of evidence of efficacy for A. The PoC Stop decision was deemed to have been achieved if the upper limit of a one-sided 80% confidence interval for δ was below 0.9.

Table 11.1: PoC design for two treatments and two periods.

Sequence	Periods	
1	A	P
2	P	A

- **Pause for A.**
If neither of the above was achieved, i.e., that there was evidence that $0.9 < \delta < 1.35$, this would be considered a "pause" decision for the novel drug program. The value of 1.35 was chosen because an improvement of at least 0.45 over the standard treatment was required.

11.2 Calculating the sample size

The sample size for the trial was calculated to ensure that the probability of a Go Forward decision was 0.80, when $\delta = 1.35$ and $\sigma = 1.5$.

Let $\hat{\delta}$ denote the estimator of δ and σ_δ its standard error. For the 2×2 design, $\sigma_\delta = \sqrt{2\sigma^2/N}$, if N is the total number of subjects ($N/2$ per group). The lower limit of the confidence interval is $\hat{\delta} - z_{0.8} * \sigma_\delta$, where $z_{0.8}$ is the upper 0.8 percentile of the standard normal distribution. If K denotes the cut-off value (0.9, here), we require that:

$$Pr\left(\hat{\delta} - z_{0.8} * \sigma_\delta > K \mid \delta = 1.35\right) \geq 0.8.$$

That is,

$$Pr\left(\frac{\hat{\delta} - \delta}{\sigma_\delta} > \frac{K - \delta}{\sigma_\delta} + z_{0.8} \mid \delta = 1.35\right) \geq 0.8.$$

Calculating this probability for a series of sample sizes determined that a sample size of 33 subjects per group ($N = 66$) would be more than adequate. (Strictly, in fact, $N = 64$ would have been sufficient.) The power curve for $N = 66$ (i.e., the above probability as a function of δ) is plotted in the left hand side of Figure 11.1. The vertical lines indicate the power when $\delta = 0.9$ and when $\delta = 1.35$. As constructed, these are 0.2 and 0.811, respectively.

In addition, we can calculate the probabilities of the other two decisions for a range of values of δ. These are plotted in Figure 11.2, where the light gray area indicates the probability of a Go Forward decision, the gray area indicates the probability of a Pause decision and the dark gray area indicates the probability of a Stop decision. For a given value of δ, on the axis below the dark gray area, the probability of a Stop decision is the vertical distance from the top of the plot to the edge of the dark gray area. The probability of a Pause decision, for a given value of δ on the axis below the gray area, is the vertical length of the line within the boundaries of the gray area. The probability of a Go

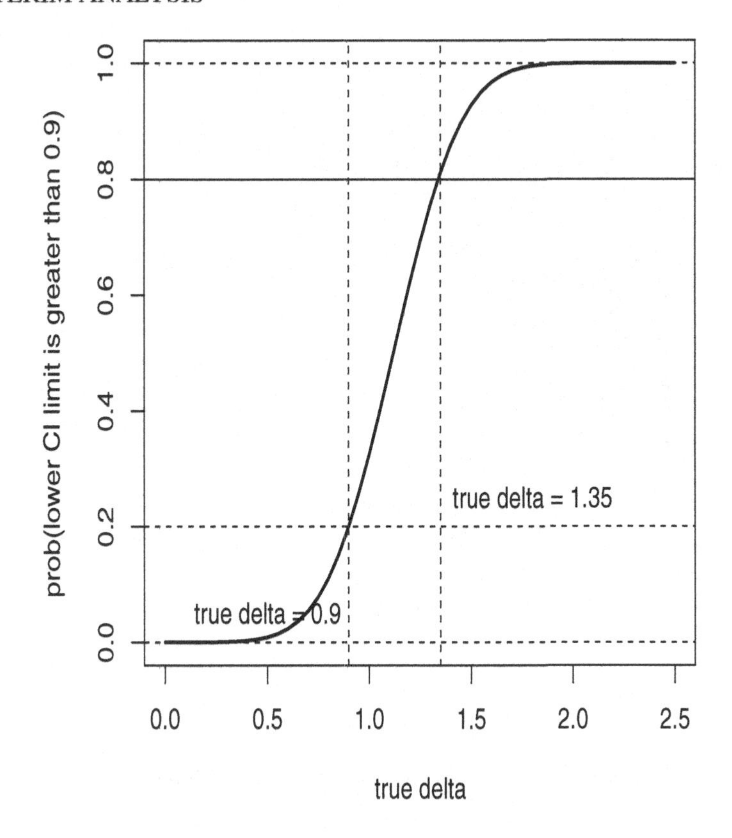

Figure 11.1: Probability of a Go Forward decision for A vs P.

Forward decision, for a given value of δ on the axis below the light gray area, is the height of the line.

We can see that when $\delta = 0.9$, a value we might term the value under the null hypothesis, the probability of a Go Forward decision is 0.2, the Type I error rate. When $\delta = 1.35$, an improvement of 0.45 of A over the standard treatment, this probability is 0.811. Conversely, if $\delta = 0.45$, the probability of a Stop decision is over 0.8.

11.3 Interim analysis

Because there was uncertainty in the estimate of σ^2, an interim analysis was done after about 25% of the subjects had completed the trial (nine in each sequence group). The aim of the interim analysis was to re-estimate σ^2 and increase the sample size if necessary. No reduction in sample size was allowed. The sample size would be increased to ensure that the probability was at least

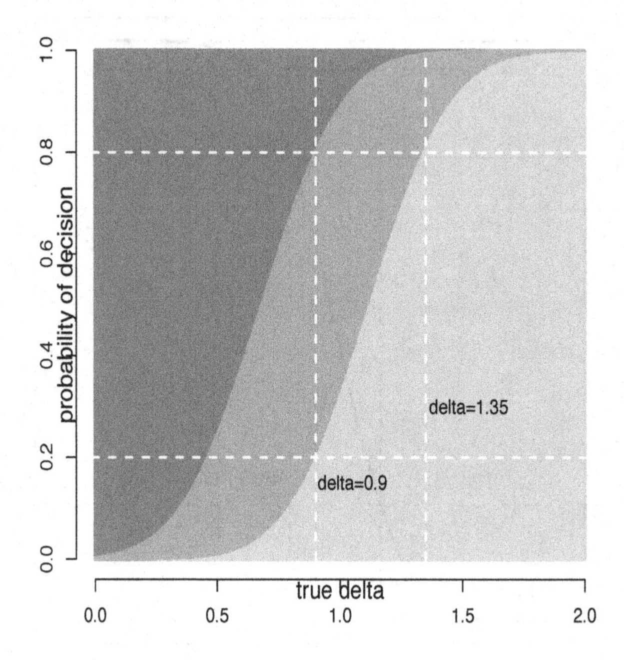

Figure 11.2: Probabilities of Go Forward, Pause and Stop decisions.

0.8 and that the estimated lower limit of an 80% confidence interval was greater than 0.9.

The re-estimation of σ can be done in a blinded or unblinded way. Here we will assume that it will be done in a blinded way. Possible approaches for allowing an unblinded analysis will be described Chapters 13 and 14.

Kieser and Friede (2003) showed that in a parallel groups design for two treatments, there is practically no inflation in the Type I error of a significance test for a treatment difference at the end of the trial if an interim blinded re-estimation of σ is done and the sample size increased if necessary. Before going any further we re-express the results of Kieser and Friede (2003) in terms of the 2×2 cross-over trial.

For simplicity, we assume that at the interim there are n subjects in each group.

Let y_{ijk} denote the response observed in period j on subject k in sequence group i, $i = 1,2; j = 1,2; k = 1,2,\ldots,n$. We assume the same linear model for y_{ijk} as used in Chapter 2, but without any carry-over effects.

Let $d_{ik} = y_{i1k} - y_{i2k}$ denote the within-subject difference for subject k in group i and let $\bar{d}_i$ denote its mean, $k = 1,2,\ldots,n$ and $i = 1,2$.

Using this model, we see that

$$E(\bar{d}_1) = \pi_1 - \pi_2 + \tau_1 - \tau_2$$

and

$$E(\bar{d}_2) = \pi_1 - \pi_2 + \tau_2 - \tau_1.$$

Further,

$$E\left(\frac{\bar{d}_1 - \bar{d}_2}{2}\right) = \tau_1 - \tau_2$$

and

$$Var\left(\frac{\bar{d}_1 - \bar{d}_2}{2}\right) = \frac{\sigma^2}{n},$$

where σ^2 is the within-subject variance.

Recognizing that the structure of the d_{ik} is the same as that of a data set from a parallel groups design with two groups (where the responses are now the d_{ik}), we can express the formulae of Kieser and Friede (2003) as follows.

Let $\Delta_1 = \pi_1 - \pi_2 + \tau_1 - \tau_2$ and $\Delta_2 = \pi_1 - \pi_2 + \tau_2 - \tau_1$; then

$$d_{1k} \sim N(\Delta_1, 2\sigma_W^2) \text{ and } d_{2k} \sim N(\Delta_2, 2\sigma_W^2).$$

Defining s_p^2 as

$$s_p^2 = \frac{\sum_{i=1}^{2}\sum_{j=1}^{n}\left(d_{ij} - \bar{d}\right)^2}{2n-1},$$

where $\bar{d} = (\bar{d}_1 + \bar{d}_2)/2$, we can easily show that

$$E((2n-1)s_p^2) = (2n-1)2\sigma^2 + \frac{n}{2}(\Delta_1 - \Delta_2)^2.$$

The blinded estimator of σ^2 is then

$$s_p^2/[2(2n-1)],$$

which has bias

$$\frac{n}{(2n-1)}\Delta_{AB}^2,$$

where $\Delta_{AB} = \tau_1 - \tau_2$. The bias can removed by assuming a correct value for Δ_{AB}. The estimator

$$s_p^2/[2(2n-1)] - \frac{n}{(2n-1)}\Delta_{AB}^2$$

is referred to as the adjusted estimator by Kieser and Friede (2003).

Table 11.2: WOMAC score.

Group PA				Group AP		
	Period				Period	
Subject	1	2		Subject	1	2
1	2.04	2.48		10	4.80	6.51
2	3.49	9.60		11	1.00	1.95
3	3.00	3.51		12	4.89	3.18
4	3.56	4.71		13	6.82	2.36
5	2.20	4.52		14	0.00	0.67
6	3.77	1.70		15	4.88	2.38
7	5.34	8.58		16	1.07	2.41
8	3.70	5.19		17	4.63	2.27
9	1.08	7.43		18	1.47	3.69

11.4 Data analysis

Due to confidentiality reasons we cannot use the actual data from this trial, so simulated data will be used for illustration. The simulated interim data set is given in Table 11.2, where we have rounded the data to two decimal places.

To obtain the blinded estimate of σ^2, we fit a linear model with fixed effects for subjects and periods only, leaving out the treatment factor. This gives a blinded, unadjusted estimate of $\hat{\sigma}^2 = 3.95$, which was higher than the value of $\sigma^2 = 1.5^2 = 2.25$, assumed when the trial was planned. If it is assumed that $\Delta_{AB} = 1.35$, as at the planning stage, the bias = 0.965, which is a considerable proportion of the assumed $\sigma^2 = 2.25$. Adjusting for this amount of possible bias will therefore cause a large reduction in the blinded estimate of 3.95. Of course, if we know that Δ_{AB} is truly 1.35, then on average (over many trials) this is the correct adjustment to make. The dilemma we face is that we do not know the true value of Δ_{AB} with certainty: if we did, we would not need to run the trial. If there truly is a nonzero treatment difference, we will certainly increase (on average) the sample size after the interim by more than is necessary if we use the unadjusted estimator. However, if the true bias is incorrectly underestimated, then we risk not increasing the sample size when it is necessary.

In our artificial example, using simulated data, we know the truth and can also unblind the data. Therefore, we can compare the three estimators of σ^2: unblinded, blinded and blinded with adjustment. In truth, the data were simulated with $\sigma^2 = 2.25$. Based on the data in Table 11.2, the three estimators are, respectively, 3.223, 3.949 and 2.984. As it turns out, the unblinded estimator and the adjusted estimator are both larger than 2.25 and will lead to an increase in sample size if a sample size re-estimation is done. However, ignoring our knowledge of the truth, the blinded estimator is at least uncontroversial in that it does not need a value of Δ_{AB} to be specified. Therefore we will continue this example using the blinded unadjusted estimator, fully realizing that we may be increasing the sample size unnecessarily, due to the presence of potential bias.

Assuming $\sigma^2 = 3.949$ and $\delta = 1.35$, the power to achieve a Go Forward decision with $N = 66$ patients is 0.677. If N is increased to 112, the power to achieve a Go Forward decision is 0.803. The power to achieve a Go Forward is 0.92 if we make the calculation again but using the originally assumed value of $\sigma^2 = 2.25$ and with $N = 112$. Given this is a simulated example, we will not continue to simulate the data from the second stage of the study and make a final choice out of the three possible decisions for PoC.

In conclusion, this example has highlighted some of the consequences of using a blinded sample size re-estimation. In Chapters 13 and 14 we consider variations on methods for an unblinded sample size re-estimation.

Chapter 12

Case study: Blinded sample size re-estimation in a bioequivalence study

12.1 Introduction

In Chapter 7 we defined average bioequivalence (ABE) and showed how to test for it using the data from a 2×2 cross-over trial. Here we will look at a method of re-estimating (i.e., recalculating) the sample size after an interim analysis. Before we do this we first define the within-subject coefficient of variation (CV).

On the logarithmic scale we assume that each of log(AUC) and log(Cmax) is normally distributed. If we consider log(AUC), for example, we assume that for a given period i and treatment j, this variate has a mean μ_{ij} and variance σ^2. On the back-transformed, natural scale, the mean of AUC is $e^{(\mu_{ij}+\frac{\sigma^2}{2})}$ and its variance is $(e^{\sigma^2}-1)e^{(2\mu_{ij}+\sigma^2)}$. The CV is the ratio of the standard deviation to the mean and is therefore equal to $\sqrt{e^{\sigma^2}-1}$. In terms of the CV, $\sigma^2 = \log(1+CV^2)$.

We know that the sample size for such a trial depends on the CV and the assumed value of the Test to Reference ratio of means on the back-transformed, i.e., natural, scale. Getting either or both of these wrong at the planning stage could result in an underpowered study and failure to declare ABE when Test and Reference are in fact bioequivalent.

One way to guard against this is to include an interim analysis part way through the trial, where either the CV and/or the true ratio of means is estimated and the sample size recalculated. Here we describe one possible approach where the re-estimation of the sample size is based on a blinded estimate of the CV. In the next two chapters we describe two alternatives that use an unblinded interim analysis.

12.2 Blinded sample size re-estimation (BSSR)

In a blinded sample size re-estimation (BSSR), the sample size is recalculated at the interim analysis using a blinded estimate of the CV and the same value for the true ratio of means as used when originally planning the study. The method or formula for the sample size calculation is the same at the interim as that used when planning the study.

It is well known (Kieser and Friede (2003)) that when testing for superiority of one treatment over another, using a parallel groups design, the Type I error rate is not inflated if a BSSR is done at a single interim analysis. However, the Type I error rate is inflated if the hypothesis test is for equivalence, rather than for superiority (Friede and Kieser (2003)). Similar results apply to cross-over trials. In particular, the Type I error rate is inflated if a BSSR is done at an interim analysis in a 2×2 cross-over trial to show ABE (Golkowski (2011), Golkowski et al. (2014)).

Here we will demonstrate how to undertake a BSSR for a 2×2 trial using a simulated set of data on log(AUC). At the planning stage for this trial there was some uncertainty in the value of the CV. The best estimate of the CV was that it was about 0.33 (i.e., as CV ≥ 0.30, the drug was borderline highly variable), but the actual CV could be higher. To guard against an underestimation of the CV, a BSSR was planned at a single interim analysis. The planned sample size of 38 subjects in total (19 in each sequence group) was chosen to ensure that there was at least a power of 0.80 to declare ABE if the ratio of the true T:R means on the natural scale was 1 (see calculations below).

For consistency with the other results that we will quote from Golkowski (2011); we state his sample size formula for the total number of subjects (n) required to give power $1-\beta$, assuming that the significance level of the two one-sided tests procedure is α and the ratio of the true T:R means on the natural scale is 1:

n is the smallest even integer that satisfies

$$n \geq \frac{2(\Phi^{-1}(1-\alpha)+\Phi^{-1}(1-\beta/2))^2\sigma^2}{\Delta^2},$$

where $\Phi(x)$ is the cumulative probability distribution of the standard normal distribution, evaluated at x, $\sigma = \sqrt{log(1+CV^2)}$ and $\Delta = log(1.25)$.

If we assume that $\sigma = 0.321$, $\alpha = 0.05$ and $\beta = 0.2$, then $n = 36$.

As the above formula uses a normal approximation to the t-distribution, the power of the TOST procedure was also estimated using simulation. The estimated powers for each of three different total sample sizes, 36, 38 and 40, were calculated using 100,000 simulated trials, with a true CV of 0.33 and a ratio of T:R true means of 1. The values of the estimated powers were, respectively, 0.7863, 0.8153 and 0.8431, suggesting that the above formula gives a slight underestimation of the sample size. Given these results, a sample size of 38 was chosen for this illustrative example.

The timing of the interim analysis was also a matter of debate. The choice was between an early look at the data (i.e., when 5 subjects in each group had completed both periods) or a later look when 10 subjects had completed both periods. Using code written in R by D. Golkowski to evaluate the Type I error rate using numerical integration, the maximum increase in the Type I error rate for the early timing of the interim analysis was calculated to be 0.065, compared to 0.05 (see Golkowski (2011) for details of the integrals).

If a BSSR is done when there are 10 completed subjects per group, the Type I error rate is maximally increased from 0.05 to about 0.061. Clearly, there is an advantage in having the interim at the later time. A simulation of 100,000 trials, with a BSSR at this later time, gave an estimated maximum Type I error rate of 0.060.

In the presence of Type I error rate inflation, the value of α used in the TOST must be reduced, so that the achieved Type I error rate is no larger than 0.05. We note that for fixed equivalence margins, the adjusted level depends only on the (known) sample size of the interim analysis. Golkowski (2011) gives a simple algorithm for determining this reduced value of α. At each step of his algorithm the value of the α used in the TOST is reduced by the amount of inflation in the achieved Type I error rate. The maximum excess (if any) of the achieved Type I error rate is then recalculated using this revised value of α. These steps are repeated until the excess over 0.05 is zero. Applying this algorithm to our planned trial gives $\alpha = 0.0405$ when the interim analysis is done when 20 subjects (10 in each group) have completed both periods. We assume that the data from subjects who have completed only one period at the time of interim will not be used in the BSSR. Using this reduced value of α in a simulation of 100,000 trials gave an estimated Type I error rate of 0.0499, confirming that using the reduced significance level has been effective.

When the sample size has been re-estimated, there are still more choices to be made. These are the minimum and maximum sizes of the trial, post interim. Golkowski (2011), following Birkett and Day (1994), constrains the minimum sample size to be the number of subjects used in the interim analysis. This means that the trial may have a final sample size that is smaller than that originally planned. An alternative would be to constrain the minimum sample size to be equal to the originally planned sample size. This means the sample size, post interim, can never be smaller than that originally planned. This latter choice means that the average total sample size (over many simulated realizations of the trial) is bound to be larger than that originally planned. Here we will adopt the rule suggested by Birkett and Day (1994).

A further consideration, when using a BSSR, is whether the Type II error rate (i.e., $1-$ power) is also controlled at the planned level. Golkowski (2011) shows that the Type II error rate is typically increased when using a BSSR, especially when the interim total sample size is 10 or less. In our illustrative example, where the true CV is 0.33, and using the adjusted significance level of $\alpha = 0.0405$, the power of the BSSR, calculated by simulation, falls to about 0.77 with an average total sample size of 36.6. To remedy this, Golkowski (2011) recommends inflating the sample size obtained from the BSSR at an interim by the following factor (first suggested by Zucker et al. (1999)):

$$\textit{inflation factor} = \left(\frac{t_{1-\alpha,\nu_1} + t_{1-\beta,\nu_1}}{\Phi^{-1}(1-\alpha) + \Phi^{-1}(1-\beta)} \right)^2,$$

where the BSSR includes a total of n_1 subjects, $\nu_1 = n_1 - 1$ are the degrees of freedom for the blinded estimate of σ^2 at the interim and $t_{1-\gamma,\nu_1}$ is the $1-\gamma$ quantile of the t-distribution.

12.3 Example

For our illustrative example, the interim sample size is $n_1 = 20$, giving an inflation factor of 1.0851. Applying this increase to the BSSR in 100,0000 simulated trials raised the power to 0.8118, with an average total sample size of 39.5 (i.e., 40 for the 2×2 trial). Given that the CV used in the planning is the same as that used in the simulations, our results suggest that when a sample size increase is not needed, the penalty, on average at least, is not high (39.5 vs 38 planned).

Of course, the advantage of a BSSR comes when the CV is underestimated at the planning stage. Suppose, in our illustrative example, the true CV was 0.40 and not 0.33. Without a BSSR, the sample size for the trial would need to be about 26 subjects per group. This is larger than the 19 per group currently planned for.

To see the effectiveness of the BSSR, 100,000 trials that included a BSSR at $n_1 = 20$ were simulated for data with CV = 0.4. The TOST procedure was again applied with an adjusted value of $\alpha = 0.0405$, as stated above. Based on simulation results, and using the inflation factor to increase the re-estimated sample size, the estimated power of the completed trial was 0.789 and the average total sample size was 56.4. Again a modest increase in the average total sample size is observed.

Let us now illustrate the calculations to be performed in an interim analysis that includes a BSSR at $n_1 = 20$. Here we will only consider the AUC.

The simulated interim AUC data are given in Table 12.1. For the purposes of this illustration, we will assume that the interim analysis is blinded, even though the data in the table are clearly not.

Table 12.1: Interim data (AUC) for ABE trial.

Group RT				Group TR		
	Period				Period	
Subject	1	2		Subject	1	2
1	378.651	195.087		11	117.959	58.757
2	94.213	75.521		12	98.642	38.214
3	109.403	70.000		13	116.086	172.217
4	54.627	86.047		14	141.519	189.386
5	46.091	115.534		15	94.859	122.682
6	39.142	58.813		16	861.083	484.664
7	116.717	96.812		17	103.272	128.985
8	97.478	102.687		18	21.710	20.950
9	20.419	41.228		19	75.497	81.664
10	124.546	129.570		20	52.003	160.478

Table 12.2: Additional post-interim data for ABE trial.

Group RT			Group TR		
	Period			Period	
Subject	1	2	Subject	1	2
21	95.458	140.784	40	51.519	37.138
22	44.884	50.444	41	16.730	13.780
23	69.974	101.397	42	83.234	194.130
24	121.891	99.202	43	323.905	309.659
25	23.411	19.728	44	20.939	23.364
26	43.648	58.350	45	107.516	91.755
27	390.265	311.951	46	54.074	82.135
28	178.143	92.506	47	153.877	84.087
29	222.559	132.397	48	45.282	39.559
30	88.751	150.988	49	26.723	36.630
31	38.197	74.594	50	51.605	36.590
32	56.073	117.833	51	283.012	160.818
33	121.242	98.176	52	37.279	85.925
34	258.457	228.396	53	175.526	224.687
35	44.084	61.106	54	68.410	72.473
36	30.629	50.592	55	99.632	119.244
37	95.699	55.377	56	41.525	90.671
38	81.309	42.483	57	65.352	177.254
39	182.205	134.586	58	58.868	86.633

The blinded estimate of σ is 0.3879, giving a CV of 0.403, which is higher than that assumed at the planning stage. Using this blinded estimate to recalculate the sample size gives a value of 51.76. The inflated total sample size (on rounding up) is then 58, i.e., 29 subjects per group.

The simulated data from the second stage are given in Table 12.2. Based on an analysis of the unblinded data from both stages, the estimate of the treatment difference, δ, on the log scale, and its associated 91.9%(i.e., $100(1-2\times 0.0405)$) confidence interval are given in Table 12.3. Also given are the back-transformed values of these quantities. We can see that the limits of the confidence interval on the natural scale are within the limits of (0.8, 1.25), confirming that there is no evidence to reject the null hypothesis that T and R are ABE on AUC.

Table 12.3: TOST procedure results.

Endpoint	$\hat{\delta}$	91.9% Confidence Interval
log(AUC)	−0.0264	(−0.1418, 0.0890)
Endpoint	$\exp(\hat{\delta})$	91.9% Confidence Interval
AUC	0.974	(0.868, 1.093)

Chapter 13

Case study: Unblinded sample size re-estimation in a bioequivalence study that has a group sequential design

13.1 Introduction

An alternative to the approach taken in the last chapter is to plan from the beginning to use a group sequential design. Although group sequential designs for testing ABE are not new, and can be traced back at least as far as Gould (1995) and Hauck et al. (1997), recent interest in two-stage designs with the possibility of stopping was prompted by methods described in Potvin et al. (2008) and, as a follow-up, in Montague et al. (2012). Indeed, regulatory agencies now seem receptive to the use of two-stage designs (e.g., see EMA (2010), FDA (2013), Health Canada (2012)), and as consequence their use is likely to increase. However, firm recommendations on which type of analysis to employ are still not agreed, and it is likely that a number of variations will find their way into everyday use. See Fuglsang (2013, 2014) and Karalis and Macheras (2013), for example, for further discussion on this topic. Here we will consider one particular design of this type: the one that uses a single interim analysis and the Pocock (Pocock (1977)) boundaries to stop or continue. In practical terms this means using a one-sided significance level of $\alpha = 0.0304$ in the TOST at the interim and $\alpha = 0.0304$ in the TOST at the final analysis, if the study completes both of the planned stages. We assume that the interim analysis takes place when half of the subjects in the trial have completed both periods. In the next chapter we will describe the methods suggested by Potvin et al. (2008).

For the example used in the previous chapter, where the CV = 0.33 and the true ratio on the natural scale is 1, the sample size needed to achieve at least 0.80 power is $N = 44$. When 100,000 ABE trials are simulated under these assumptions, the power of the study is about 0.83. When the simulation study was repeated under the null hypothesis, the Type I error rate was 0.046.

Before we continue, it is useful to note that the TOST procedure can be quite conservative, i.e., the achieved Type I error rate may be lower than the nominal 0.05 significance level. To demonstrate this, we show in Figure 13.1 a plot of the joint distribution of the two one-sided t-test statistics, obtained from simulating 100,000 trials for a design with 12 subjects per group and a

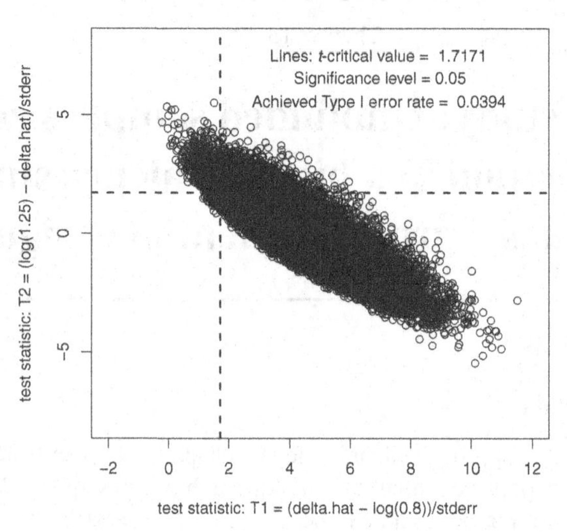

Figure 13.1: Joint distribution of TOST statistics.

CV = 0.40, and where there is no interim analysis. The coordinates of each particular point in the figure correspond to the two observed t-statistics (T1, T2) in that particular simulated trial. Here the achieved Type I error rate is 0.0394. To understand why this is lower than 0.05, we note that the points above the horizontal line correspond to the significant t-values under the null hypothesis that the true ratio of means on the original scale = 1.25. The proportion of these points (corresponding to T2) out of the 100,000 is 0.05007. However, not all the points are to the right of the vertical line, which means that those to the left correspond to nonsignificant t-statistics (for T1). The achieved significance level is the proportion of points that are both above the horizontal line and to the right of the vertical line. This is 0.05007 − 0.01071 = 0.03936, where 0.01071 is the proportion of points above the horizontal line and to the left of the vertical line.

13.2 Sample size re-estimation in a group sequential design

Here we will make an unblinded sample size re-estimation after the interim analysis if BE is not declared at the interim. If the estimated power, based on the estimated CV and the treatment difference used in the planning of the trial (i.e., not the treatment difference observed at the interim analysis), is not at least 0.80, the total sample size of the study will be increased, so that a power of 0.80 will be achieved, based on the current estimate of the CV. The minimum sample size after the interim will be the size of the trial at the interim (as recommended by Birkett and Day (1994)). We add a slight variation in that the minimum sample size increase will be two subjects in each group, to allow estimation of the variance in the second stage of the trial. The power is calculated using the R package PowerTOST (Labes (2013)) with the "exact" option.

However, if we increase the sample size without modification of the test statistics of the TOST procedure, the Type I error rate will be inflated. The modification we use is to replace each of the one-sided t-statistics with a z-statistic defined, respectively, as

$$z_1 = \sqrt{w}\Phi^{-1}(1-p_{11}) + \sqrt{1-w}\Phi^{-1}(1-p_{21})$$

and

$$z_2 = \sqrt{w}\Phi^{-1}(1-p_{12}) + \sqrt{1-w}\Phi^{-1}(1-p_{22}),$$

where $0 \leq w \leq 1$, p_{11} is the P-value for testing H_{01}, as defined in Chapter 7, obtained from the data in the first stage, p_{21} is the P-value for testing H_{01} in the second stage, p_{12} is the P-value for testing H_{02} in the first stage and p_{22} is the P-value for testing H_{02} in the second stage. $\Phi^{-1}(1-p)$ is the inverse of the cumulative standard normal distribution for quantile $1-p$ and w is a prespecified weight (Lehmacher and Wassmer (1999)). We refer to this test as the Combination Test.

The weight w is chosen to reflect the assumed proportion of patients in the the first stage. In this section we have assumed that $w = 0.5$. This is also in accordance with the choice of the Pocock boundaries (equally spaced intervals between the interim and final analysis).

The results, obtained from a million simulated trials for each combination of a range of values of N, the total sample size and CV, are given in Table 13.1. Here the true ratio of means on the natural scale is 1.25. The column headed "Combination" gives the results when the Combination Test is used and the column headed "t-tests" gives the results for the usual TOST procedure at the end of the trial.

It should be recalled that the weights used in the Combination Test do not vary and are fixed at 0.5 each. The results under the heading of "No SSR" are for the case where there is no sample size re-estimation at the interim and the results under the heading of "With SSR" are for the case with a sample size re-estimation at the interim. We should also not forget that even for the regular TOST procedure there might be some actual slight inflation (even in the "No SSR" case) since the Pocock boundaries are computed under the assumption of a bivariate normal distribution and not of a bivariate t-distribution.

Looking at the achieved Type I error rates for "No SSR," the majority of rates for both the regular TOST and the Combination Test are all below or just above 0.05 (the excess being caused by simulation variability). However, there are some cases where this rate is as low as about 0.04 and one case (N = 24, CV = 0.40) where the rate is as low as about 0.02. This case corresponds to that illustrated in Figure 13.1 (which has no interim analysis) where we noted that

Table 13.1: Type I error rates for the group sequential design.

		No SSR		With SSR	
N	100×CV	Combination	t-tests	Combination	t-tests
24	10	0.04994	0.05078	0.05010	0.05088
48	10	0.05016	0.05065	0.05013	0.05050
72	10	0.05003	0.05025	0.05025	0.05050
96	10	0.05020	0.05042	0.05047	0.05064
120	10	0.04990	0.05010	0.04992	0.05002
24	20	0.04983	0.05074	0.04940	0.05026
48	20	0.05009	0.05048	0.04953	0.04723
72	20	0.05014	0.05032	0.04993	0.05009
96	20	0.04980	0.05001	0.04965	0.04977
120	20	0.05023	0.05041	0.04985	0.05001
24	30	0.03972	0.04105	0.04058	0.04504
48	30	0.04975	0.05018	0.04957	0.04944
72	30	0.05018	0.05036	0.05011	0.04525
96	30	0.05005	0.05023	0.04986	0.04643
120	30	0.05005	0.05016	0.05009	0.04972
24	40	0.01949	0.02027	0.03242	0.03555
48	40	0.04127	0.04196	0.04208	0.04500
72	40	0.04957	0.04983	0.04968	0.05057
96	40	0.04953	0.04982	0.05007	0.04736
120	40	0.04973	0.04985	0.05017	0.04418

Note: Fixed weight $w = 0.5$. Significance level for both stages = 0.0304. First stage has $N/2$ subjects.

the achieved Type I error rate was much lower than 0.05. Apart from the issue of the potential conservatism of the TOST procedure, the group sequential design performs as expected.

Turning now to the results for "With SSR," we see that these are quite similar to those obtained for "No SSR," suggesting that the introduction of the sample size re-estimation, at least for the combination of values of N and CV considered here, does not inflate the Type I error rate sufficiently to exceed 0.05. Of course, using the Combination Test guarantees that the Type I error rate is not inflated, and so is our preferred method.

In Table 13.2 we give the achieved powers of the "No SSR" and "With SSR" options for the same set of combinations of N and CV as considered above where the true ratio of means on the natural scale is 0.95. Again the results are obtained from a million simulated trials for each combination. The ratio of 0.95 was chosen to enable a comparison with some published results to be discussed in the next chapter. For some combinations of a low N and a high CV, the powers without a sample size re-estimation are quite low, especially for $N = 24$ and CV = 0.4. The effect of the sample size re-estimation is to

Table 13.2: Estimated power for the group sequential design.

		No SSR			With SSR	
N	100×CV	Combination	t-tests		Combination	t-tests
24	10	0.99994	0.99994		0.99911	0.99935
48	10	1	1		1	1
72	10	1	1		1	1
96	10	1	1		1	1
120	10	1	1		1	1
24	20	0.84458	0.85638		0.84639	0.86124
48	20	0.98999	0.99068		0.95984	0.95983
72	20	0.99950	0.99953		0.99909	0.99909
96	20	0.99999	0.99999		0.99997	0.99998
120	20	1	1		0.99999	0.99999
24	30	0.41466	0.43849		0.75466	0.78533
48	30	0.83495	0.84011		0.82871	0.83473
72	30	0.94984	0.95126		0.87239	0.86834
96	30	0.98584	0.98622		0.94461	0.94140
120	30	0.99621	0.99630		0.99131	0.99087
24	40	0.10141	0.10802		0.69742	0.75000
48	40	0.55334	0.56410		0.78082	0.80319
72	40	0.78794	0.79196		0.81682	0.82386
96	40	0.89323	0.89490		0.83519	0.83209
120	40	0.94656	0.94739		0.85590	0.84786

Note: Fixed weight $w = 0.5$. Significance level for both stages = 0.0304. First stage has $N/2$ subjects.

ensure that the power is close to or above 0.80 for almost all cases. For CV = 0.2 a total sample size of N = 24 is already large enough to give very high power.

In summary, we have demonstrated, for the cases considered here, that the Combination Test, while guaranteeing to preserve the Type I error rate, does not lead to a significant loss of power.

13.3 Modification of sample size re-estimation in a group sequential design

A feature of the Combination Test, as used in the previous section, is that the weight w remains fixed (at 0.5) even though the size of the second stage in the trial may be increased or decreased as a result of the sample size re-estimation. In other words, where the sample size has been increased, the second stage results are given lower weight in proportion to their sample size. Looking back to Table 13.2, this does not seem to have had a major impact on the achieved power.

Table 13.3: Estimated Type I error rate and power for the group sequential design and using the Combination Test with variable weights.

		No SSR		With SSR	
N	100×CV	Type I	Power	Type I	Power
24	10	0.04991	0.99994	0.04992	0.99938
48	10	0.05014	1	0.05010	1
72	10	0.05000	1	0.05022	1
96	10	0.05017	1	0.05044	1
120	10	0.04987	1	0.04990	1
24	20	0.04980	0.84446	0.05040	0.85193
48	20	0.05007	0.98997	0.04890	0.96543
72	20	0.05011	0.99950	0.04986	0.99921
96	20	0.04979	0.99999	0.04963	0.99997
120	20	0.05020	1	0.04983	0.99999
24	30	0.03969	0.41435	0.03974	0.75825
48	30	0.04972	0.83484	0.05026	0.83249
72	30	0.05015	0.94980	0.05018	0.88204
96	30	0.05003	0.98583	0.04934	0.95185
120	30	0.05003	0.99620	0.04988	0.99241
24	40	0.01946	0.10125	0.02868	0.71539
48	40	0.04124	0.55311	0.04085	0.78199
72	40	0.04954	0.78781	0.04998	0.81839
96	40	0.04949	0.89313	0.05053	0.84016
120	40	0.04970	0.94651	0.05017	0.86670

Note: Significance level for first stage = 0.0304. Second-stage significance level may vary. First stage has $N/2$ subjects.

A modification that might address this is to recalculate the weights after the interim to reflect the new sample size proportions in stages 1 and 2, and to alter the significance level used for the TOST procedure at the end of the trial. The new significance level must be such that, conditional on the Type I error rate already spent (0.0304), the total Type I error rate spent at the end of the trial is maintained at 0.05. To do this recalculation of the significance level, we use the R code give in the appendix of Chapter 5 of Proschan et al. (2006). Of course, we can no longer guarantee that the Type I error rate will not be inflated. Our motivation is that it may not be increased too much above 0.05, and the resulting power will be greater than when fixed weights are used. The corresponding results to those given in Tables 13.1 and 13.2 are given in Table 13.3.

Comparing Table 13.3 with Tables 13.1 and 13.2, we see that the Type I error rates are quite similar, suggesting that using variable weights does not cause a significant inflation. The powers are slightly higher when variable weights are used, but not significantly so. In conclusion, it seems that using variable weights does not bring any significant benefits in terms of either Type I error rate control or the power.

Chapter 14

Case study: Various methods for an unblinded sample size re-estimation in a bioequivalence study

14.1 Introduction

Here we will describe the four methods proposed by Potvin et al. (2008). For each method it is assumed that an interim analysis will be done after a pre-specified number of subjects (n_1) have completed both periods. At the interim, the unblinded log-transformed data are analyzed and an estimate of the treatment difference and within-subject variance is obtained. Depending on the method, one or more of the following are done: the TOST procedure is applied; the power of the study is recalculated; the sample size is recalculated, and the study stops or continues. If the study continues, with or without a sample size re-estimation, the TOST procedure is applied to the complete set of data from the study. Potvin et al. (2008) compared the methods using simulation under the assumption that the true ratio of the Test and Reference means on the natural scale was either 0.95 (a value consistent with approximate ABE) or 1.25 (i.e., a value consistent with the null hypothesis).

14.1.1 Methods

Method A:

1. At the interim, calculate the power to declare ABE (using the same calculation formula as when planning the study and $\alpha = 0.05$).
2. If the power is ≥ 0.80, apply the TOST procedure with $\alpha = 0.05$ and declare whether ABE is achieved or not. Do not continue to stage 2.
3. If the power is < 0.80, recalculate the sample size so that the power is at least 0.80 for the given estimates of the treatment difference on the log scale and within-subject variance. Continue to stage 2 assuming the revised sample size.
4. At the end of stage 2, apply the TOST procedure with $\alpha = 0.05$ to the combined data from stages 1 and 2 and declare whether ABE is achieved or not.

Potvin et al. (2008) show that the Type I error rate of Method A is inflated for some combinations of n_1 and within-subject coefficient of variation (CV). Taking the illustration in the previous chapter as an example, i.e., $n_1 = 10$ or 20 and a CV of 0.4, the Type I error rate obtained from 100,000 simulated trials was 0.0550 and 0.0546, respectively.

Their Method A is basically an extension of the method described in Chapter 12, but with an unblinded interim analysis and the possibility to stop after the interim and declare whether ABE is achieved or not. Not surprisingly, this method inflates the Type I error rate.

Their Method B is a variation on a group-sequential design with two groups and a significance level for the TOST procedure taken from the Pocock spending function (Pocock (1977)) at each stage. The simulation results of Potvin et al. (2008) indicate that this method is conservative. For our example with $n_1 = 10$ or 20 and a CV of 0.4, the Type I error rate obtained from 100,000 simulated trials was about 0.0339 and 0.0381, respectively.

Method B:

1. Apply the TOST procedure to the first stage data using $\alpha = 0.0294$. If ABE is achieved, then stop and declare ABE.
2. If ABE is not achieved at first stage, evaluate the power to declare ABE using $\alpha = 0.0294$. If power ≥ 0.80, then stop and declare that ABE is not achieved.
3. If power < 0.80, recalculate the samples size to achieve a power of 0.80 with $\alpha = 0.0294$.
4. Apply the TOST procedure to the data from the first and second stages using $\alpha = 0.0294$ and declare if ABE is achieved or not.

Their Method C is a variation on Method B, where $\alpha = 0.05$ is used in the first stage and $\alpha = 0.0294$ is used in the second stage.

Method C:

1. Evaluate the power at the end of the first stage using $\alpha = 0.05$.
2. If power ≥ 0.80, apply the TOST procedure to the first stage data using $\alpha = 0.05$. Declare if ABE is achieved or not and stop.
3. If power < 0.80, apply the TOST procedure to the first stage data using $\alpha = 0.0294$. If ABE is achieved, then stop.
4. If ABE is not achieved using $\alpha = 0.0294$, recalculate the sample size to achieve a power of 0.80 with $\alpha = 0.0294$.
5. Apply the TOST procedure to the data from the first and second stages using $\alpha = 0.0294$ and declare if ABE is achieved or not.

Of course, this variation has the potential to inflate the Type I error rate compared to Method B. Potvin et al. (2008) noted that inflation occurred for CV = 0.1 and 0.20, but not for higher values of the CV. These results are reflected in our example with $n_1 = 10$ or 20 and a CV of 0.4, where the Type I error rate obtained from 100,000 simulated trials was about 0.0315 and 0.0325, respectively.

The power (obtained by simulation) of the Methods B and C, as applied to our example, were, respectively, 0.709 and 0.708 for $n_1 = 10$ and 0.790 and 0.777, respectively, for $n_1 = 20$. The corresponding average sample sizes were 62.77 and 62.98, respectively, for $n_1 = 10$ and 61.90 and 62.88, respectively, for $n_1 = 20$.

Potvin et al. (2008) also introduced a Method D, which is the same as Method C but uses a slightly more conservative $\alpha = 0.028$ instead of $\alpha = 0.0294$. Overall, Potvin et al. (2008) recommended Method C, given its minimal amount of Type I error rate inflation (i.e., a rate no greater than 0.052).

In a follow-up paper, Montague et al. (2012) repeated the simulation study of Potvin et al. (2008) but with an assumed true ratio of means equal to 0.90, instead of 0.95, as used in Potvin et al. (2008). One conclusion from this later study was that for CV $\leq$ 0.5, Methods B and C had Type I error rates that exceeded 0.052. In addition, the Type I error rates for Method D were no larger than 0.052 for any of the values of CV (0.10 to 1.0) used in the simulation study.

In conclusion, we recommend that before using any of the methods suggested by Potvin et al. (2008), their operating characteristics should be evaluated for a range of values of n_1, CV and true ratio of means that are of interest, in order to decide if the Type I error rate is controlled, the power is adequate and the potential maximum total sample size is not too great. Of course, we should not forget that the adaptive group sequential design that uses the Combination Test (see previous chapter) is a simple alternative that guarantees control of the Type I error rate.

14.2 Example

As an illustration, we will apply Methods B and C to the interim data set given in Table 12.1 in Chapter 12. The unblinded estimate of σ at the interim is 0.397, i.e., a CV of 0.413.

If we use Method B, then we first apply the TOST procedure with $\alpha = 0.0294$. The corresponding 94.12% confidence interval for the true ratio of means is (0.814, 1.350), so ABE is not achieved at the interim. Using the PowerTost (Labes (2013)) R library function, the power, for a true ratio of 1, for this estimated CV and a total sample size of 20 is just over 0.04. Hence we must continue to recalculate the sample size and generate data for stage 2. Again, using the PowerTost R library with $\alpha = 0.0294$, the recalculated sample size, for a true ratio of 1, is a total of 66 subjects. So the second stage will require

Table 14.1: Additional post-interim data for ABE trial.

Group RT				Group TR		
	Period				Period	
Subject	1	2		Subject	1	2
59	127.028	78.841		63	51.796	87.500
60	44.549	58.087		64	62.571	79.687
61	226.697	157.255		65	187.575	155.026
62	29.372	67.988		66	110.383	77.101

46 subjects. This is larger than the total of 58 subjects required after the BSSR described in Chapter 12.

We add the simulated data in Table 14.1 to that in Table 12.2 to give the complete second-stage data for the Potvin Method B analysis. The 94.12% confidence interval obtained using the combined data from both stages is (0.871, 1.098) and ABE is achieved for AUC.

If we apply Method C, then we first calculate the power using $\alpha = 0.05$. This is much lower than 0.80 and so we must test for ABE using $\alpha = 0.0294$. We already know that ABE is not achieved with $\alpha = 0.0294$, so we would proceed as for Method B, i.e., recalculate the sample size, complete stage 2 and test for ABE.

Appendix A

Least squares estimation

In this book we have generally been concerned with inference about effects associated with treatments, such as direct treatment and carry-over effects. On those occasions when we need explicit expressions for estimators of these effects, to be able to compare designs for example, we want to obtain them by the simplest route. In this appendix we show how the correct expressions can be derived in several ways using different models for the expectations of (continuous) cross-over data. In this context the use of different models is an artifice to obtain simple derivations of estimators of effects; it does not imply that analyses based on different models would be equivalent. In particular, it is easier to manipulate models with sequence (group) effects rather than subject effects, and we show below how each leads to equivalent estimators, but analyses based on the two types of models would not lead to the same estimates of error. We demonstrate equivalences for the following three cases:

1. a model that contains a different parameter for each subject (fixed subject effects);
2. a model with sequence effects but no subject effects;
3. a model for the contrasts between the means for each period in each sequence group.

We will be deriving expressions for **Generalized Least Squares (GLS)** estimators under a general covariance matrix Σ for the repeated measurements from a subject. This general framework contains as a special case, **Ordinary Least Squares (OLS)** estimation and includes the analyses described in Chapter 5. It is assumed that we have a cross-over design with s sequence groups, p periods and n_i subjects in each group and let $n = \sum n_i$.

A.0.1 Case 1

Let ϕ_{ik} denote the subject *parameter* for subject k on sequence i. In terms of the intercept μ and subject effects s_{ik} used in Chapter 5,

$$\phi_{ik} = \mu + s_{ik}.$$

Set $\phi_i = [\phi_{i1}, \phi_{i2}, \ldots, \phi_{in_i}]^T$ and $\phi = [\phi_1^T, \phi_2^T \ldots, \phi_s^T]^T$. We can then write

$$\mathrm{E}(\mathbf{Y}) = [\mathbf{I}_n \otimes \mathbf{j}_p, \mathbf{X}] \left[\begin{array}{c} \phi \\ \beta \end{array} \right] = \mathbf{X}_* \psi_1,$$

say, where $\otimes$ is the right Kronecker product, $\mathbf{j}_p$ is a $(p \times 1)$ vector of 1's, and the $(v \times 1)$ vector

$$\beta = \begin{bmatrix} \pi \\ \xi \end{bmatrix}$$

consists of period *effects* π and treatment and other treatment-related *effects* ξ, with associated full rank design matrix $\mathbf{X}$. If $\mathbf{X}_i$ is the $(p \times v)$ design matrix that applies to each subject in group i, then we can write,

$$\mathbf{X} = [\mathbf{j}_{n_1}^T \otimes \mathbf{X}_1^T, \ldots, \mathbf{j}_{n_s}^T \otimes \mathbf{X}_s^T].$$

Also we have

$$\mathrm{V}(\mathbf{Y}) = \mathbf{V} = \mathbf{I}_n \otimes \Sigma.$$

Now, in this case, the GLS estimator of ψ_1 is

$$\begin{aligned} \hat{\psi}_1 &= \begin{bmatrix} \hat{\phi} \\ \hat{\beta}_1 \end{bmatrix} = (\mathbf{X}_*{}^T \mathbf{V}^{-1} \mathbf{X}_*)^{-1} \mathbf{X}_*{}^T \mathbf{V}^{-1} \mathbf{Y} \\ &= \begin{bmatrix} \mathbf{A}_1 & \mathbf{B}_1 \\ \mathbf{B}_1^T & \mathbf{C} \end{bmatrix}^{-1} \begin{bmatrix} \mathbf{Q}_1 \\ \mathbf{P} \end{bmatrix}, \end{aligned}$$

where

$$\begin{aligned} \mathbf{A}_1 &= \mathbf{j}_p^T \Sigma^{-1} \mathbf{j}_p \mathbf{I}_n, \\ \mathbf{B}_1 &= [\mathbf{j}_{n_1}^T \otimes \mathbf{X}_1^T \Sigma^{-1} \mathbf{j}_p, \ldots, \mathbf{j}_{n_s}^T \otimes \mathbf{X}_s^T \Sigma^{-1} \mathbf{j}_p], \\ \mathbf{C} &= \sum_{i=1}^{s} n_i \mathbf{X}_i^T \Sigma^{-1} \mathbf{X}_i, \\ \mathbf{Q}_1 &= [\mathbf{j}_p^T \Sigma^{-1} \mathbf{Y}_{11}, \ldots, \mathbf{j}_p^T \Sigma^{-1} \mathbf{Y}_{sn_s}], \text{ and} \\ \mathbf{P} &= \sum_{i=1}^{s} n_i \mathbf{X}_i^T \Sigma^{-1} \overline{\mathbf{Y}}_i. \end{aligned}$$

for $\mathbf{Y}_{ik} = [Y_{i1k}, Y_{i2k}, \ldots, Y_{ipk}]^T$.

We are directly interested in the estimator $\hat{\beta}_1$. Using standard matrix results we have

$$\begin{aligned} \hat{\beta}_1 &= (\mathbf{C} - \mathbf{B}_1^T \mathbf{A}^{-1} \mathbf{B}_1)^{-1} (\mathbf{P} - \mathbf{B}_1^T \mathbf{A}_1^{-1} \mathbf{Q}_1) \\ &= \left(\sum_{i=1}^{s} n_i \mathbf{X}_i^T \mathbf{H}_\Sigma \mathbf{X}_i \right)^{-1} \sum_{i=1}^{s} n_i \mathbf{X}_i^T \mathbf{H}_\Sigma \overline{\mathbf{Y}}_{i,\cdot}, \end{aligned} \tag{A.1}$$

where

$$\mathbf{H}_\Sigma = \Sigma^{-1} - \Sigma^{-1} \mathbf{j}_p (\mathbf{j}_p^T \Sigma^{-1} \mathbf{j}_p)^{-1} \mathbf{j}_p^T \Sigma^{-1}.$$

Using a standard matrix equality we can also write

$$\mathbf{H}_\Sigma = \mathbf{K} (\mathbf{K}^T \Sigma \mathbf{K})^{-1} \mathbf{K}^T \tag{A.2}$$

where $\mathbf{K}$ is any $p \times (p-1)$ matrix of full rank satisfying

$$\mathbf{K}^T \mathbf{j}_p = \mathbf{0}.$$

In other words, the columns of $\mathbf{K}$ constitute a complete set of contrasts among the p periods.

A.0.2 *Case 2*

To obtain the required model for Case 2 we replace ϕ_{ik} by the corresponding sequence parameter γ_i. We then have

$$\mathrm{E}(\mathbf{Y}) = \mathbf{X}_G \phi_2,$$

where $\mathbf{X}_G = [\mathrm{diag}(j_{pn_1}, \ldots, j_{pn_s}), \mathbf{X}]$ and $\phi_2 = [\gamma^T, \beta^T]^T$, for $\gamma = [\gamma_1, \ldots, \gamma_s]^T$. The GLS estimator of ϕ_2 is

$$\begin{aligned} \hat{\psi}_2 &= \begin{bmatrix} \hat{\phi} \\ \hat{\beta}_2 \end{bmatrix} = (\mathbf{X}_G^T \mathbf{V}^{-1} \mathbf{X}_G)^{-1} \mathbf{X}_G^T \mathbf{V}^{-1} \mathbf{Y} \\ &= \begin{bmatrix} \mathbf{A}_2 & \mathbf{B}_2 \\ \mathbf{B}_2^T & \mathbf{C} \end{bmatrix}^{-1} \begin{bmatrix} \mathbf{Q}_2 \\ \mathbf{P} \end{bmatrix}, \end{aligned}$$

where

$$\begin{aligned} \mathbf{A}_2 &= \mathrm{diag}[n_1 \mathbf{j}_p^T \Sigma^{-1} \mathbf{j}_p, \ldots, n_s \mathbf{j}_p^T \Sigma^{-1} \mathbf{j}_p], \\ \mathbf{B}_2 &= [n_1 \mathbf{X}_1^T \Sigma^{-1} \mathbf{j}_p, \ldots, n_1 \mathbf{X}_s^T \Sigma^{-1} \mathbf{j}_p], \text{ and} \\ \mathbf{Q}_2 &= [n_1 \mathbf{j}_p^T \Sigma^{-1} \overline{\mathbf{Y}}_{1\cdot}, \ldots, n_s \mathbf{j}_p^T \Sigma^{-1} \overline{\mathbf{Y}}_{s\cdot}] \end{aligned}$$

From this we obtain,

$$\hat{\beta}_2 = \left(\sum_{i=1}^{s} n_i \mathbf{X}_i^T \mathbf{H}_\Sigma \mathbf{X}_i \right)^{-1} \sum_{i=1}^{s} n_i \mathbf{X}_i^T \mathbf{H}_\Sigma \overline{\mathbf{Y}}_{i\cdot},$$

the same expression as in (A.1) above, that is, $\hat{\beta}_1 = \hat{\beta}_2$.

A.0.3 *Case 3*

Instead of modeling the raw data, $\mathbf{Y}$, we now obtain GLS estimators directly from sets of within-subject contrast means defined by $\mathbf{K}^T \overline{\mathbf{Y}}_{i\cdot}$, for $\mathbf{K}$ the matrix defined above in Case 1. Because $\mathbf{K}^T \mathbf{j}_p = \mathbf{0}$, we have

$$\mathrm{E}(\mathbf{K}^T \overline{\mathbf{Y}}_{i\cdot}) = \mathbf{K}^T \mathbf{X}_i \beta$$

under the models defined in both Cases 1 and 2 above. Also we have,

$$\mathrm{V}(\mathbf{K}^T\overline{\mathbf{Y}}_{i\cdot}) = \frac{1}{n_i}\mathbf{K}^T\Sigma\mathbf{K}.$$

Defining

$$\mathbf{X}_K = \begin{bmatrix} \mathbf{K}^T\mathbf{X}_1 \\ \vdots \\ \mathbf{K}^T\mathbf{X}_s \end{bmatrix}, \quad \overline{\mathbf{Y}}_K = \begin{bmatrix} \mathbf{K}^T\overline{\mathbf{Y}}_{1\cdot} \\ \vdots \\ \mathbf{K}^T\overline{\mathbf{Y}}_{s\cdot} \end{bmatrix},$$

and

$$\mathbf{V}_K = \mathrm{diag}[n_1^{-1}\mathbf{K}^T\Sigma\mathbf{K},\ldots,n_s^{-1}\mathbf{K}^T\Sigma\mathbf{K}],$$

we can write the GLS estimator of β as

$$\begin{aligned} \hat{\beta}_3 &= (\mathbf{X}_K^T\mathbf{V}_K^{-1}\mathbf{X}_K)^{-1}\mathbf{X}_K^T\mathbf{V}_K^{-1}\overline{\mathbf{Y}}_K \\ &= \left(\sum_{i=1}^{s} n_i\mathbf{X}_i^T\mathbf{K}(\mathbf{K}^T\Sigma\mathbf{K})^{-1}\mathbf{K}^T\mathbf{X}_i\right)^{-1} \sum_{i=1}^{s} n_i\mathbf{X}_i^T\mathbf{K}(\mathbf{K}^T\Sigma\mathbf{K})^{-1}\mathbf{K}^T\overline{\mathbf{Y}}_{i\cdot}, \end{aligned}$$

which is equivalent to the expression for $\hat{\beta}_1$ is (A.1) with $\mathbf{H}_\Sigma$ as defined in (A.2). We would also obtain the same GLS estimator by modeling the contrasts from each subject, $[\mathbf{I}_n \otimes \mathbf{K}^T]\mathbf{Y}$ with covariance matrix $[\mathbf{I}_n \otimes \mathbf{K}^T\Sigma\mathbf{K}]$.

Bibliography

Afsarinejad, K. (1983). Balanced repeated measurements designs. *Biometrika*, 70:199–204.

Afsarinejad, K. (1990). Repeated measurement designs — A review. *Communication in Statistics — Theory and Methods*, 19(11):3985–4028.

Afsarinejad, K. and Hedayat, A. S. (2002). Repeated measurements designs for a model with self and simple mixed carryover effects. *Journal of Statistical Planning and Inference*, 106:449–459.

Agresti, A. (1989). A survey of models for repeated ordered categorical response data. *Statistics in Medicine*, 8:1029–1224.

Agresti, A. and Lang, J. B. (1993). Quasi-symmetric latent class models, with application to rater agreement. *Biometrics*, 49:131–139.

Agresti, A., Lang, J. B., and Mehta, C. R. (1993). Some empirical comparisons of exact, modified exact, and higher-order asymptotic tests of independence for ordered categorical variables. *Communications in Statistics, Simulation and Computation*, 22:1–18.

Altan, S., McCartney, M., and Raghavarao, D. (1996). Two methods of analyses for a complex behavioural experiment. *Journal of Biopharmaceutical Statistics*, 4:437–447.

Altham, P. M. E. (1971). The analysis of matched proportions. *Biometrika*, 58:561–676.

Anderson, I. and Preece, D. A. (2002). Locally balanced change-over designs. *Utilitas Mathematica*, 62:33–59.

Ansersen, E. B. (1977). Sufficient statistics and latent trait models. *Psychometrika*, 42:69–81.

Archdeacon, D. S., Dinitz, J. H., Stinson, D. R., and Tillson, T. W. (1980). Some new row-complete Latin squares. *Journal of Combinatorial Theory, Series A*, 29:395–398.

Armitage, P. (1955). Tests for linear trends in proportions and frequencies. *Biometrics*, 11:375–386.

Armitage, P. (1996). Design and analysis of clinical trials. In Gosh, S. and Rao, C. R., editors, *Handbook of Statistics 13: Design and Analysis of Clinical Trials*, pages 63–90. Elsevier Science B.V., Amsterdam.

Armitage, P. and Berry, G. (1987). *Statistical Methods in Medical Research.* Blackwell Scientific Publications: Oxford.

Atkinson, G. F. (1966). Designs for sequences of treatments with carry-over effects. *Biometrics*, 22:292–309.

Bailey, R. A. (1984). Quasi-complete Latin squares: construction and randomization. *Journal of the Royal Statistical Society, Series B*, 46:323–334.

Balaam, L. N. (1968). A two-period design with t^2 experimental units. *Biometrics*, 24:61–73.

Bate, S. T. and Jones, B. (2006). The construction of nearly balanced and nearly strongly balanced uniform cross-over designs. *Journal of Statistical Planning and Inference*, 136:3248–3267.

Bate, S. T. and Jones, B. (2008). A review of uniform cross-over designs. *Journal of Statistical Planning and Inference*, 138:336–351.

Bellavance, F., Tardif, S., and Stephens, M. A. (1996). Tests for the analysis of variance of crossover designs with correlated errors. *Biometrics*, 52:608–612.

Berenblut, I. I. (1964). Change-over designs with complete balance for first residual effects. *Biometrics*, 20:707–712.

Berenblut, I. I. (1967a). A change-over design for testing a treatment factor at four equally spaced levels. *Journal of the Royal Statistical Society, Series B*, 29:370–373.

Berenblut, I. I. (1967b). The analysis of change-over designs with complete balance for first residual effects. *Biometrics*, 23:578–580.

Berenblut, I. I. (1968). Change-over designs balanced for the linear component of first residual effects. *Biometrika*, 55:297–303.

Birkett, M. A. and Day, S. J. (1994). Internal pilot studies for estimating sample size. *Statistics in Medicine*, 13:2455–2463.

Bishop, S. H. and Jones, B. (1984). A review of higher order crossover designs. *Journal of Applied Statistics*, 11(1):29–50.

Biswas, N. (1997). *Some results on residual effects designs.* PhD thesis, Temple University, Philadelphia, PA.

Biswas, N. and Raghavarao, D. (1998). Construction of rectangular and group divisible partially balanced residual effects designs by the method of differences. *Journal of Combinatorics, Information and System Sciences*, 23:135–141.

Blaisdell, E. A. (1978). *Partially balanced residual effects designs.* PhD thesis, Temple University, Philadelphia, PA.

Blaisdell, E. A. and Raghavarao, D. (1980). Partially balanced changeover designs based on m-associate class pbib designs. *Journal of the Royal Statistical Society, Series B*, 42:334–338.

Bornkamp, B., Bretz, F., and Pinhiero, J. (2014). R package: Dosefinding. *CRAN.*

Bornkamp, B., Pinheiro, J., and Bretz, F. (2009). MCPMod: An R package for the design and analysis of dose-finding studies. *Journal of Statistical Software*, 29:1–23.

Bose, M. and Dey, A. (2009). *Optimal Crossover Designs.* World Scientific, Singapore.

Bose, M. and Dey, A. (2013). Developments in crossover designs. *http://www.isid.ac.in/ statmath/2013/isid201307.pdf.*

Bose, R. C. and Shimamoto, T. (1952). Classification and analysis of partially balanced incomplete block designs. *Journal of the American Statistical Association*, 47:151–184.

Box, G. E. P. (1954a). Some theorems on quadratic forms applied in the study of analysis of variance problems. Effect of inequality of variance in the one-way classification. *Annals of Mathematical Statistics*, 25:290–302.

Box, G. E. P. (1954b). Some theorems on quadratic forms applied in the study of analysis of variance problems. Effects of inequality of variance and of correlations between errors in the two way classification. *Annals of Mathematical Statistics*, 25:484–498.

Bradley, J. V. (1958). Complete counterbalancing of immediate sequential effects in a Latin square design. *Journal of the American Statistical Association*, 53:525–528.

Brandt, A. E. (1938). Tests of significance in reversal or switchback trials. *Research Bulletin No. 234, Iowa Agricultural Experimental Station.*

Breslow, N. E. and Day, N. E. (1980). *Statistical Methods in Cancer Research – Volume 1.* International Agency for Cancer Research: Lyon.

Bretz, F., Pinheiro, J. C., and Branson, M. (2005). Combining multiple comparisons and modelling techniques in dose-response studies. *Biometrics*, 61:738–748.

Carlin, B. P. and Louis, T. A. (1996). *Bayes and Empirical Bayes Methods for Data Analysis.* Chapman and Hall/CRC: New York.

Carpenter, J. R. and Kenward, M. G. (2008). *Missing Data in Randomised Controlled Trials – A Practical Guide.* UK NHS (NCCRM), Birmingham, UK.

Chassan, J. B. (1964). On the analysis of simple cross-overs with unequal numbers of replicates. *Biometrics*, 20:206–208.

Cheng, C. S. and Wu, C. F. (1980). Balanced repeated measurements designs. *Annals of Statistics*, 8:1272–1283, 11:349.

Ciminera, J. L. and Wolfe, R. K. (1953). An example of the use of extended cross-over designs in the comparison of NPH insulin mixtures. *Biometrics*, 9:431–446.

Clatworthy, W. H. (1973). Tables of two-associate partially balanced designs. *National Bureau of Standards Applied Mathematics Series No. 63, U.S. Department of Commerce.*

Cochran, W. G. (1939). Long-term agricultural experiments (with discussion). *Journal of the Royal Statistical Society, Series B*, 6:104–148.

Cochran, W. G., Autrey, K. M., and Cannon, C. Y. (1941). A double change-over design for dairy cattle feeding experiments. *Journal of Dairy Science*, 24:937–951.

Collombier, D. and Merchermek, I. (1993). Optimal cross-over experimental designs. *Indian Journal of Statistics Series B*, 55:249–161.

Conaway, M. R. (1989). Analysis of repeated categorical measurements with conditional likelihood methods. *Journal of the American Statistical Association*, 84:53–62.

Cook, R. D. and Weisberg, S. (1982). *Residuals and Influence in Regression.* Chapman and Hall: New York.

Cornell, R. G. (1980). Evaluation of bioavailability data using non-parametric statistics. In Albert, K. S., editor, *Drug Absorption and Disposition: Statistical Considerations*, pages 51–57. American Pharmaceutical Association.

Cornell, R. G. (1991). Nonparametric tests of dispersion for the two-period crossover design. *Communications in Statistics, A*, 20:1099–1106.

Cotter, S. C., John, J. A., and Smith, T. M. F. (1973). Multi-factor experiments in non-orthogonal designs. *Journal of the Royal Statistical Society, Series B*, 35:361–367.

Cotton, J. W. (1998). *Analyzing Within-Subjects Experiments.* Lawrence Erlbaum Associates: Mahwah, New Jersey.

Cox, D. R. (1972). Regression models and life tables (with discussion). *Journal of the Royal Statistical Society, Series B*, 34:187–220.

Cox, D. R. (1984). Interaction. *International Statistical Review*, 52:1–31.

Cox, D. R. and Reid, N. (2000). *The Theory of the Design of Experiments.* Chapman and Hall/CRC: London.

Cox, D. R. and Snell, E. J. (1989). *Analysis of Binary Data.* Chapman and Hall: London.

Cramer, J. S. (1991). *The Logit Model — An Introduction for Economists.* Edward Arnold: London.

Crowder, M. (1995). On the use of a working correlation matrix in using generalised linear models for repeated measures. *Biometrika*, 82:407–410.

Cui, L., Hung, H. M. J., and Wang, S.-J. (1999). Modification of sample size in group sequential trials. *Biometrics*, 55:853–857.

Curtin, F. C., Elbourne, D., and Altman, D. G. (1995). Meta-analysis combining parallel and cross-over clinical trials. II: Binary outcomes. *Biometrika*, 82:407–410.

Cytel (1995). *StatXact 3 for Windows: Statistical Software for Exact Nonparametric Inference (User Manual).* Cytel Software Corporation, Cambridge, MA.

Davis, A. W. and Hall, W. B. (1969). Cyclic change-over designs. *Biometrika*, 56(2):283–293.

Dean, A. M., Lewis, S. M., and Chang, J. Y. (1999). Nested changeover designs. *Journal of Statistical Planning and Inference*, 77(2):337–351.

DeMets, D. (2002). Clinical trials in the new millennium. *Statistics in Medicine*, 21:2779–2787.

Diggle, P. J., Heagerty, P., Liang, K. Y., and Zeger, S. L. (2002). *Analysis of Longitudinal Data, Second Edition.* Oxford University Press: Oxford.

Donev, A. N. (1997). An algorithm for the construction of crossover trials. *Applied Statistics*, 46(2):288–298.

Donev, A. N. and Jones, B. (1995). Construction of A-optimal designs. In Kitsos, C. P. and Mueller, W. G., editors, *MODA4 — Advances in Model-Oriented Data Analysis*, pages 165–171. Heidelberg, Physica-Verlag.

Dunsmore, I. R. (1981). Growth curves in two-period change-over models. *Applied Statistics*, 30:575–578.

Ebbutt, A. F. (1984). Three-period crossover designs for two treatments. *Biometrics*, 40:219–224.

Eccleston, J. and Street, D. (1994). An algorithm for the construction of optimal or near optimal change-over designs. *Australian Journal of Statistics*, 36(3):371–378.

Eccleston, J. and Whitaker, D. (1999). On the design of optimal change-over experiments through multi-objective simulated annealing. *Statistics and Computing*, 9(1):37–41.

EMA (2010). CHMP Guideline on the Investigation of Bioequivalence. *European Medicines Agency.*

EMA (2014). Draft Qualification Opinion of MCP-Mod as an efficient statistical methodology for model-based design and analysis of Phase II dose finding studies under model uncertainty. *European Medicines Agency (EMA).*

Farewell, V. T. (1985). Some remarks on the analysis of cross-over trials with a binary response. *Applied Statistics*, 34:121–128.

Fay, M. P. and Graubard, B. I. (2001). Small-sample adjustments for Wald-type tests using sandwich estimators. *Biometrics*, 57:1198–1206.

FDA (1992). FDA Guidance: Statistical procedures for bioequivalence studies using a standard two treatment cross-over design.

FDA (1997). FDA Draft Guidance: In vivo bioequivalence studies based on population and individual bioequivalence approaches.

FDA (1999a). FDA Draft Guidance: Average, population, and individual approaches to establishing bioequivalence.

FDA (1999b). FDA Draft Guidance: BA and BE studies for orally administered drug products: General considerations.

FDA (2000). FDA Guidance: Bioavailability and bioequivalence studies for orally administered drug products: General considerations.

FDA (2001). FDA Guidance: Statistical approaches to establishing bioequivalence.

FDA (2002). FDA Revised Guidance: Bioavailability and bioequivalence studies for orally administered drug products: General considerations.

FDA (2013). Draft Guidance on Loteprednol Etabonate. *USA Food and Drug Administration.*

Federer, W. T. (1955). *Experimental Design – Theory and Application.* Macmillan: New York.

Federer, W. T. and Atkinson, G. F. (1964). Tied-double-change-over designs. *Biometrics*, 20:168–181.

Fedorov, V. V., Jones, B., and Leonov, S. L. (2002). PK cross-over model with cost constraints. Presentation at Joint Statistical Meetings, New York, 2002.

Fieller, E. C. (1940). The biological standardization of insulin (with discussion). *Supplement of the Journal of the Royal Statistical Society*, 7:1–64.

Finney, D. J. (1956). Cross-over designs in bioassay. *Proceedings of the Royal Society, Series B*, 145:42–60.

Finney, D. J. and Outhwaite, A. D. (1955). Serially balanced sequences. *Nature*, 176:748.

Finney, D. J. and Outhwaite, A. D. (1956). Serially balanced sequences in bioassay. *Proceedings of the Royal Society, Series B*, 145:493–507.

Fisher, L. D. (1998). Self-designing clinical trials. *Statistics in Medicine*, 17:1551–1562.

Fleiss, J. L. (1986). On multiperiod crossover studies. Letter to the editor. *Biometrics*, 42:449–450.

Fletcher, D. and John, J. (1985). Changeover designs and factorial structure. *Journal of the Royal Statistical Society, Series B*, 47:117–124.

Fletcher, D. J. (1987). A new class of change-over designs for factorial experiments. *Biometrika*, 74:649–654.

Fluehler, H., Grieve, A. P., Mandallaz, D., Mau, J., and Moser, H. A. (1983). Bayesian approach to bioequivalence assessment: an example. *Journal of Pharmaceutical Sciences*, 72:1178–1181.

Ford, I., Norrie, J., and Ahmadi, S. (1995). Model inconsistency, illustrated by the Cox proportional hazards model. *Statistics in Medicine*, 14:735–746.

France, L. A., Lewis, J. A., and Kay, R. (1991). The analysis of failure time data in crossover studies. *Statistics in Medicine*, 10:1099–1113.

Freeman, P. (1989). The performance of the two-stage analysis of two treatment, two period crossover trials. *Statistics in Medicine*, 8:1421–1432.

Friede, T. and Kieser, M. (2003). Blinded sample size reassessment in non-inferiority and equivalence trials. *Statistics in Medicine*, 22:995–1007.

Friedman, L. M., Furberg, C. D., and DeMets, D. L. (1998). *Fundamentals of Clinical Trials (3rd edition).* Springer-Verlag: Heidelberg.

Fuglsang, A. (2013). Sequential bioequivalence trial designs with increased power and control of type I error rates. *The AAPS Journal*, 15:659–661.

Fuglsang, A. (2014). Futility rules in bioequivalence trials with sequential designs. *The AAPS Journal*, 16:79–82.

Gail, M. H., Wineand, S., and Piantadosi, S. (1984). Biased estimates of treatment effect in randomized experiments with non linear regressions. *Biometrika*, 71:431–444.

Gamerman, D. and Lopes, H.F. (2006). *Markov Chain Monte Carlo. Second Edition.* Chapman and Hall/CRC: London.

Gart, J. J. (1969). An exact test for comparing matched proportions in crossover designs. *Biometrika*, 56:75–80.

Gelman, A., Carlin, J. B., Stern, H. S., and Rubin, D. B. (1995). *Bayesian Data Analysis.* Chapman and Hall/CRC: New York.

Gibbons, J. D. (1985). *Nonparametric Statistical Inference.* Marcel Dekker: New York.

Gilks, W. R., Richardson, S., and Spiegelhalter, D. J. (1996). *Markov Chain Monte Carlo in Practice.* Chapman and Hall/CRC: London.

Golkowski, D. (2011). Blinded sample size re-assessment in cross-over bioequivalence trials. *Diploma Thesis in Mathematics, University of Heidelberg.*

Golkowski, D., Friede, T., and Kieser, M. (2014). Blinded sample size re-estimation in crossover bioequivalence trials. *Pharmaceutical Statistics*, 13:157–162.

Gould, A. L. (1995). Group sequential extensions of a standard bioequivalence testing procedure. *Journal of Pharmacokinetics and Biopharmaceutics*, 23:57–86.

Grieve, A. P. (1982). The two-period changeover design in clinical trials. Letter to the editor. *Biometrics*, 38:517.

Grieve, A. P. (1985). A Bayesian analysis of the two-period changeover design in clinical trials. *Biometrics*, 41:979–990.

Grieve, A. P. (1986). Corrigenda to Grieve (1985). *Biometrics*, 42:459.

Grieve, A. P. (1987). Application of Bayesian software: two examples. *The Statistician*, 36:282–288.

Grieve, A. P. (1990). Crossover vs parallel designs. In Berry, D. A., editor, *Statistical Methodology in the Pharmaceutical Sciences*, pages 239–270. Marcel Dekker: New York.

Grieve, A. P. (1994a). Bayesian analyses of two-treatment crossover studies. *Statistical Methods in Medical Research*, 3:407–429.

Grieve, A. P. (1994b). Extending a Bayesian analysis of the two-period crossover to allow for baseline measurements. *Statistics in Medicine*, 13:905–929.

Grizzle, J. E. (1965). The two-period change-over design and its use in clinical trials. *Biometrics*, 21:467–480.

Grizzle, J. E. (1974). Corrigenda to Grizzle (1965). *Biometrics*, 30:727.

Grizzle, J. E., Starmer, C. F., and Koch, G. G. (1969). Analysis of categorical data by linear models. *Biometrics*, 25:189–195.

Hauck, W. W., Hyslop, T. F., Anderson, S., Bois, F. Y., and Tozer, T. N. (1995). Statistical and regulatory considerations for multiple measures in bioequivalence testing. *Clinical Research and Regulatory Affairs*, 12:249–265.

Hauck, W. W., Preston, P. E., and Bois, P. E. (1997). A group sequential approach to crossover trials for average bioequivalence. *Journal of Biopharmaceutical Statistics*, 7:87–96.

Health Canada (2012). Guidance Document: Conduct and Analysis of Comparative Bioavailability Studies. *Health Canada*.

Hedayat, A. S. and Afsarinejad, K. (1975). Repeated measurements designs. I. In Srivastava, J. N., editor, *A Survey of Statistical Design and Linear Models*, pages 229–242. North-Holland:Amsterdam.

Hedayat, A. S. and Afsarinejad, K. (1978). Repeated measurements designs, II. *Annals of Statistics*, 6:619–628.

Hedayat, A. S. Jacroux, M., and Majumdar, D. (1988). Optimal designs for comparing test treatments with controls. *Statistical Science*, 3:462–491.

Hedayat, A. S. and Zhao, W. (1990). Optimal two-period repeated measurements designs. *Annals of Statistics*, 18:1805–1816.

Hills, M. and Armitage, P. (1979). The two-period cross-over clinical trial. *British Journal of Clinical Pharmacology*, 8:7–20.

Ho, W.-K., Matthews, J. N. S., Henderson, R., Farewell, D. M., and Rogers, L. R. (2013). Two-period, two-treatment crossover designs subject to non-ignorable missing data. *Statistics in Medicine*, 31:1675–1687.

Hodges, J. L. and Lehman, E. L. (1963). Estimates of location based on rank tests. *Annals of Mathematical Statistics*, 34:598–611.

Hollander, M. and Wolfe, D. A. (1999). *Nonparametric Statistical Methods.* Wiley: New York.

Hunter, K. R., Stern, G. M., Lawrence, D. R., and Armitage, P. (1970). Amantadine in Parkinsonism. *Lancet*, i:1127–1129.

Iqbal, I. and Jones, B. (1994). Efficient repeated measurements designs with equal and unequal period sizes. *Journal of Statistical Planning and Inference*, 42(1-2):79–88.

Isaac, P. D., Dean, A. M., and Ostrum, A. (1999). Sequentially counterbalanced Latin squares. *Technical Report No. 644. The Ohio State University, Columbus.*

Jennison, C. and Turnbull, B. W. (2003). Mid-course sample size modification in clinical trials based on the observed treatment effect. *Statistics in Medicine*, 22:971–993.

John, J. A. (1973). Generalized cyclic designs in factorial experiments. *Biometrika*, 60:55–63.

John, J. A. and Russell, K. G. (2002). A unified theory for the construction of crossover designs. Unpublished manuscript.

John, J. A. and Russell, K. G. (2003). Optimising changeover designs using the average efficiency factors. *Journal of Statistical Planning and Inference*, 113:259–268.

John, J. A. and Whitaker, D. (2002). CrossOver: An algorithm for the construction of efficient crossover designs. Unpublished manuscript.

John, P. W. (1971). *Statistical Design and Analysis of Experiments.* Macmillan: New York.

Jones, B. (1985). Using bricks to build block designs. *Journal of the Royal Statistical Society, Series B*, 47:349–356.

Jones, B. and Deppe, C. (2001). Recent developments in the design of cross-over trials: a brief review and bibliography. In Altan, S. and Singh, J., editors, *Recent Advances in Experimental Designs and Related Topics*, pages 153–173. Nova Science Publishers, Inc.: New York.

Jones, B. and Donev, A. N. (1996). Modelling and design of cross-over trials. *Statistics in Medicine*, 15:1435–1446.

Jones, B. and Kenward, M. G. (1989). *Design and Analysis of Cross-over Trials.* Chapman and Hall: London.

Jones, B., Kunert, J., and Wynn, H. P. (1992). Information matrices for mixed effects models with applications to the optimality of repeated measurements designs. *Journal of Statistical Planning and Inference*, 33:361–274.

Jones, B. and Wang, J. (1999). Constructing optimal designs for fitting pharmacokinetic models. *Computing and Statistics*, 9:209–218.

Jung, J. W. and Koch, G. G. (1999). Multivariate non-parametric methods for Mann-Whitney statistics to analyse cross-over studies with two treatment sequences. *Statistics in Medicine*, 18:989–1017.

Kalbfleish, J. D. and Prentice, R. L. (1980). *The Statistical Analysis of Failure Time Data.* Wiley: Chichester.

Karalis, V. and Macheras, P. (2013). An insight into the properties of a two-stage design in bioequivalence studies. *Pharmaceutical Research*, 30:1824–1835.

Kauermann, G. and Carroll, R. J. (2001). A note on the efficiency of sandwich covariance estimation. *Journal of the American Statistical Association*, 96:1387–1396.

Kempthorne, O. (1983). *The Design and Analysis of Experiments.* Krieger: Malabar, Florida.

Kenward, M. G. (1987). A method for comparing profiles of repeated measurements. *Applied Statistics*, 36:296–308.

Kenward, M. G. and Jones, B. (1987). The analysis of data from 2×2 cross-over trials with baseline measurements. *Statistics in Medicine*, 6:911–926.

Kenward, M. G. and Jones, B. (1988). Crossover trials. In Kotz, S., Read, C. B., and Banks, D. L., editors, *Encyclopedia of Statistical Sciences, Update Volume 2*, pages 167–175. Wiley: New York.

Kenward, M. G. and Jones, B. (1991). The analysis of categorical data from cross-over trials using a latent variable model. *Statistics in Medicine*, 10:1607–1619.

Kenward, M. G. and Jones, B. (1992). Alternative approaches to the analysis of binary and categorical repeated measurements. *Journal of Biopharmaceutical Statistics*, 2:137–170.

Kenward, M. G. and Jones, B. (1994). The analysis of binary and categorical data from cross-over trials. *Statistical Methods in Medical Research*, 3:325–344.

Kenward, M. G. and Roger, J. H. (1997). Small sample inference for fixed effects estimators from restricted maximum likelihood. *Biometrics*, 53:983–997.

Kenward, M. G. and Roger, J. H. (2009). An improved approximation to the precision of fixed effects from restricted maximum likelihood. *Computational Statistics and Data Analysis*, 53:2583–2595.

Kenward, M. G. and Roger, J. H. (2010). The use of baseline covariates in cross-over studies. *Biostatistics*, 11:1–17.

Kenward, M. G., White, I. R., and Carpenter, J. R. (2010). Letter to the Editor on 'Should baseline be a covariate or dependent variable in analyses of change from baseline in clinical trials?' by Liu G.F. et al. (2009), *Statistics in Medicine*, 28, 2509–2530. *Statistics in Medicine*, 29:1455–1456.

Kershner, R. P. and Federer, W. T. (1981). Two-treatment crossover designs for estimating a variety of effects. *Journal of the American Statistical Association*, 76:612–618.

Kiefer, J. (1975). Construction and optimality of generalised Youden designs. In Srivastava, J. N., editor, *A Survey of Statistical Design and Linear Models*, pages 333–353. Amsterdam: North Holland.

Kieser, M. and Friede, T. (2003). Simple procedures for blinded sample size adjustment that do not affect the type I error rate. *Statistics in Medicine*, 22:3571–3581.

Koch, G. G. (1972). The use of non-parametric methods in the statistical analysis of the two-period changeover design. *Biometrics*, 28:577–584.

Koch, G. G., Gitomer, S., Skalland, L., and Stokes, M. (1983). Some nonparametric and categorical data analysis for a changeover study and discussion of apparent carryover effects. *Statistics in Medicine*, 2:397–412.

Koch, G. G., Landis, J. R., Freeman, J. L., Freeman, D. H., and Lehnen, R. G. (1977). A general methodology for the analysis of experiments with repeated measurement of categorical data. *Biometrics*, 33:133–158.

Kunert, J. (1983). Optimal designs and refinement of the linear model with applications to repeated measurements designs. *Annals of Statistics*, 11:247–257.

Kunert, J. (1984). Optimality of balanced uniform repeated measurements designs. *Annals of Statistics*, 12:1006–1017.

Kunert, J. (1987). On variance estimation in cross-over designs. *Biometrics*, 43:833–845.

Kunert, J. (1991). Cross-over designs for two treatments and correlated errors. *Biometrika*, 78:315–324.

Kunert, J. and Stufken, J. (2002). Optimal crossover designs in a mixed model with self and mixed carryover effects. *Journal of the American Statistical Association*, 97:898–906.

Kushner, H. B. (1997a). Optimal repeated measurements designs: the linear optimality equations. *Annals of Statistics*, 25:2328–2344.

Kushner, H. B. (1997b). Optimality and efficiency of two treatment repeated measurements designs. *Biometrika*, 84:455–468.

Kushner, H. B. (1998). Optimal and efficient repeated measurement designs for uncorrelated observations. *Journal of the American Statistical Association*, 93(443):1176–1187.

Kushner, H. B. (1999). H-symmetric optimal repeated measurements designs. *Journal of Statistical Planning and Inference*, 76:235–261.

Labes, D. (2013). R package PowerTost: Power and sample size based on two one-sided t-tests (TOST) for (bio) equivalence studies, Version 1.1-06.

Lall, R., Campbell, M. D., Walters, S. J., and Morgan, K. (2002). A review of ordinal regression models applied on health-related quality of life assessment. *Statistical Methods in Medical Research*, 21:49–67.

Lancaster, H. O. (1961). Significance tests in discrete data. *Journal of the American Statistical Association*, 56:223–234.

Laska, E. M. and Meisner, M. (1985). A variational approach to optimal two-treatment crossover designs: applications to carry-over effect models. *Journal of the American Statistical Association*, 80:704–710.

Laska, E. M., Meisner, M., and Kushner, H. B. (1983). Optimal crossover designs in the presence of crossover effects. *Biometrics*, 39:1089–1091.

Lawes, J. B. and Gilbert, J. H. (1864). Report of experiments on the growth of wheat for twenty years in succession on the same land. *Journal of the Agricultural Society of England*, 25:93–185, 449–501.

Lehmacher, W. and Wassmer, G. (1999). Adaptive sample size calculations in group sequential designs. *Biometrics*, 55:1286–1290.

Lewis, S. M., Fletcher, D. J., and Matthews, J. N. S. (1988). Factorial cross-over designs in clinical trials. In Dodge, Y., Fedorov, V. V., and Wynn, H. P., editors, *Optimal Design and Analysis of Experiments*, pages 133–140. North-Holland: Amsterdam.

Lewis, S. M. and Russell, K. G. (1998). Crossover designs in the presence of carry-over effects from two factors. *Applied Statistics*, 47(3):379–391.

Liang, K.-Y. and Zeger, S. L. (1986). Longitudinal data analysis using generalized linear models. *Biometrika*, 73:13–22.

Liang, K.-Y., Zeger, S. L., and Qaqish, B. (1992). Multivariate regression models for categorical data (with discussion). *Journal of the Royal Statistical Society, Series B*, 54:3–40.

Liebig, J. (1847). In Playfair, L. and Gregory, W., editors, *Chemistry in its Application to Agriculture and Physiology (4th edition). In English.* Taylor and Walton: London.

Lin, X. and Carroll, J. (2009). Non-parametric and semi-parametric regression methods for longitudinal data. In Fitzmaurice, G., Davidian, M., Verbeke, G., and Molenberghs, G., editors, *Longitudinal Data Analysis*, , pages 199–222, Chapman & Hall/CRC Press: Boca Raton, FL.

Lindsey, J. K., Byrom, W. D., Wang, J., Jarvis, P., and Jones, B. (2000). Generalized nonlinear models for pharmacokinetic data. *Biometrics*, 56:30–36.

Linnerud, A. C., Gates, C. E., and Donker, J. D. (1962). Significance of carryover effects with extra period change-over design (abstract). *Journal of Dairy Science*, 45:675.

Lipsitz, S. R. and Fitzmaurice, G. M. (1994). Sample size for repeated measures studies with binary responses. *Statistics in Medicine*, 13:1233–1239.

Littell, R. C., Milliken, G. A., Stroup, W. W., and Wolfinger, R. D. (1996). *SAS System for Mixed Models.* SAS Institute Inc.: Cary, NC.

Longford, N. T. (1998). Count data and treatment heterogeneity in 2×2 crossover trials. *Applied Statistics*, 47:217–229.

Lucas, H. L. (1957). Extra-period Latin-square change-over designs. *Journal of Dairy Science*, 40:225–239.

Lund, R. E. (1975). Tables for an approximate test for outliers in linear models. *Technometrics*, 17:473–476.

Lunn, D., Jackson, C., Best, N., Thomas, A., and Spiegelhalter, D. (2013). *The BUGS Book: A Practical Introduction to Bayesian Analysis.* CRC Press: New York.

Mainland, D. (1963). *Elementary Medical Statistics (2nd ed.).* Saunders: Philadelphia.

Mancl, L. A. and DeRouen, T. A. (2001). A covariance estimator for GEE with improved small-sample properties. *Biometrics*, 57:126–134.

Mantel, N. (1963). Chi-square tests with one degree of freedom: Extension of Mantel-Haenszel procedure. *Journal of the American Statistical Association*, 58:690–700.

Marks, H. P. (1925). The biological assay of insulin preparations in comparison with a stable standard. *British Medical Journal*, ii:1102–1104.

Martin, R. J. and Eccleston, J. A. (1998). Variance-balanced change-over designs for dependent observations. *Biometrika*, 85(4):883–892.

Matthews, J. N. S. (1987). Optimal crossover designs for the comparison of two treatments in the presence of carryover effects and autocorrelated errors. *Biometrika*, 74:311–320.

Matthews, J. N. S. (1988). Recent developments in crossover designs. *International Statistical Review*, 56:117–127.

Matthews, J. N. S. (1990). Optimal dual-balanced two treatment crossover designs. *Sankhya Ser. B*, 52:332–337.

Matthews, J. N. S. (1994a). Modelling and optimality in the design of crossover studies for medical applications. *Journal of Statistical Planning and Inference*, 42:89–108.

Matthews, J. N. S. (1994b). Multiperiod crossover designs. *Statistical Methods in Medical Research*, 3:383–405.

Matthews, J. N. S. and Henderson, R. (2013). Two-period, two-treatment crossover designs subject to non-ignorable missing data. *Biostatistics*, 14:626–638.

Matthews, J. N. S., Henderson, R., Farewell, D. M., Ho, W.-K., and Rogers, L. R. (2013). Dropout in crossover and longitudinal studies: Is complete case so bad? *Statistical Methods in Medical Research*, 23:60–73.

McCullagh, P. (1980). Regression models for ordinal data (with discussion). *Journal of the Royal Statistical Society, Series B*, 42:109–142.

McCullagh, P. and Nelder, J. A. (1989). *Generalized Linear Models, Second Edition.* Chapman and Hall: London.

McNemar, Q. (1947). Note on the sampling error of the difference between correlated proportions or percentages. *Psychometrika*, 12:153–157.

McNulty, P. A. (1986). *Spatial Velocity Induction and Reference Mark Density.* PhD thesis, University of California, Santa Barbara, CA.

Millard, S. and Krause, A. (2001). *Applied Statistics in the Pharmaceutical Industry with Case Studies using S-Plus.* Springer-Verlag: New York.

Molenberghs, G. and Kenward, M. G. (2007). *Missing Data in Clinical Studies.* Wiley: Chichester.

Molenberghs, G. and Verbeke, G. (2000). *Models for Distrete Longitudinal Data.* Springer Verlag: New York.

Molenberghs, G., Verbeke, G., Demétrio, C., and Vieira, A. (2010). A family of generalized linear models for repeated measures with normal and conjugate random effects. *Statistical Science*, 25:325–347.

Montague, T. H., Potvin, D., DiLiberti, C. E., Hauck, W. W., Parr, A. F., and Schuirmann, D. J. (2012). Additional results for 'Sequential design apraoches for bioequivalence studies with crossover designs'. *Pharmaceutical Statistics*, 11:8–13.

Nam, J. (1971). On two tests for comparing matched proportions. *Biometrics*, 27:945–959.

Namboordiri, K. N. (1972). Experimental design in which each subject is used repeatedly. *Psychological Bulletin*, 77:54–64.

Newcombe, R. G. (1996). Sequentially balanced three-squares cross-over designs. *Statistics in Medicine*, 15:2143–2147.

Newhaus, J. M., Kalbfleisch, J. D., and Hauck, W. W. (1991). A comparison of cluster-specific and population-averaged approaches for analyzing correlated binary data. *International Statistical Review*, 59:25–35.

Oakes, D. (1986). Semiparametric inference, in a model for association in bivariate survival data. *Biometrika*, 73:353–361.

Pan, W. and Wall, M. (2002). Small-sample adjustments in using the sandwich variance estimator in generalized estimating equations. *Statistics in Medicine*, 21:1429–1441.

Parkes, K. R. (1982). Occupational stress among student nurses. *Journal of Applied Psychology*, 67:784–796.

Patel, H. I. (1983). Use of baseline measurements in the two period cross-over design. *Communications in Statistics — Theory and Methods*, 12:2693–2712.

Patterson, H. D. (1950). The analysis of change-over trials. *Journal of Agricultural Science*, 40:375–380.

Patterson, H. D. (1951). Change-over trials. *Journal of the Royal Statistical Society, Series B*, 13:256–271.

Patterson, H. D. (1952). The construction of balanced designs for experiments involving sequences of treatments. *Biometrika*, 39:32–48.

Patterson, H. D. (1970). Non-additivity in change-over designs for a quantitative factor at four levels. *Biometrika*, 57:537–549.

Patterson, H. D. (1973). Quenouille's change-over designs. *Biometrika*, 60:33–45.

Patterson, H. D. and Lucas, H. L. (1962). Change-over designs. *North Carolina Agricultural Experimental Station, Tech. Bull. No. 147.*

Patterson, S. D. and Jones, B. (2006). *Bioequivalence and Statistics in Clinical Pharmacology.* Chapman and Hall/CRC Press: Boca Raton.

Pepe, M. S. and Anderson, G. L. (1994). A cautionary note on inference for marginal regression models with longitudinal data and general correlated response data. *Communications in Statistics — Simulation and Computation*, 23:939–951.

Peterson, B. and Harrell, F. E. (1990). Partial proportional odds models for ordinal response variables. *Journal of the Royal Statistical Society, Series A*, 39:205–217.

Pigeon, J. G. (1984). Residual effects designs for comparing treatments with a control. *PhD dissertation. Temple University, Philadelphia, PA.*

Pigeon, J. G. and Raghavarao, D. (1987). Crossover designs for comparing treatments with a control. *Biometrika*, 74:321–328.

Pinheiro, J., Bornkamp, B., Glimm, E., and Bretz, F. (2014). Multiple comparisons and modelling for dose finding using general parametric models. *Statistics in Medicine*, 33:1646–1661.

Pocock, S. J. (1983). *Clinical Trials.* Wiley: Chichester.

Pocock, S. J. (1977). Group sequential methods in the design and analysis of clinical trials. *Biometrika*, 64:191–199.

Pocock, S. J., Assmann, S. E., Enos, L. E., and Kasten, L. E. (2002). Subgroup analysis, covariate adjustment and baseline comparisons in clinical trial reporting: curent practice and problems. *Statistics in Medicine*, 21:2917–2930.

Potvin, D., DiLiberti, C. E., Hauck, W. W., Parr, A. F., Schuirmann, D. J., and Smith, R. A. (2008). Sequential design approaches for bioequivalence studies with crossover designs. *Pharmaceutical Statistics*, 7:245–262.

Prescott, P. (1999). Construction of sequentially counterbalanced designs formed from two Latin squares. *Utilitas Mathematica*, 55:135–152.

Prescott, R. J. (1979). On McNemar's and Gart's tests for cross-over trials. Letter to the editor. *Biometrics*, 35:523–524.

Prescott, R. J. (1981). The comparison of success rates in cross-over trials in the presence of an order effect. *Applied Statistics*, 30:9–15.

Proschan, M., Lan, K. K. G., and Wittes, J. T. (2006). *Statistical Monitoring of Clinical Trials.* Springer: New York.

Quenouille, M. H. (1953). *The Design and Analysis of Experiments.* Griffin: London.

Racine, A., Grieve, A. P., Fluehler, H., and Smith, A. F. M. (1986). Bayesian methods in practice: Experiences in the pharmaceutical industry (with discussion). *Applied Statistics*, 35:93–150.

Raghavarao, D. (1971). *Constructions and Combinatorial Problems in Design of Experiments.* Wiley: New York.

Raghavarao, D. (1989). Crossover designs in industry. In Gosh, S., editor, *Design and Analysis of Experiments, with Applications to Engineering and Physical Sciences*. Marcel Dekker: New York.

Raghavarao, D. and Xie, Y. (2003). Split-plot type residual effects designs. *JSPI*, 116:197–207.

Rohmeyer, K. (2014). R package: Crossover. *CRAN.*

Rohmeyer, K. and Janes, B. (2015). Examples of using the R package *Crossover*, In preparation.

Rosenkranz, G. K. (2014). Analysis of cross-over studies with missing data. *Statistical Methods in Medical Research*, 24:000–000.

Rowland, M. and Tozer, T. N. (1995). *Clinical Pharmacokinetics Concepts and Applications, Third Edition.* Lippincott, Williams and Wilkins: Philadelphia.

Ruppert, D., Wand, M. P., and Carroll, R. J. (2003). *Semiparametric Regression.* Cambridge University Press: Cambridge.

Russell, K. G. (1991). The construction of good change-over designs when there are fewer units than treatments. *Biometrika*, 78:305–313.

Russell, K. G. and Dean, A. M. (1998). Factorial designs with few subjects. *Journal of Combinatorics, Information and System Sciences*, 23:209–235.

Sampford, M. R. (1957). Methods of construction and analysis of serially balanced sequences. *Journal of the Royal Statistical Society, Series B*, 19:286–304.

SAS (2014). *SAS/STAT User's Guide, Version 9.3.* SAS Insitute Inc: Cary, NC.

Satterthwaite, F. E. (1946). An approximate distribution of estimates of variance components. *Biometrics Bulletin*, 2:110–114.

Schuirmann, D. J. (1987). A comparison of the two one-sided tests procedure and the power approach for assessing the equivalence of average bioavailability. *Journal of Pharmacokinetics and Biopharmaceutics*, 15:657–680.

Seath, D. M. (1944). A 2×2 factorial design for double reversal feeding experiments. *Journal of Dairy Science*, 27:159–164.

Selwyn, M. R., Dempster, A. R., and Hall, N. R. (1981). A Bayesian approach to bioequivalence for the 2×2 changeover design. *Biometrics*, 37:11–21.

Sen, M. and Mukerjee, R. (1987). Optimal repeated measurement designs under interaction. *Journal of Statistical Planning and Inference*, 17:81–91.

Senn, S. J. (1993). *Cross-over Trials in Clinical Research.* Wiley: Chichester.

Senn, S. J. (1996). The AB/BA cross-over: How to perform the two-stage analysis if you can't be persuaded that you shouldn't. In Hansen, B. and de Ridder, M., editors, *Liber Amicorum Roel van Strik*, pages 93–100. Erasmus University: Rotterdam.

Senn, S. J. (1997a). Cross-over trials. In Armitage, P. and Colton, T., editors, *Encyclopedia in Biostatistics,* **2**, pages 1033–1049. Wiley: New York.

Senn, S. J. (1997b). The case for cross-over trials in Phase III. Letter to the Editor. *Statistics in Medicine*, 16:2021–2022.

Senn, S. J. (2000). Crossover design. In Chow, S. C., editor, *Encyclopedia of Biopharmaceutical Statistics*, pages 142–149. Marcel Dekker: New York.

Senn, S. J. (2002). *Cross-over Trials in Clinical Research. Second Edition*. Wiley: Chichester.

Sharples, K. and Breslow, N. (1992). Regression analysis of binary data: Some small sample results for the estimating equation approach. *Journal of Statistical Computation and Simulation*, 42:1–20.

Sheehe, P. R. and Bross, I. D. J. (1961). Latin squares to balance immediate residual and other effects. *Biometrics*, 17:405–414.

Sheppard, L. (2003). Insights on bias and information in group-level studies. *Biostatistics*, 4:265–278.

Simpson, T. W. (1938). Experimental methods and human nutrition (with discussion). *Journal of the Royal Statistical Society, Series B*, 5:46–69.

Skene, S. and Kenward, M. G. (2010a). The analysis of very small samples of repeated masaurements. II. A modified Box correction. *Statistics in Medicine*, 29:2838–2856.

Skene, S. and Kenward, M. G. (2010b). The analysis of very small samples of repeated measurements. I. An adjusted sandwich estimator. *Statistics in Medicine*, 29:2825–2837.

Spiegelhalter, D., Thomas, N., and Best, N. (2000). WinBUGS. Version 1.3 User Manual. MRC Biostatistics Unit, Cambridge, UK.

Stokes, M. S., Davis, C. S., and Koch, G. G. (2012). *Categorical Data Analysis Using the SAS System, 3rd Edition.* SAS Institute Inc.: Cary, NC.

Struthers, C. A. and Kalbfleisch, J. D. (1986). Misspecified proportional hazards models. *Biometrika*, 73:363–369.

Stufken, J. (1991). Some families of optimal and efficient repeated measurement designs. *Journal of Statistical Planning and Inference*, 27:75–83.

Stufken, J. (1996). Optimal crossover designs. In Gosh, S. and Rao, C. R., editors, *Handbook of Statistics 13: Design and Analysis of Experiments*, pages 63–90. North Holland: Amsterdam.

Tudor, G. E. and Koch, G. G. (1994). Review of nonparametric methods for the analysis of crossover studies. *Statistical Methods in Medical Research*, 3:345–381.

Tudor, G. E., Koch, G. G., and Catellier, D. (2000). Statistical methods for crossover designs in bioenvironmental and public health studies. In Sen, P. K. and Rao, C. R., editors, *Handbook of Statistics, Vol 18*, pages 571–614. Elsevier Science B.V., Amsterdam.

Vartak, M. N. (1955). Review of nonparametric methods for the analysis of crossover studies. *Annals of Mathematical Statistics*, 26:420–438.

Verbeke, G. and Molenberghs, G. (2000). *Linear Mixed Models for Longitudinal Data.* Springer Verlag: New York.

Wallenstein, S. (1979). Inclusion of baseline values in the analysis of crossover designs (abstract). *Biometrics*, 35:894.

Welham, S. J. (2009). Smoothing spline models for longitudinal data. In Fitzmaurice, G., Davidian, M., Verbeke, G., and Molenberghs, G., editors, *Longitudinal Data Analysis*, pages 253–290. Chapman & Hall/CRC Press: Boca Raton, FL.

Welling, P. G. (1986). *Pharmacokinetics: Processes and Mathematics.* American Chemical Society.

White, H. (1982). Maximum likelihood estimation of misspecified models. *Econometrika*, 50:1–25.

Willan, A. R. and Pater, J. L. (1986). Using baseline measurements in the two-period crossover clinical. *Controlled Clinical Trials*, 7:282–289.

Williams, E. J. (1949). Experimental designs balanced for the estimation of residual effects of treatments. *Australian Journal of Scientific Research*, 2:149–168.

Williams, E. J. (1950). Experimental designs balanced for pairs of residual effects. *Australian Journal of Scientific Research*, 3:351–363.

Yates, F. (1938). The gain in efficiency resulting from the use of balanced designs. *Journal of the Royal Statistical Society, Series B*, 5:70–74.

Zeger, S. L. (1988). Commentary on papers on the analysis of repeated categorical response. *Statistics in Medicine*, 7:161–168.

Zeger, S. L. and Liang, K.-Y. (1986). Longitudinal data analysis for discrete and continuous outcomes. *Biometrics*, 42:121–130.

Zeger, S. L., Liang, K. Y., and Albert, P. S. (1988). Models for longitudinal data: a generalized estimating equation approach. *Biometrics*, 44:1049–1060.

Zucker, D. M., Wittes, J. T., Schabenberger, O., and Brittain, E. (1999). Internal pilot studies. II. Comparison of various procedures. *Statistics in Medicine*, 18:3493–3509.

Index

Printed in the United States
by Baker & Taylor Publisher Services

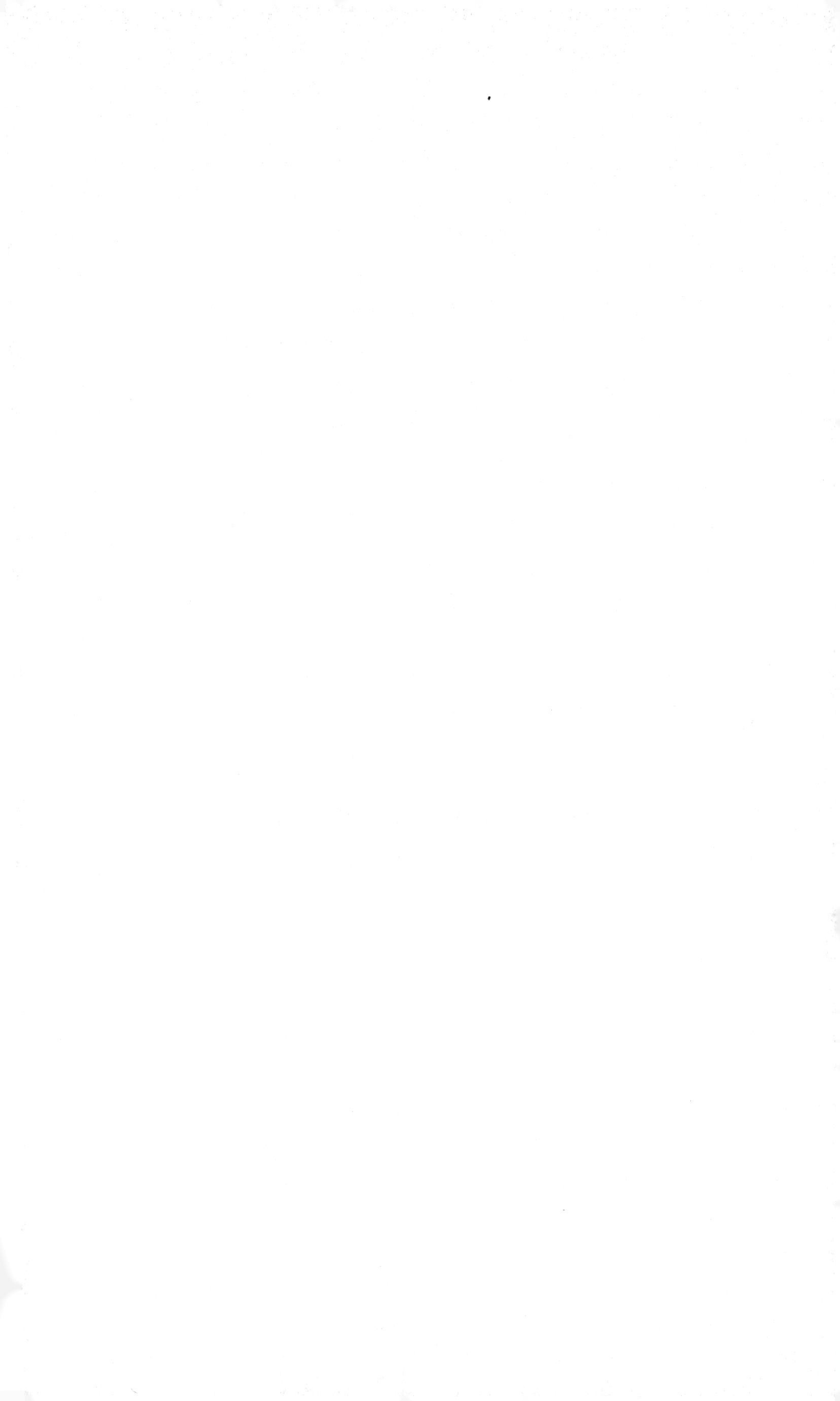